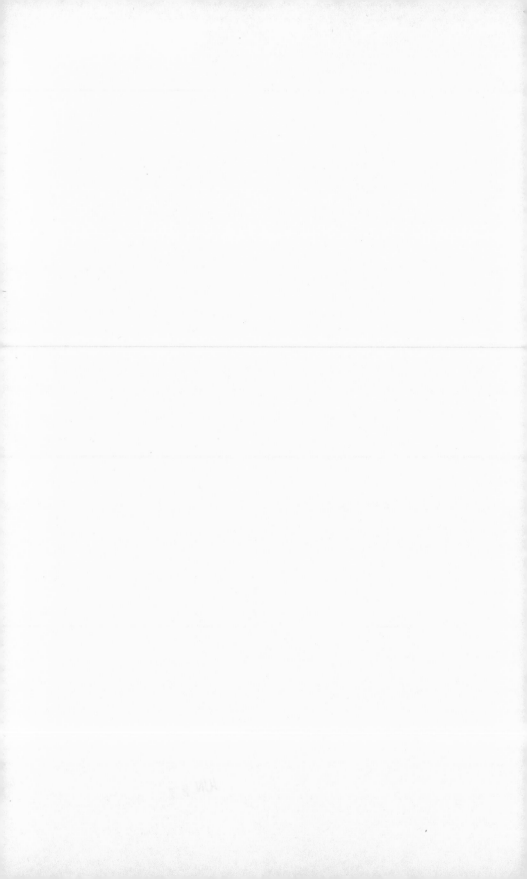

NEUROBIOLOGY OF INFANT VISION

Edited by Brian Hopkins
and Scott P. Johnson

Advances in Infancy Research

PRAEGER

Westport, Connecticut
London

ISBN: 1–56750–691–7

First published in 2003

Praeger Publishers, 88 Post Road West, Westport, CT 06881
An imprint of Greenwood Publishing Group, Inc.
www.praeger.com

Printed in the United States of America

The paper used in this book complies with the
Permanent Paper Standard issued by the National
Information Standards Organization (Z39.48–1984).

10 9 8 7 6 5 4 3 2 1

Copyright Acknowledgment

Contents

Introduction

Brian Hopkins and Scott P. Johnson

Since first appearing in 1981, Advances in Infancy Research has become a major source of reference for students of infant development. In no small way, the success of this monograph series has been due to the outstanding and dedicated work of its founding editors, Carolyn Rovee-Collier and Lewis P. Lipsitt. Under their astute guidance, each volume consisted of contributions covering a variety of topics written by individuals whose work was considered to be at the forefront of infancy research. The present volume marks both a continuation and a break with this editorial policy. Thus, we invited contributions from noted researchers, all of which would focus on a particular domain of interest to infancy researchers. In this instance, we felt that the theme of infant vision was a timely choice, especially when addressed from a neurobiological perspective.

In recent years, our understanding of infant visual cognition and perception has been advanced by the emergence of developmental cognitive neuroscience and by breakthroughs in revealing the cellular and molecular mechanisms underpinning visual development. Traditionally, the visual system has been regarded as a testing ground par excellence for examining general issues concerning the nature of ontogenetic development. Certainly, it is organized throughout most of its development in ways that are conducive to both neurobiological and psychological research, with, for example, inputs to both eyes being separated up to and including the visual cortex. Perennial issues that continue to be addressed encompass the role of activity-dependent experience and when it becomes potent as well as those relating to whether there are "windows of opportunity" for modifying or even transforming visual development both structurally and functionally. Others that come to mind are how development and evolution conspire to ensure the achievement of species-characteristic end states and matters that need to be clarified with regard to whether object and face recognition involve similar or different neural circuits. More recent issues have been triggered by the distinction between dorsal and ventral streams and thus the question of how they might codevelop. At the molecular level, they include the prospect of achieving the immunocytochemical identification of immediate (or early) genes (e.g., *fos*), thus enabling one to trace the neural circuits associated with infant vision. Despite the progress made, certain aspects of visual development still suffer from relative neglect. A prime example is how the visual perception of object movement direction develops during infancy. Another concerns the development of perceptual binding.

This volume covers most, if not all, of these issues. Add to this the inclusion of modeling by computer simulations of how the visual system develops at the cellular and behavioral levels, then we can begin to appreciate the richness of material on offer. However, there is no pretense that we have accounted for *all* topics that pertain to infant vision. Selections had to be made, but in doing so we hope that the reader will come to appreciate how the growing, multidisciplinary field of infant vision is beginning to challenge some cherished ideas about the nature of (visual) development in general.

The opening contribution by Barbara Finlay, Barbara Clancy, and Marcy Kingsbury, Chapter 1, sets the standard for the rest of the monograph. It provides a breathtaking overview that takes into account both the structural and functional development of the visual system from prenatal life into early infancy. One of the main points they make is that the structural development of the mammalian visual system is initially highly constrained and then increasingly relies on activity-dependent processes of self-organization to establish its functional architecture during prenatal life. As such, it is marked by the involvement of a multiplicity of redundant mechanisms at the molecular and cellular levels that ensure the achievement of species-characteristic functional outcomes such as binocular vision and orientational selectivity.

Two other selections from the rich array of material presented by Finlay and colleagues concern human neural development. One involves a statistical model that enables predictions about the timing of visual neural events in the human to be derived from findings based on other mammalian species. What emerges is that these events are very predictable in terms of ages of first appearance, peaks in development, and end states relative to those occurring in other brain systems. From the model's application flows a more controversial claim: Human neural development is relatively advanced at birth—a claim that has been diametrically opposed by others in the past (e.g., see Prechtl, 1984). While much of visual neurogenesis may be complete at birth, visual functions in the human newborn such as grating and Vernier acuity, contrast sensitivity, and movement perception as detected by event-related potentials (ERPs) undergo protracted periods of development postnatally that last years rather than months (see Daw, this volume). In addition, connections between cells with oriented receptive fields within the visual cortex, assumed to be essential for the development of perceptual differentiation and integration, can take up to 6 years after birth before they become fully established (Burkhalter, Bernardo, & Charles, 1993). While Finlay et al. rightly challenge a cherished notion, it would appear that the human newborn presents a mosaic pattern of altricial and precocial neural functions that is perhaps unique among mammalian species.

A theme addressed by Finlay, Clancy, and Kingsbury (viz., plasticity in the development of the visual cortex) reoccurs in the contribution by Nigel Daw, Chapter 2, but now allied to the notion of critical periods. Seemingly first introduced by Stockard (1921) in the context of embryology and then transported to research on imprinting and the development of song in avian species, it soon gained the status of a central concept across the developmental sciences in general. Inevitably, it became surrounded by semantic confusion (Bateson, 1979). However, it has retained its status in the study of visual neurogenesis as amply illustrated by Daw in his thorough and very informative review of a complex body of literature. His main thesis is that there is no such thing as *the* critical period in the development of the visual system. Rather, there are critical periods for "a particular function in a particular part of the nervous system after a particular history of visual exposure with a particular kind of visual deprivation."

This important qualification is amplified in another cornerstone of Daw's contribution. This is that, broadly speaking, visual development consists of three critical periods: an initial period of development (during which particular properties emerge), a second when functions can be disrupted (and which will degenerate if not stimulated in an age-appropriate manner), and a third one during which recovery from degeneration is possible (thus providing a plastic period for treatment). Evidence in support of the existence of these periods is sought from animal research involving eyelid suturing, retinal lesions, and artificial scotomas as well as from clinical studies of human infants with, for example, cataracts, anisometropia, and strabismus. One general principle to arise from this tripartite classification is that critical periods for the disruption of a function can last longer than those for initial development, while that for recovery can endure longest of all. For all the visual functions considered, recovery can be achieved when disruption ends, with the possible exception of contrast sensitivity. This points to the problem of knowing the degree to which a particular function involves cortical areas with their inherent plastic properties. The review ends with a helpful identification of three topics that suffer from lacunas in our knowledge and all of which have important implications for the practice of visual therapeutics: crowding effects on the development of Snellen acuity, the development of coarse as against fine stereopsis, and the development of suppression mechanisms (e.g., binocular rivalry) in normal children.

Daw mentions that the inferotemporal cortex (IT) retains plasticity for longer than the primary visual cortex. IT, and its role in the development of visual object recognition, receives detailed coverage in the thought-provoking contribution by Hillary Rodman, Chapter 3. As she emphasizes, more is known about the functional development of object recognition compared to how its neural substrates may develop. At the functional level, this ability is evident in a rudimentary form early in postnatal life but then undergoes a gradual and protracted development beyond the period of infancy. In accounting for this ontogenetic scenario, Rodman proposes that there is a developmental delay in achieving the neural plasticity typifying the functioning of the adult temporal lobe and that this delay results in the establishment of a circuitry dedicated to the recognition of objects. Any discussion of IT circuitry brings with it the two visual systems hypothesis in which the ventral stream is ascribed to "vision for perception" and the dorsal stream to "vision for action." Referred to by other authors in this volume (Gilmore, de Haan), this distinction in visual information processing pathways rests largely on studies with the macaque, and it is still an open question as to whether the same neural structures and pathways can be found in the human. This problem is exemplified by the finding that area V2 in the macaque consists of an orderly arrangement of thin and thick cytochrome oxidase stripes, while its homologue in the human displays a jumble of patches (Tootell & Taylor, 1995). Moreover, little is known about how the two systems codevelop in the human, notwithstanding Rodman's suggestion that the dorsal stream becomes functional before its ventral counterpart—a suggestion faced with contradictory findings and that Rodman attempts to resolve.

At the heart of Rodman's contribution is a model she offers to account for the development of object recognition in terms of underlying neural mechanisms. It contains two key features: first, the achievement of a relatively dedicated circuitry in which neurons within processing units are mainly engaged in analyzing a particular class of objects; second, that this achievement is ensured by a delay in the plasticity of IT together with what is referred to as an early bootstrapping operation. The latter is portrayed as a mechanism by which visual recognition is established in rudimentary form by means of neurons that are inherently (and weakly) responsive to object properties and in which feedback from eye movements plays an increasingly important role. The model lends itself to a number of testable predictions (e.g., that the dorsal stream becomes operational before the ventral stream). While this well-formulated model embraces a number of neural substrates, there are others that could be implicated in the development of object recognition. For example, on the basis of functional Magnetic Resonance Imaging (fMRI) findings, it was suggested that the LO region in the human (which has topographical similarities with V4 in the macaque) may serve as an intermediate staging post between V1 and higher-order stages of object recognition (Malach et al., 1995). If so, then LO/V4 could be a crucial structure in the development of object recognition.

Do object and face recognition share the same neural substrates during development? This was a question tackled by Michelle de Haan in Chapter 4. Answers to the question, she stresses, are stymied by a lack of studies comparing face and object recognition in infants. In fact, most of those concerned with newborns have only employed facelike displays. However, research with brain-damaged patients and the poorer performance of neurologically intact adults in identifying inverted versus upright faces compared to objects in the same orientations implicate distinct neural pathways in the ventral stream for the two types of visual recognition (see Farah, 1996). Developmentally, the inversion effect does not become evident until about 4 months of age (Fagan, 1972), while the face-responsive ERP component in infants (P400), assumed to be a precursor to that in adults (N170), has not been shown to be affected by inversion until 6 months. These, and other, findings converge on the conclusion that the visual system is broadly tuned to faces early in infancy and that subsequent development is facilitated by experience-dependent processes. As yet there is no clear answer to the question of whether the development of face and object recognition is subserved by different neural mechanisms during the period of infancy.

While face processing during infancy is addressed by de Haan, her review concerns the broader issue of how (delayed) visual recognition memory develops. In doing so, she provides a valuable coverage of the techniques devised for studying this ability in infants. An important conclusion is that evidence in favor of recognition memory is to a large extent dependent on the testing procedures used in any technique. Thus, the delayed nonmatch-to-sample task reveals a slow development of remembering in contrast to other techniques (e.g., those based on looking time measures). Such differences appear to indicate that the development of visual memory undergoes qualitative change during infancy and is mediated by different brain structures than in the adult. The need for models more explicitly geared toward accounting for the mechanisms of developmental change is emphasized by de Haan. In this respect, she does an excellent job of evaluating the strengths and weaknesses of currently available models, which focus on the development of the hippocampus, parahippocampal regions, or the inferotemporal cortex. Adult studies suggest other structures need to be accounted for such as the amygdala and the middle fusiform gyrus in the right hemisphere (Nelson, 2001).

In Chapter 5, Rick Gilmore considers the neglected issue of how infants acquire the ability to perceive the direction of objects moving in the environment (i.e., heading or self-motion perception). He contrasts this dynamical form of perception with perceiving static direction (i.e., where objects are located in space relative to oneself)—a topic that has received considerably more attention from infancy researchers. The latter focuses on the distinction between eye-centered and body-centered coding of object location. Based on an ingenious adaptation of the double-step saccade paradigm, he was able to show in his own studies a shift from the use of eye- to body-centered position information occurring at about 5 months of age. As with changes in face recognition, the neural mechanisms involved remain obscure and Gilmore speculates that they reflect the development of extrastriate areas and thus the dorsal stream.

In turning to the development of dynamic perception, Gilmore is concerned with how the sensitivity of infants to optical flow patterns changes with age. He contends that the development of such sensitivity may not constitute a rate-limiting factor in the visual control of posture. In this, he is supported by Jouen et al. (2000) who cast this constraint in terms of achieving the ability to apply the appropriate force in responding to the velocity of the optical flow. Gilmore then reports four of his own experiments concerned with the perception of dynamic direction and once again based on clever experimentation, this time using infant-controlled habituation and the forced-choice preferential looking technique. In summary, these studies reveal that, relative to adults, infants up to about 5 months of age are not able to discriminate simulated flow patterns indicative of quite large changes in heading direction. Given that the infants in these studies were not moved, the logical next step is to investigate if increased sensitivity to changes in heading obtains when they move through space (thus providing additional information about self-motion from the vestibulum and/or mechanoreceptors). In a final set of comments, Gilmore argues for a distinction between active and passive visual experience and suggests that the latter is predominant early in development as young infants do not generate much optical flow via their own movements. Certainly, there are dramatic increases in the availability of self-induced experience as sitting and the ability to locomote are achieved (see Campos et al., 2000). We note also that even newborns can adjust their posture to optical flow velocity (Jouen et al., 2000). Perhaps, then, this ability provides the foundation from which further active responses to visual input emerge.

In the final contribution, Chapter 6, Stephen Grossberg leads us through the computational modeling of how cortical processes give rise to visual perception and in particular to binocular vision, selective attention, and perceptual grouping. In reading this, one is richly rewarded with challenging ideas about how the visual system might develop, linking as they do neurophysiological and behavioral data. In a nutshell, Grossberg reviews three interrelated models, each of which is designed to account for particular features of visual development. One (the Triple-O model) deals with how cortical maps in VI of ocular dominance and orientational selectivity develop from opponent simple cells. Another (the disparity-tuning model) attempts to account for the development of complex cell receptive fields that receive inputs from simple cells and that subserve 3-D vision and figure-ground separation. The third partner (the LAMINART model), which is discussed in most detail, is directed toward explaining how intra- and interlaminar circuits in the visual cortex develop connections that enable selective attention and perceptual grouping. As such, it offers a resolution of the binding problem and how it can be addressed from a developmental perspective.

The LAMINART model assumes that classical receptive fields of simple and complex cells have already developed (presumably due to the mechanisms dictated by the disparity-tuning model). An interesting finding with regard to these fields is that they are susceptible to the attentional state of the organism such that state can "resize" them to give them smaller ones that enable selectivity in visual attention (Martinez et al., 1999). Such state-related effects are not a part of the LAMINART model, but they might prove to be a useful addendum in accounting for top-down developmental changes in infant attention. As it stands, the model can offer an explanation of the development of object unity and thus the problem of how an early manifestation of perceptual grouping is acquired (i.e., why newborns perceive a partly occluded object as two separate ones, while 2 to 4 months later it is seen as a complete object). The explanation rests on the selectionist principle of "cells that fire together, wire together." Accordingly, during early development, cells in layer 2/3 of the visual cortex that abide by this principle come to form the dominant grouping and in turn inhibit the activities of other cells via the layer 6-to-4 off-surround. With further development, cells in the winning group become connected, resulting in increases in their projection ranges and orientational selectivity, and thereby more capable of completing the perceptual grouping that imposes the most coherence on a particular visual display. This is but one example of the power of Grossberg's modeling approach that can help us further understand brain-behavior relationships in the development of the visual system. We await with interest his promise of unifying the three models into one overarching developmental model.

We gratefully acknowledge the invaluable help of Velma Dobson, Denis Mareschal, and Ruxandra Sireteanu in reviewing the chapters contained in this volume.

REFERENCES

Bateson, P. (1979). How do sensitive periods arise and what are they for? *Animal Behaviour, 27,* 470–486.

Burkhalter, A., Bernardo, K.L., & Charles, V. (1993). Development of local circuits in human visual cortex. *Journal of Neuroscience, 13,* 1916–1931.

Campos, J.J, Anderson, D.I., Barbu-Roth, M.A., Hubbard, E.M., Hertenstein, M.J., & Witherington, D. (2000). Travel broadens the mind. *Infancy, 1,* 149–219.

Fagan, J. (1972). Infants' recognition memory for faces. *Journal of Experimental Child Psychology, 14,* 453–476.

Farah, M.J. (1996). Is face recognition special? Evidence from neuropsychology. *Behavioural Brain Research, 76,* 181–189.

Jouen, F., Lepecq, J-C., Gapenne, O., & Bertenthal, B.I. (2000). Optic flow sensitivity in neonates. *Infant Behavior and Development, 23,* 271–284.

Malach, R., Reppas, J.B., Benson, R.R., Kwong, K.K., Jiang, H., Kennedy, W.A., Ledden, P.J., Brady, T.J., Rosen, B.R., & Tootell, R.B.H. (1995). Object-related activity revealed by functional magnetic resonance imaging in human occipital cortex. *Proceedings of the National Academy of Sciences (USA), 92,* 8135–8139.

Martinez, A., Anllo-Vento, L., Sereno, M.I., Frank, L.R., Buxton, R.B., Dubowitz, D.J., Wong, E.C., Hinrichs, H., Heinze, H.J., & Hillyard, S.A. (1999). Involvement of striate and extrastriate visual cortex areas in spatial attention. *Nature Neurosciences, 2,* 364–369.

Nelson, C.A. (2001). The development and neural bases of face recognition. *Infant and Child Development, 10,* 3–18.

Prechtl, H.F.R. (Ed.). (1984). *Continuity of neural functions from prenatal to postnatal life.* Oxford: Blackwell.

Stockard, C.R. (1921). Developmental rate and structural expression: An experimental study of twins, "double monsters" and single deformities, and the interaction among embryonic organs during origin and development. *American Journal of Anatomy, 28,* 115–275.

Tootell, R.B., & Taylor, J.B. (1995). Anatomical evidence for MT and additional cortical visual areas in humans. *Cerebral Cortex, 5,* 39–55.

Chapter 1

The Developmental Neurobiology
of Early Vision

Barbara L. Finlay, Barbara Clancy,
and Marcy A. Kingsbury

ABSTRACT

The early structural and functional development of the eye, retina, and visual system is best understood in a broad phylogenetic context to see the generality of the developmental mechanisms that specify the developing visual system. The sequence of generation of cell classes in the retina, the control of eye size and conformation, the pathfinding of the optic nerve, and the generation of retinotopic maps all demonstrate the complex interplay of experience-dependent and -independent effects. The generation of the visual cortex, including both primary visual cortex and extrastriate areas, from deployment of the first neurons, specification of cortical areas, and the organization of features like ocular dominance columns and single neuron response properties is a further example of this interplay. New analysis shows that the human visual system is surprisingly mature at birth, ready to assimilate experience. Overall, visual system development employs multiple and apparently redundant mechanisms in production of every adult feature that in concert produce robust and reliable functional outcomes.

The developing human visual system is a spatially distributed assemblage of optical and neural components. These components come informed by evolution as to which must be preformed, which may make use of environmental predictability to inform their own construction, or which might utilize a variable, learning-based organizational strategy. We will briefly review the mechanics of the early generation and specification of the visual system, from eyes to isocortex. The eye particularly is a unique case of a physical structure directly molded by its own activity. We will contrast generalities with specializations of the visual system by comparing the visual system to the structure of other developing neural systems and by comparing the structure of the human or primate visual system to that of other vertebrates. We will review the contribution of genetic specification, activity-dependent self-organization, and environmental activity–dependent organization to various features of visual system organization including retinotopic map formation, binocular organization, and receptive field structure. Using new information about the relative timing of neural events across species, we predict when visual events occur in the developing human brain and point out some surprising features of the human nervous system at birth.

Overall, we will argue that the process of visual system development is a highly constrained and redundant one, with every well-studied feature showing multiple overlaid production mechanisms that together produce robust and reliable functional outcomes. This redundancy may be understood in the context of "evolvability": Our eyes and brains carry the informational legacy of millions of years of our diverse ancestors' evolution, including those that developed rapidly or slowly, informed by environmental structure or required to develop independently of experience, and those that took their form in daylight or in darkness.

BASIC VISUAL SYSTEM STRUCTURE: EVOLUTION, GENOMICS, AND MECHANICS OF INITIAL DEPLOYMENT

Conservation of Segmentation Genes

Eyes are ancient. Not long ago, the very surprising report was made that the Pax-6 gene, which controls development of the vertebrate eye in the mouse, if transplanted to the genome of a developing fruit fly, *Drosophila*, would cause the production of a *Drosophila*-appropriate compound eye in whatever embryo segment received the transplant (Quiring et al., 1994). Pax-6 is one of a limited and distinct set of genes conserved across vertebrates and invertebrates that are involved in the differentiation of the early embryo into head, body, and appendages, each with their appropriate specializations (reviewed in Callaerts, Halder, & Gehring, 1997). These genes are expressed in an overlapping and nested fashion. They do not control the direct expression of the proteins relevant to visual system function, such as opsin (the protein component of the light-absorbing molecular complex in the retina) or crystalline lens proteins, but rather control the order and coordination of their expression. Subsequently, Pax-6 was found to be important in the coordinated expression of photoreceptor-cell complexes ubiquitously, including those in jellyfish and mollusks, raising the previously unsuspected possibility that eyes are "monophyletic"—meaning the essential photoreceptor mechanism arose just once in evolution and was elaborated into all its diverse present forms (Callaerts, Halder, & Gehring, 1997). Current debate centers on just what assemblage the Pax-6 gene controls, a multiple-cell complex (Callaerts, Halder, & Gehring, 1997) or just those cells producing opsin (Fernald, 2000).

Phototransduction, the process in which photopigments composed of a retinal-opsin complex react directly to light, is also highly conserved across invertebrates and vertebrates. This is a generality of particular interest for those primarily concerned with human vision—for example, the fact that the opsin complex has a limited number of functional isoforms in all species constrains the kinds of trichromatic color vision that primates may have (Nathans, 1999). In addition, the Pax-6 gene is involved in the development of the olfactory bulb, a structure with which the eye shares many features of molecular biology and embryonic structure. These few examples of many conserved features of molecular biology should serve as cautions to take a very long and evolutionary view when considering anything that might appear to be a specialized feature in mammalian or human eyes—it's probably been done before.

Development of the Eye

The eye primordium everts from the lateral part of the diencephalon (the portion of the forebrain that also includes the thalamus and hypothalamus) and interacts with tissue in the head end that will become the lens (Figure 1.1). As in all parts of the nervous system, neurons are generated in a "ventricular zone" directly adjacent to the ventricle of the primordial neural tube, then migrate toward the outer limiting membrane, most typically in the immediate radial direction. In mammalian retinas, the order of generation is quite stable and may be thought of (with some oversimplification) as occurring in two spatially overlaid bouts (Cepko et al., 1996; LaVail, Rapaport, & Rakic, 1991; Polley, Zimmerman, & Fortney, 1989). The first bout produces components of the diurnal eye, whereas the second produces the nocturnal eye; their combination produces the mature duplex retina. This sequence is depicted in Figure 1.2, using a timetable based on predicted dates for human neurogenesis. The statistical modeling technique that produced these dates will be described in a later section. Retinal ganglion cells that transmit visual information to the brain; cones, the photoreceptors of daylight vision; cone bipolar cells, which connect the cones to the retinal ganglion cells; and horizontal and amacrine cells, which support lateral information transfer within the retina—these begin production first. They are followed by rod bipolar cells, which connect the low-light photoreceptors, the rods to retinal output, additional amacrine cells, Muller cells (the supporting cells of the retina), and finally the rods themselves.

Although the center of the retina is often considered to be the "most

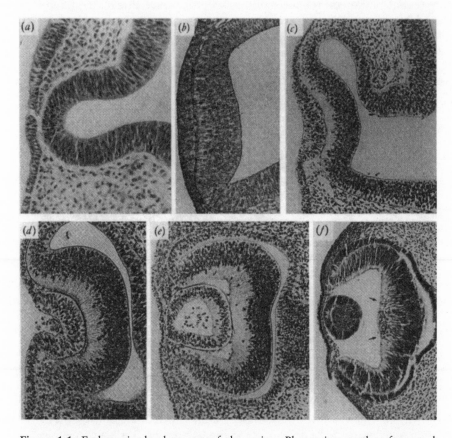

Figure 1.1. Embryonic development of the retina. Photomicrographs of coronal sections passing through the developing eyecup of human (**b–e**) and quokka (a rabbit-sized marsupial) (**a, f**) embryos. Dorsal is toward the top of the page. (**a**) The optic vesicle of a 16 postconceptional day (PCD) embryo, showing the neuroectoderm contacting the surface ectoderm. (**b**) Section through a 32-somite human embryo showing the intimate relation between the lens ectoderm and optic vesicle. Note that both tissues are beginning to thicken along the zone of contact. (**c**) The optic vesicle in a 28 PCD human embryo is just beginning to invaginate to form the optic cup. (**d**) Section through a human embryo at about 31 PCD showing the optic cup and lens cup in the process of invaginating. (**e**) A human retina at about 34 PCD. The lens has now detached from the surface ectoderm but still contacts the central part of the retina. (**f**) Section through a quokka retina aged 22 PCD. The central region of the retina is thicker and is developmentally advanced compared with other parts of the retina. The developmentally advanced region is characterized by the appearance of the first ganglion cells (between the arrows). Reprinted with permission from Robinson, S.R. (1991). Development of the mammalian retina. In B. Dreher & S.R. Robinson (Eds.), *Neuroanatomy of the visual pathways and their development* (vol. 3, pp. 69–128). London: Macmillan.

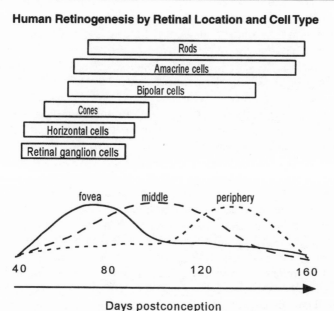

Figure 1.2. Human retinogenesis. The order of genesis of retinal cells occurs in two spatially overlaid bouts. The first produces the components of the diurnal eye, while the second burst produces the nocturnal eye. The dates, which are listed as human postconception (PC) dates, are based on macaque retinogenesis reported by Rakic and colleagues (Angevine & Sidman, 1961) and "translated" into human time from a general comparative database (Clancy, Darlington, & Finlay, 2000, 2001; Darlington, Dunlop, & Finlay, 1999; Finlay & Darlingon, 1995). The curves indicate the timing of production of cells over the entire retinal area (RGC = retinal ganglion cells).

mature," it attains this status in a nonintuitive way (Rapaport & Stone, 1982). Neurogenesis begins with the generation of the first ganglion cells and cones over the entire retina, not just the center (Sengelaub, Dolan, & Finlay, 1986). But, as illustrated by the curves in Figure 1.2, cell generation in the primate central retina (not the "fovea," which has not yet formed) barely makes it to the production of the very first nocturnal components (the rod bipolars and rods) before production ceases there, and so a very high central ganglion cell and cone density is stabilized (LaVail, Rapaport, & Rakic, 1991). Photoreceptors and other retinal neurons are continually added in a gradient increasing toward the peripheral retina, thus diluting the relative density of cones and ganglion cells in the periphery and also increasing the convergence of the photoreceptors (cones and rods both) onto ganglion cells. In all retinal areas, the differentiated cells rapidly develop interconnections and also send axons back toward the diencephalon (Maslim, Webster, & Stone, 1986). Some of the elaboration, lamination, and specification of connections between the cells of the retina depends on the normal electrophysiological activity of retinal cells, while some does not (Bodnarenko, Jeyarasasingam, & Chalupa, 1995; Gunhan-Agar, Kahn, & Chalupa, 2000; Wong, Hermann, & Shatz, 1991). This aspect of retinal development has as yet been little studied.

The retina begins its development as an inhomogeneous incomplete sphere, a balloon with areas of greater or lesser thickness, and these physical attributes determine the way the eye will grow in the embryo, fetus, and early childhood (Kelling et al., 1989; Reichenbach, Eberhardt et al., 1991; Reichenbach, Schnitzer et al., 1993). As noted above, the central retina contains a high-density region of cells undisturbed by the continual interposition of new elements—it is both thicker and more mature than the periphery, with more internally connective elements. The peripheral retina is thinner, more elastic, and less mature; in addition, there is a very substantial programmed "apoptotic" loss of cells from the peripheral retina ("apoptosis" refers to an orchestrated program of cell death, not a disorganized dissolution of the cell; Finlay, 1992; Provis & Penfold 1988). As the production of photoreceptors and neurons is concluding, the eye and retina begin to grow and stretch just like a balloon, requiring intraocular pressure for "inflation" (Coulombre & Coulombre, 1956). Because of its inhomogeneous initial condition, the retina undergoes a pronounced differential stretch, with the peripheral retina stretching the most; this will continue in humans into the first year after birth. Note that this fact *absolutely requires* plasticity in intramodal topographic mapping in the central nervous system, as the visual angle corresponding to a particular set of retinal cells will undergo substantial change from birth to the first birthday (Aslin, 1993).

Superimposed upon this mammalian general plan of growth, in primates we find construction of a specialized feature for high-acuity vision, the fovea, studied in detail by Hendrickson and her collaborators (Curcio & Hendrickson, 1992; Hendrickson, 1994). The word *fovea* refers to the half-millimeter pit created by the displacement of the cell bodies of photoreceptors and all other neurons away from the photoreceptive elements of the cones. During development, the outer segments of the cones are reduced in diameter, resulting in a greater absolute and angular density of photoreceptors as the cell processes are pulled to the side. In humans, this process is under way at birth (Curcio & Hendrickson, 1992; Hendrickson, 1994; Hendrickson & Drucker, 1992; Provis et al., 1985a, 1985b) and continues until about the first birthday, thus requiring ongoing topographic reorganization of the retina. Interestingly, the absolute size of the foveal specialization is conserved from the very smallest to largest primates, even though the size of the eye itself may vary greatly. This suggests that the fovea, with its extended fiber processes and unusually limited vascularization, might be at some physiological limit, an idea that receives some support from the high incidence of macular (essentially foveal) degeneration in aging humans (Franco et al., 2001).

Thus, in human infants, we find an eye whose neurons and photoreceptors have been generated and establishing connectivity for at least 6 months prior to birth but whose topological conformation is very much in flux during the first year or so, both in the center of gaze and in the retinal periphery. The quality of the image an infant sees also undergoes substantial change during the first year after birth (see Daw, this volume).

Growing the Eye into Focus

"Emmetropization," the process of matching the length of the eye to the optical power of the lens and cornea, has been the object of much study, both the phenomenon and the mechanisms behind it (reviewed in Troilo, 1992). At birth, human eyes show substantial astigmatism and more variability in focusing an image on the retina than they will after they have had some visual experience (Howland, 1983; Howland & Sayles, 1985). Experience itself is necessary for the improvement. Major changes in eye size, optics, and accommodative ability will occur in the first year or so after birth and continue into early childhood. Prenatal genetic programs, loosely defined as the interaction of the genome and tissues without any corrective effects of experience, delivers a roughly functioning eye to the world, capable of such things as resolving faces, but thereafter experience will direct the details.

How can a developing eye tell that the optical power of the lens and cornea match the length of the eye? The answer lies in the activity of the neural elements in the retina. High-contrast (focused) images produce maximum activity in photoreceptors and their associated neural elements. If the eye has such activity, the optics and length of the eye are matched, and a signal is given to limit growth (Wallman, 1992). However, if the neural elements of the eye are relatively inactive, this creates the problem of determining the nature and direction of the defocus, and the answer to this problem is complex. If the eye is attached to the brain, the brain can produce an accommodative signal to the intraocular musculature to bring an image into focus and thus induce high retinal activity. Evidence exists that the nature of the accommodative signal itself might produce a growth-inhibiting or -enhancing signal (Schaeffel & Howland, 1991).

Independent of a connection to the brain, however, the eye can change its growth rate in response to its activity, though sometimes maladaptively (Troilo, Gottlieb, & Wallman, 1987). If the eye is prevented from forming a focused image at all, it will fail to check its growth, and the condition "deprivation myopia" will ensue, basically forming an eye too long for its optics (Miles & Wallman, 1990). The effect is local—if just part of the retinal image is defocused, only that part of the eye will show enhanced growth or greater elasticity. Although the full mechanism is not yet understood, evidence points to direct local effects of the retina on cytogenesis or on scleral elasticity (stretching of the tough part of the outer eyeball). There are other potential complications—eye conformation could be thought of as a contest between the requirements of night and day vision, each with different growth requirements. Minimally, it is crucial that low light levels at night not be taken as evidence that the diurnal eye is out of focus, and so the process of emmetropization is also gated by circadian rhythms (Erskine et al., 2000).

Crossing the Chiasm

After the optic nerves, composed of retinal ganglion cell axons, make their way across the diencephalic surface of the eye to the diencephalon proper, there is the problem of getting the information from the two eyes to the proper side of the brain, and from there, into spatial register with one another. To solve this problem, a molecular solution is employed that is similar to the one used to produce commissures in fruitflies and zebra fish. Basically, axons in each optic nerve are attracted to the midline of the diencephalon through interactions with attractant molecules (e.g., netrin, reviewed in Cook, Tannahill, & Keynes, 1998). Once attracted, however, the optic nerves must be induced to leave. The attractant molecule then induces expression of new receptor proteins for the cellular recognition mechanisms, and the initial attraction is turned into repulsion. In most mammals, the situation is complicated in that some axons will leave the midline after crossing to the contralateral side, while others will remain on the ipsilateral side before moving away. Similar to the attraction/repulsion interactions at the midline, the process of selective crossing is also accomplished by specific molecular recognition molecules. Even with such mechanisms, errors of crossing do occur, although typically at a low rate. The aberrantly projecting retinal ganglion cells are later removed by activity-dependent cell death (Sengelaub & Finlay, 1981).

Distribution to Targets

In all vertebrates (e.g., fish, frogs, and mammals) the eye distributes itself to a collection of targets of various functions. These include a hypothalamic structure involved in the maintenance of circadian rhythms (the suprachiasmatic nucleus in mammals); at least two diencephalic structures that transmit visual information forward to the telencephalon (in mammals, these are the visual thalamic nuclei termed the lateral geniculate nucleus [LGN] and the nucleus lateralis posterior or pulvinar, the latter of which also

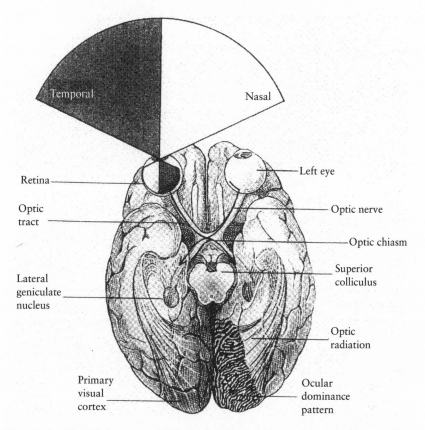

Figure 1.3. General diagram of the visual system. A view of the components of the visual system as viewed from beneath the brain, which has been partially cut away to reveal the internal components. Images detected by the rods or cones in the nasal (inside) halves of each retina reach ganglion cells whose nerve fibers cross over at the optic chiasm to reach their level-two target neurons in the lateral geniculate and the superior colliculus. Reprinted with permission from Bloom, F.E., & Lazerson, A. (1988). *Brain, mind and behavior* (2nd ed.). New York: Freeman.

receives midbrain input), a midbrain structure (the superior colliculus in mammals), and a complex of structures related to the vestibulocerebellum and the oculomotor system (Butler & Hodos, 1996). Most of these targets of retinal input contain topographic (point-to-point) representation of the visual field, often referred to as a visual or retinotopic "map" (Figure 1.3).

We emphasize here the ancient nature of the developmental problems addressed by the visual system. As a result, developmental neurobiologists may select as "model systems" animals distributed widely across the vertebrate spectrum, with good confidence in the ubiquity of the mechanisms they will discover. In the case of retinotopic mapping, the frog, the goldfish, and the current workhorse of developmental neurobiology, the zebra fish (Easter & Nicola, 1996; Karlstrom, Trowe, & Bonhoeffer, 1997), have been the species of choice.

Retinotopic Mapping

A central and conspicuous feature of brain organization is the topographic representation of sensory surfaces and the preservation of topographic order as one brain structure "maps" to the next. In the visual system, neighboring points in visual space are represented as neighboring points in the thalamus, midbrain, primary visual cortex, and cortical regions beyond. Retinotopic map formation was first investigated systematically by Roger Sperry in the developing optic tectum of the frog beginning in the 1940s (Sperry, 1963). How might such maps be formed? A remarkable number of independent mechanisms can be imagined: (1) The spatial layout of elements in connecting maps could be passively mapped, nearest neighbor to nearest neighbor; (2) temporal gradients could map one element to another in an organized sequence; (3) neighboring elements in a map could actively recognize one another so that the map might travel in a coherent pattern of axons to its target; (4) different parts of the map might have different "road maps" to find different parts of the target; (5) the elements in the first map might recognize locations in the target map at varying degrees of specificity; (6) statistical regularities in the activity pattern of the input array could be used to confer order in the target array; (7) the map might develop from trial and error, based on motor experience in target acquisition.

While a description of each of these mechanisms is beyond the scope of this review, all of these logical possibilities have been shown to contribute to the formation or features of the adult map, sometimes in different species and cases (Fraser & Perkel, 1990; Udin & Fawcett, 1988). Unsurprisingly (given the multiplicity of mechanisms), multiple genes are required for the successful development of a map (Karlstrom et al., 1996). Different features solve the mapping problem at different developmental times; for example, molecular cues are more important early, and activity-dependent organization late. As a whole, this apparent redundancy of mechanisms may be responsible for the robust nature of map formation. That such a host of mechanisms might bear on such an essentially simple problem might be good to keep in mind when developmental scientists in other domains have debates that imply singular mechanisms—"the" mechanism of language acquisition, for example.

At the time of eye opening (in humans, this occurs around the sixth month of gestation, well before birth), the topographic map of the retina is already established in the thalamus and midbrain, and the inputs from the two eyes are already sorted out in the layers of the LGN and the midbrain (Figure 1.3; Rakic, 1976; Shatz & Sretavan, 1986). Studies investigating the intermodal perception of spatial location have demonstrated that a crude multimodal map of space, to be sharpened by experience, is also represented in the midbrain (Knudsen, 1994; Stein, 1984). As with emmetropization, where a roughly useable optics/eye length ratio emerges before the onset of experience, we find an initial mapping of the relationship of auditory, visual, and motor space also appearing prior to experience but one that can be quite substantially altered by experience.

HOW "VISUAL" DOES THE VISUAL CORTEX START OUT? EVO-DEVO EVIDENCE

The Overall Nature of the Cortex

There can be no controversy that the eye is directly adapted to its visual function. But what about the parts of the brain that the retina sends its information to? The most obvious question concerns the primary visual cortex, where both generic and specialized accounts can be offered. For the whole cortex, two kinds of organization have typically been contrasted. At one extreme, the cortex might begin equipotential throughout (O'Leary, 1989), a uniformly connected neural net that will take its adult local specificity from the information and activity relayed via inputs from specific thalamic nuclei and from the negotiations made between the derived cortical areas via their intracortical connectivity. Alternatively, the cortex might begin as a mosaic of specific regions right from the start (Rakic, 1988); that is, cortical areas might begin with specified features particularly suitable for the input they will receive or the functions they will perform. For example, visual cortex might have a complement of neurotransmitters and generate lengths of axonal processes uniquely matched for the temporal and spatial character of visual information, or have a recognition process specific to segregating binocular input (Crowley & Katz, 1999; see also Grossberg, this volume). Inferotemporal cortex might come prewired with the cell assemblies useful for detecting faces in their characteristic orientation and size (see Rodman, this volume). Does the literature on comparative organization of the forebrain, or the early genetic instructions expressed in the developing cortex, suggest that the primary visual cortex or other visual cortices have any special genetic identity that would allow them unique information-processing properties, independent of instruction from visual experience?

COMPARATIVE EVIDENCE THAT VISUAL CORTEX MIGHT BE UNIQUE

From comparative information, primary visual cortex presents the strongest case for unique, area-specific identity of all the cortical areas. As noted earlier, the primary visual cortex in mammals (also called striate cortex, or area 17) gets its major input from the LGN and contains one visuotopic map. In birds, the area of the telencephalon that receives input from the thalamic homologue of the LGN is called the visual Wulst, which is one part of the "dorsal cortex" (Butler & Hodos, 1996). The Wulst has a layered organization and response properties very similar to mammalian visual cortex (Pettigrew & Konishi, 1976) and appears to be developmentally, connectionally, and functionally homologous to it. Reptiles have a similar organization of the visual system, although nomenclature varies (i.e., the reptilian homologue of primary visual cortex is the dorsal lateral cortex [DLC] rather than the Wulst). The DLC or Wulst is different in structure from the rest of the telencephalon thought to be homologous with isocortex (the six-layered cortex also called the neocortex)—the remaining telencephalon that receives thalamic input consists of nuclear masses without layered organization (Northcutt & Kaas, 1995). Thus, the structural homologue of mammalian visual cortex in birds and reptiles is organized a bit differently than other telencephalic areas. Mammalian visual cortex also has a noticeable peculiarity of organization—although other cortical regions divide into topographically distinct subdivisions as brains enlarge, primary visual cortex does not.

The fact that evolution has selected out and elaborated the visual cortex (in mammals) and its homologues (in other vertebrates) in several different directions suggests that the embryonic precursor of the visual cortex has some feature that makes it easily "visible" to natural selection. For example, a segmentation gene (or genes) unique to the visual cortex but present across species might come to control various other genes involved in the development of particular cortical cell connectivity or neurotransmitter patterns.

DEVELOPMENTAL EVIDENCE THAT VISUAL CORTEX MIGHT HAVE SOME UNIQUE INSTRUCTIONS

Brief Overview of Cortical Development

Similar to the neurons of the retina, the neurons of the cerebral cortex are generated from precursor cells formed in a ventricular zone (Fujita, 1963; Rakic, 1974; Sauer, 1935). Although early cell division in the ventricular zone serves simply to expand the pool of precursor (or progenitor) cells, later divisions of precursors give rise to cortical neurons. The first generation of cortical cells migrates from the ventricular zone into overlying tissue to form the preplate, an early scaffold for later-migrating neurons (Marin-Padilla, 1978). The next generation of cortical cells, which will become layers II to VI, migrates into the preplate and splits it into a superficial layer (layer I) and a deep layer (subplate). Subsequent cortical development is characterized by an inside-out gradient as younger neurons occupy progressively more superficial positions in the cortex (Angevine & Sidman, 1961).

Similar to migration trajectories in the eye, the majority of cortical neurons travel radially from the ventricular zone (Rakic, 1972), although nonradial migration has also been observed (O'Rourke et al., 1992; Walsh & Cepko, 1988). Embedded within the fundamental laminar structure of the cortex are differences in the tangential plane that emerge during development to give rise to the discrete areas that characterize adult isocortex. For example, in primates, layer IV of the primary visual cortex matures into a thick band of dense stellate cells and myelinated axons. The resulting striped (or striated) appearance of this region, even to the naked eye, is the reason primary visual cortex is also known as "striate" cortex.

Proliferation Rates

Cortical areas may also be distinguished from one another based on differences in the rate of cell proliferation. In primates, the rate of neuronal production in the neuroepithelium underlying primary visual cortex is greater than the rate of production underlying "extrastriate" visual cortical areas, such that the number of neurons in a "unit column" or primary visual area of the adult is twice that of surrounding cortex, principally due to the large number of stellate cells in layer 4 (Dehay et al., 1993).

Transcription Factors

Molecules or proteins known as transcription factors are produced from regulatory genes and serve to activate or repress gene expression by binding to DNA. Transcription factors show unique patterns of expression across the developing cortical plate; most are expressed in gradients (Bulfone et al., 1995; Donoghue & Rakic, 1999; Nakagawa, Johnson, & O'Leary, 1999), and some show striking localization to individual cortical layers (Frantz, Bohner et al., 1994; Frantz, Weimann et al., 1994; Neuman et al., 1993). One developmental regulatory gene, Otx2, is localized to lower layer 4 and/or upper layer V of the visual cortex during development (Nothias, Fishell, & Ruiz i Altaba, 1998).

Although no single expression pattern seems to be confined to a specific cortical modality, the combined expression patterns of various transcription factors do appear to distinguish some cortical boundaries. The combined expression of Lhx2, Emx1, and SCIP distinguishes presumptive visual cortex from presumptive auditory cortex (Nakagawa, Johnson, & O'Leary, 1999), while the combined expression of Id-2 and Tbr-1 marks the boundary between rat somatosensory and motor cortex (Bulfone et al., 1995; Rubenstein et al., 1999). More cortical transcription factors will undoubtedly be discovered; it may (or may not) prove noteworthy that several of those currently identified appear to mark the boundaries of visual cortex.

Cellular Communication Molecules

Cell surface–bound receptors and their ligands (molecules that bind to and activate a receptor) also demarcate some cortical boundaries (Donoghue & Rakic, 1999; Gao et al., 1998; Mackarehtschian et al., 1999; Rubenstein et al., 1999). Some of the receptors and ligands specifically identified in cortex are the Eph receptor tyrosine kinases and ephrins, respectively. In primate visual cortex, the early nested expression of the EphA3 and EphA6 receptors delineate primary and secondary visual areas—EphA6 is expressed in both cortices, while EphA3 is expressed only in presumptive extrastriate (secondary visual) cortex (Donoghue & Rakic, 1999). These molecules, similar to those at the visual midline, are believed to serve as guidance cues for developing axons (Flanagan & Vanderhaeghen, 1998). Because the combination of an Eph receptor and its ligand is inhibitory, the expression of one of these molecules in a target may serve to repel axons expressing the other molecule (Cheng et al., 1995; Drescher et al., 1995; Gao et al., 1996). It is likely that the patterns of Eph receptors and ephrins in the visual cortex, as well as in the thalamus, contribute to the establishment of visual-specific thalamocortical projections, as has also been suggested for somatosensory thalamocortical projections (Gao et al., 1998; Mackarehtschian et al., 1999).

INTERACTIONS OF THE VISUAL SYSTEM—EXPERIENCE AND PLASTICITY

The evidence cited above can only give the visual cortex the potential to generate visual perception–specific wiring independent of experience (we use the term *experience* at this point in its widest possible sense to mean any internally or externally generated activity pattern). It should be emphasized that there is little evidence tying genetic instruction of the visual cortex to any particular feature of its wiring. Moreover, it is worth recalling that primary visual cortex retains all of the stereotypical features that make up a typical cortex (layers, connections, and columns). Visual cortex also shows extensive plasticity.

As the visual cortex is generated, it begins to arrange the various overlaid features of adult organization that Hubel and Wiesel (1962) first characterized. These features have been the subject of extensive study and include retinotopy (mapping) (Naegele, Jhaveri, & Schneider, 1988), ocular dominance (a pattern of left-right alternation in thalamic input to layer IV of primary visual cortex [Figure 1.3; Katz & Shatz, 1996; Miller & Stryker, 1990]), binocularity, and orientation selectivity (Wiesel & Hubel, 1974).

The latter feature is "multiscaled"; that is, it includes a range of spatial frequencies. As noted earlier, the LGN initially innervates the cortex in a point-to-point manner (Miller, Chou, & Finlay, 1993; Naegele, Jhaveri, & Schneider, 1988), though there is evidence here, as in most cases, that the map "sharpens" with visual experience.

Activity

Retinal activity, and indeed activity in the entire visual system, begins well before external visual experience. As noted earlier, retinal ganglion cells are the first cells of the retina to be generated, and they extend axons soon after generation—these axons show "spike" activity very early on. Although the inputs from the two eyes will for the most part be noncorrelated, the activity from closely adjoining cells in the retina is more correlated (see Grossberg, this volume). In addition, prior to eye opening, the retina generates systematic waves of activity, "hypercorrelating" the activity of neighboring cells (Wong, 1999; Wong, Meister, & Shatz, 1993). These waves may be a potential source of information for the formation of retinotopy, orientation-sensitive cells, and ocular dominance columns. The details of the timing of many of these events in human development will be discussed more fully later.

Binocular Vision

The case of merging the input from the two eyes has a complex account—the now-familiar multicausal one. Before embarking on a description of development of binocular vision, it would be useful to describe the potential uses of binocularity and how anatomy might reflect them. One use of binocular vision is the redundancy it provides for nocturnal vision (the initiating step for frontal eyes in our primate lineage) whereby two sensory surfaces are used to capture light. In this case, identifying which eye is the source of the information is not necessary. Additionally, binocularity allows the input from the two eyes to be segregated and compared in order to discover contours present in only one eye, sources of object contour information, or depth contours in scenes. In these cases, identifying which eye the signal comes from is of importance. Finally, there is the familiar binocular disparity cue to depth, in which a difference must be computed. Two physical features are tracked when looking at binocular interaction in the visual cortex: (1) the responses of single neurons to visual information derived from either eye and (2) the supraordinate grouping of those neurons into ocular dominance columns. The function of ocular dominance columns distinct from the cell-by-cell convergence of information from the two eyes is not known—intuitively, it would seem useful for those cases where the eye of origin should be tracked for the computation. However, to our knowledge, there has never been any study linking psycho-physical capabilities in binocular vision to the specific properties of ocular dominance columns.

In monkeys and cats, the projections from the two eyes are initially over-laid in the LGN and self-segregate in early development, before birth. A competitive process is implicated, as removal of one eye allows the stabi-lization of projections to those layers where the remaining eye would not normally project (Rakic, 1981; Shatz, 1990). Endogenous activity of the two eyes (e.g., uncorrelated spontaneous activity or retinal waves) or mo-lecular cues could be the basis of this segregation (Crowley & Katz, 1999, 2000; Wong, 1999). In the developing monkey or cat cortex, the projec-tions from the eye-specific layers of the LGN to layer IV of the visual cortex are already overlaid by the time of birth. The perinatal response properties of individual cortical cells do not differ from those in the adult—there are fully binocular cells, monocular cells, and intermediates, but these cells are not spatially segregated into the ocular dominance column responses seen in the adult. If one eye is made inactive at birth, the other eye retains its spread throughout layer IV and retains physiological influence on the cor-tical cells. If activity is reduced (e.g., if both eyes are experimentally closed) the segregation into ocular dominance columns is retarded (Hubel & Wie-sel, 1965; LeVay, Wiesel, & Hubel, 1980; Stryker & Harris, 1986). If the two eyes are made spatially incongruent and their input is never correlated (i.e., the animal is strabismic), few or no physiologically binocular cells remain (Hubel & Wiesel, 1965). This activity-dependent correlational pro-cess is dependent on transmitter/receptor mechanisms in the cortex, and physiological plasticity and transmitter/receptor-mediated plasticity covary (Hensch & Stryker, 1996; Katz & Shatz, 1996).

Recent reports of segregation of LGN projections in the visual cortex of the ferret have been made very early in development, in situations where the role of activity is minimized (Crowley & Katz, 1999, 2000). These studies implicate a molecular mechanism of segregation as well as an activity-dependent one. It is not yet clear if this contradiction with previous studies that have implicated activity-dependence alone might reflect species differences, tracer sensitivity differences, or some other factor. However, if the molecular component turns out to be generally the case, this would make the segregation of ocular dominance columns seem very similar to the other visual functions we have discussed so far (i.e., development of retinotopic maps, control of eye size), in that they depend on both molec-ular recognition components and activity-dependent mechanisms. No single mechanism "trumps" the others in early development, but rather all con-tribute to the final conformation.

Orientation Selectivity

On eye opening, cats and monkeys have orientation-selective cells in their cortex, though not so responsive as those found in the adult. However, the complex pinwheel organization of varying orientation selectivity seen in the adult appears very early, before substantial visual experience (Chapman, Stryker, & Bonhoeffer, 1996). It is not really known if the deployment of LGN projections that are slightly more spatially extensive on one axis than another (e.g., giving rise to an oriented cortical cell) is dependent on molecular instructions or on endogenous activity. Experience with natural images alone is adequate to develop a neural net with the oriented, multiscale properties of visual cortex (Olshausen & Field, 1996); it is not yet known if retinal waves alone are adequate to produce this organization. However, every other piece of information we have about cortex development suggests that a model combining both molecular and activity-driven mechanisms would be a good bet.

In addition to the "classical" receptive field, the axons and dendrites of cortical cells may extend past the immediate cortical column; for example, they may link up extended orientation columns over a wider range of the visual field than that represented by a single orientation column (Fitzpatrick, 2000; Weliky et al., 1995). Initial axon outgrowth is circularly symmetrical and does not show the patchiness and anisotropies of axonal spread that can link oriented contours over several orientation columns (i.e., linking vertically oriented receptive fields along the vertical axis of the entire visual field, and horizontally oriented receptive field along the horizontal axis). Development of these asymmetries is a visual-experience concurrent event and seems highly likely to be directly related to infants' abilities to link object contours and motion over progressively more distant parts of the visual field. It should also be noted that dynamic changes in nonclassic receptive field structure and extent are experience dependent throughout life (Gilbert et al., 1996).

Visual Response Properties in Auditory Cortex

Interesting demonstrations of the ability of a robust developmental process to survive an extreme "dislocation" are the experiments of Sur, Pallas, and others, who were able to induce retinal projections into the medial geniculate (auditory) nucleus of the thalamus of ferrets at birth (Pallas, Roe, & Sur, 1990; Sur, Pallas, & Roe, 1990; von Melchner, Pallas, & Sur, 2000). Removal of auditory input to the medial geniculate coupled with destruction of the lateral geniculate causes a subset of retinal projections to redirect their projections to medial geniculate. The medial geniculate neurons faithfully transmit visual information to formerly auditory cortex, where the cortical neurons are then driven by stimulation of the eyes.

There is a topological feature of the visual system that the auditory system does not share, seen on both a macro- and microlevel of analysis. The macro map of the LGN onto the visual cortex is two dimensional, reflecting the retina (i.e., up/down; nasal/temporal), while the cochlea/medial geniculate typically maps only one dimension (tonotopic) in auditory cortex. At the level of single cells, the microlevel of two-dimensionality in vision is seen in the oriented receptive fields of the visual cortex. Does the experimentally induced medial geniculate representation of visual information in the auditory cortex reflect normal auditory one-dimensionality or visual two-dimensionality? The rerouting studies indicate that at both the macrolevel of retinotopy (Pallas, Roe, & Sur, 1990) and the microlevel of orientation selectivity (Roe et al., 1992) the two-dimensional properties of the retina do appear in the conventionally one-dimensional auditory cortex. It is not known precisely when these dimensional properties are formed, although it is known that alterations in intracortical connectivity are critical (Gao & Pallas, 1999; Pallas, Littman, & Moore, 1999). However, in the ferret rerouting experiments, the manipulation is done pre-eye opening, yet postnatally, so both endogenous and visual experience–related activity might contribute to their expression. Nevertheless, this is strong evidence that activity is adequate to produce some major features of cortical visual map organization, independent of any genetic instructions the visual cortex may have on its own. But note that this *does not* signify that there are no predisposing genetic or molecular instructions in the visual cortex that might normally contribute to the organization of the visual map— almost certainly there are such. The message, as always, is that there are multiple, redundant, cospecifying mechanisms for important organizational features.

Other Visual Cortical Areas

The "Van Essen diagram" (Felleman & Van Essen, 1991), a notoriously complicated-looking map showing all the interconnections of the multiple areas of the visual system, is a map of the adult macaque visual cortex. We know very little about the variability of this map: Do all adult macaques have the same conformation and type of visual areas? Given that primary visual cortex itself can be relatively variable in size from one individual macaque to the next (Van Essen, Newsome, & Maunsell, 1984), the likelihood of variability in the number and type of cortical fields is also very high. We don't know yet if secondary visual cortical areas start out with the retinotopic precision that has been described for primary visual cortex or whether substantial self-organization occurs, as the rewired ferret experiments suggest. We don't know if the partial segregation of the M- and P- pathways that code aspects of temporal and spatial frequency selectivity in adult primates and that show partial segregation in the adult is segregated as well in their early projections. Nor do we know if or when the precise response properties of adult extrastriate cortex, such as the motion selectivity cells of area MT, the face-specific cells of the inferotemporal cortex, or the retinal/ocular position integrating cells of posterior parietal cortex, appear in the relevant cortical areas with or without experience, or at what time. The technical difficulties that these questions pose are extreme, although imaging studies may soon begin to make headway on some of the grosser aspects of these fundamental questions.

HUMAN NEURAL DEVELOPMENT

So far we have been concerned with the multiplicity of mechanisms that produce the various features of developing visual system organization. We have discussed studies that, of necessity, have been accomplished for the most part in the visual systems of nonhuman primates, carnivores, and rodents. However, we do know that in the human infant many of the events discussed above, including eye opening, will occur prenatally (although visual development will extend well into the postnatal period). How can we predict the timing of various neural events in the developing human brain? Virtually no empirical studies are available that can pinpoint such timing. Neurobiologists are severely hampered in this regard because access to human neural tissue is limited and empirical studies that determine when neurons of the retina or cortex are born require invasive techniques. Nevertheless, in this section, we would like to turn attention to timing of events in the human brain, in the particular context of understanding the relationship of structural maturation to behavioral and perceptual maturation.

The Timing of Human Neural Events

We have recently developed a comparative mammalian model (Finlay & Darlington, 1995) that can be used for translating the maturational schedules of other mammals onto human brain development (Clancy, Darlington, & Finlay, 2000, 2001). This modeling approach is possible because (1) the literature on perinatal brain development in mammals has grown so rich in the past decade that our basis for correlation and inference to human development is strong and (2) we have been able to document a striking predictability in the order and duration of neural events across developing mammalian species. Adapting a statistical approach based on general linear models, and using a data set that currently includes 95 different neural events from nine species including mouse, hamster, rat, spiny mouse, rabbit, ferret, cat, monkey, and human, we are able to generate predictions for the timing of developmental events within the human brain, including many aspects of neurogenesis and axonal outgrowth in the visual system (see Table 1.1; also Clancy, Darlington, & Finlay, 2000, 2001).

Table 1.1
Predicted Postconceptional Dates of Developing Human Visual Neural Events

Human Visual Events	Predicted PC Day	(ref.)
Gestational Month 2		
retinal ganglion cell generation begins	38.3	
superficial SC laminae begin	42.0	
dorsal LGN begins	43.1	
RGC axons in optic stalk	46.9	51.0[2]
visual cortex—subplate begins	47.1	
ventral LGN—peak	48.0	
dorsal LGN—peak	50.2	
optic axons at chiasm of optic tract	51.0	
rapid axon generation/optic nerve—begins	52.2	
retinal horizontal cells—peak	52.6	
external capsule appears	52.8	56.0[1]
visual cortex—subplate peak	53.3	
superior colliculus—peak	54.0	
dorsal LGN—ends	54.6	
retinal ganglion cells—peak	55.8	
visual cortex—layer VI begins	56.9	
optic axons reach doral LGN and SC	60.0	
internal capsule appears	60.2	63.0[1]
Month 3		
superficial SC laminae ends	63.0	
cones—peak	66.6	
visual cortex—layer V begins	67.1	
visual cortex—subplate ends	68.5	
visual cortex—layer VI—peak	68.9	
retinal amacrine cells—peak	69.7	
retinal ganglion cell generation ends	72.8	
optic axons invade visual centers	75.2	60.0[1]
visual cortex—layer V peaks	78.0	
visual cortex—layer VI ends	79.1	
visual cortex—layer IV begins	79.9	
optic nerve axon number—peak	81.8	
visual cortex—layer II/III begins	85.8	

Table 1.1 (continued)

Human Visual Events	Predicted PC Day	(ref.)
Month 3 (continued)		
visual cortex—layer V ends	86.4	
visual cortex—layer IV peaks	87.6	
Month 4		
corpus callosum appears	90.9	87.5[1]
LGN axons in subplate	93.1	
cortical axons reach dLGN	95.4	
visual cortex—layer II/III—peak	98.4	
visual cortex—layer IV ends	99.6	
retinal waves begin	107.0–136.0	
superficial SC—start of lamination	106.4	
rods—peak	107.6	
visual cortex—layer II/III ends	108.6	
retinal bipolar cells—peak	116.0	
cortical axons innervate dLGN	116.9	
Month 5		
ipsi/contra segregation in LGN and SC	125.6	175.0[4]
adultlike cortical innervation of dLGN	128.5	
rapid axon loss in optic nerve ends	129.8	
LGN axons in layer IV of visual cortex	130.2	
visual cortical axons in SC	142.6	
Month 6		
eye opening	159.9	182.0[1,2]
Month 9		
synapses surge to 85% of value at puberty		259.0[3]

The timing of various visual neural events, predicted based on comparative mammalian modeling (Clancy, Darlington, & Finlay, 2000; Darlington, Dunlop, & Finlay, 1999; Finlay & Darlington, 1995), is divided into months during human gestation. Note that the second column cites very few empirically derived human events—predictions for the dates of events listed here are made possible only by utilizing comparative modeling.
[1]Ashwell, Waite, & Marotte (1996); [2]Dunlop et al. (1997); [3]Huttenlocher et al. (1982); [4]Robinson & Dreher (1990).

Interestingly, in statistical comparisons with components such as "limbic system," "motor system," and so forth, the visual events across all the species in our data set show the least variability (Clancy, Darlington, & Finlay, 2000). In other words, visual neural events are the most predictable across all species. This suggests that the manner in which the problem of visual function is solved across species is especially conserved, even when comparing rodents, often considered a somewhat nonvisual species, and highly visual mammals such as cats and primates. The absence of statistical variability offers support for the concept that there is something particularly rigid or constrained about the visual system, which forces construction in exactly the same order across mammalian species, even if visual systems as a whole don't end up identical. It also gives us considerable confidence in the predicted dates reported below. Except where noted, these dates (and those in Figures 1.2 and 1.4 and Table 1.1) are based on the "translation" of nonhuman mammalian developmental time into human time using this comparative modeling approach first presented by Finlay and Darlington (1995). The model was subsequently refined as more information became available (Darlington, Dunlop, & Finlay, 1999) and recently adjusted to account for a systematic deviation in timing of neurogenesis in limbic and cortical structures for primates versus other mammals (Clancy, Darlington, & Finlay, 2000).

First Trimester

It is startling to realize how much of the fundamental brain morphology and organization, including almost the entire visual system, is accomplished during the 3 months following conception (Table 1.1). Virtually every neuron in the nervous system is generated in the first trimester, with the exception of the tail of the distribution of the last layer of the isocortex, the external granular layer of the cerebellum, and those few areas in which neurons are generated throughout life. The differentiation of cells into different subtypes and the migration of cells from their birthplace to their ultimate destinations in the retina, cortex, and brainstem occur in the first trimester. The "type" (specification) of a neuron includes many aspects—what shape it has, what information it receives, what transmitters and receptors it produces, and so forth. Some of these features can be specified by location, such that the path taken by a cell as it migrates and its ultimate arrival in a certain brain region will fix some aspects of its "type," while others are set on, or immediately after, generation in the ventricular zone (Cepko, 1999). For example, cells may begin to express various complements of signaling chemicals (neurotransmitters and neuromodulators) before migration, as soon as they are born in the ventricular zone (Lidow & Rakic, 1995).

Second Trimester

This is the period in which the basic patterns of connectivity develop between neural regions. This picture is confirmed in humans by looking for molecular markers that reflect the activity of building axonal and dendritic arbors (Honig, Herrmann, & Shatz, 1996). From a developmental point of view, one of the most important events is the establishment of connections from the thalamus to all regions of the isocortex, including those from the LGN to the visual cortex. These connections are set up during the second trimester in a pattern that resembles the adult pattern from the start, with animal studies showing that visual, somatosensory, auditory, and limbic areas of cortex all receive projections fairly exclusively from those thalamic nuclei that will project to them in adulthood (Miller, Chou, & Finlay, 1993; Molnar et al., 1998; O'Leary et al., 1994). Intracortical pathways (connections from one cortical region to another) also begin to establish their mature connectivity patterns in the second trimester. The corpus callosum makes its first appearance around postconceptional (PC) day 90 and lays down a pattern of homotopic connections (connections between one area of cortex and its corresponding contralateral cortex; reviewed in Innocenti, 1991). The long-range axonal connections start to produce synapses in their target structures in short order, although the bulk of synapse production will occur later (Bourgeois & Rakic, 1993).

Neural development is characterized at many levels and at many points in time by exuberance or overproduction of elements (an additive event), followed by a large-scale elimination of the same elements (a subtractive or regressive event). In addition to the events listed in Table 1.1, most of which are additive, a particular kind of regressive event occurs in the second trimester—apoptosis. This developmental cell death usually occurs in close association with the establishment of major axon pathways between regions and can contribute to removal of errors in axonal connections and numerical matching of connecting populations of cells (Finlay, 1992). Apoptosis can be quite extensive and rapid, often resulting in the loss of the majority of the neurons originally generated. For example, the retina, which establishes connections with subcortical targets in the second month postconception (PC 60), reaches the peak number of axons in the optic nerve less than a month later (PC 82). By the end of the second semester, retinal ganglion cell loss is over, removing as much as 80% of the originally generated cell population (a process that has been directly demonstrated in humans; Provis & Penfold, 1988; Provis et al., 1985a, 1985b). Such cell loss also occurs in isocortex, particularly in the subplate and the upper cortical layers (Shatz, Chun, & Luskin, 1988; Woo, Beale, & Finlay, 1991). Though subplate loss is prenatal, isocortical death in the upper layers may extend into the first couple of postnatal months (O'Kusky & Colonnier, 1982). Overall, this type of early neuronal death seems to serve to grossly fix cell numbers in interconnecting populations and to fine-tune topographic projections between structures and does not contribute to the fine-tuning of connectional anatomy associated with learning.

The second trimester is also the period in which activity-dependent self-organization of the nervous system begins (PC 107–136), a process best studied in the visual system. In the retina, waves of activity begin to be propagated across the retinal surface, generated by amacrine cells, beginning (in cats and ferrets) after basic connectivity is established and stopping before eye opening (reviewed in Wong, 1999). This organized activity could be a basis for various kinds of categorization in which correlated inputs remain together, while dissimilar (uncorrelated) inputs dissociate, perhaps aiding in establishment of ocular dominance columns prior to extrauterine experience, as suggested by the ferret studies discussed earlier (Crowley & Katz, 1999, 2000). Because retinal waves produce a hypercorrelation of the activity of spatially adjacent cells in the retina, this information might also be used to fine-tune topographically mapped projections or produce more detailed spatial structures like orientation sensitivity in visual cortical neurons. This self-organizing process has some very interesting theoretical implications for developmental psychologists: Activity-dependent organization occupies a middle ground in the nature-nurture debate, where some of the same mechanisms that will be used later for learning from the outside world (i.e., response to correlations in the input) are used in utero to set up the basic functional architecture of the brain.

Third Trimester

By the beginning of the seventh month of gestation, a remarkably large number of human neural events are already complete. The human fetus has matured to the point where the eyes move and remain open for measurable periods of time. Reciprocal connectivity from higher-order cortical areas to primary areas has also begun (Burkhalter, 1993). Pathways exhibit the initial process of myelination (Yakovlev & Lecours, 1967) in which axons are "insulated" by glial cells in order to transmit information more efficiently. Large descending pathways from the cortex continue to develop. Aside from the more obvious role of descending pathways in motor control, the appearance of descending pathways also means that the cortex can already "talk back" to its input regions. In the eighth and ninth months of gestation, a massive and coordinated birth of synaptic connections begins in the isocortex and related structures, which we will discuss in detail in the next section. In general, however, it is fair to say that the human infant is born with a nervous system whose working components are in place and organized. All cells are generated, all major incoming sensory pathways are in place and have already gone through a period of refinement of their total number of cells, connections, and topographic organization. Intracortical and interhemispheric pathways are well developed, though output pathways to such points as the midbrain, pons, and spinal cord lag behind. The primary receptive fields coding such features as motion and orientation selectivity in the visual system are already present, though linkages across receptive fields remain to be elaborated. The primary sensory and motor regions have their adult input and topography, although we do not know yet if all of the multiple subareas described for the primate visual cortex (Felleman & Van Essen, 1991) have sorted themselves out.

SYNAPTOGENESIS

Synapses, the transmitter/receptor complex through which neurons communicate, are central components of neuronal signaling. The production of these synapses (synaptogenesis) and their elimination co-occur over most of early postnatal development, and continue to co-occur throughout life. It is important to note that chemical synapses are only one of a number of ways neurons may communicate—there can be direct coupling between cells (these "electrical synapses" or "gap junctions" are particularly prominent in early development); cells can also communicate through the release of gases, notably nitric oxide (Cudeiro & Rivadulla, 1999; Wu, Williams, & Mcloon, 1994; but see Finney & Shatz, 1998) or by altering the extracellular environment through any means. However, synaptogenesis will greatly intensify during the immediate perinatal period—the surge is recognizable and countable and hence has been much studied.

Although the number of synapses is often used as an index for the amount and complexity of information transfer in a structure, and even though this might be useful in some comparisons (e.g., synapse numbers will increase after certain kinds of experience; Greenough, 1984), it would be misleading to discuss synaptic numbers during development in only this way. "More" in development does not necessarily mean better, more complex, or more mature; it might well mean the opposite. There has long been a controversy about just what the patterns of synaptogenesis are and what they might mean.

Conflicting Views of the Synapse Surge?

Data obtained from the macaque and the human literature have resulted in two hypotheses that are typically presented as conflicting views of synaptogenesis (Bourgeois, Goldman-Rakic, & Rakic, 1994; Granger et al., 1995; Huttenlocher & Dabholkar, 1997; Rakic et al., 1986; Zecevic, Bourgeois, & Rakic, 1989; Zecevic & Rakic, 1991). In one series of studies, Rakic and colleagues described a rapid increase around birth in the number of synapses that seems to take place almost simultaneously across a number of macaque cortical areas, reaching a peak at around the same time in frontal, cingulate, somatosensory, and visual cortical areas (Bourgeois, Goldman-Rakic, & Rakic, 1994; Granger et al., 1995; Rakic et al., 1986; Zecevic, Bourgeois, & Rakic, 1989; Zecevic & Rakic, 1991). In contrast, Huttenlocher, working with human neural tissue, found that the peak of synaptic density varies between visual, auditory, and somatosensory regions, with the frontal regions not reaching their peak until 3 to 4 years after birth, while the visual and auditory regions peak more closely to birth (Huttenlocher & Dabholkar, 1997).

However, it appears that the story these two investigators tell is actually not very different if the timetables of development in humans and monkeys are appropriately compared. Figure 1.4 depicts replotted data on synapses production in the cortex of the macaque (obtained from tables in Bourgeois, Goldman-Rakic, & Rakic, 1994; Granger et al., 1995; Zecevic & Rakic, 1991) and the cortex of the human (obtained from tables in Huttenlocher & Dabholkar, 1997). To facilitate comparison between the two primates, which have over a 100-day difference in gestation (macaque, 165 days; human, 270 days), the human days were translated into macaque days using our comparative model.

It is clear that what Rakic and Huttenlocher have both shown is that the ratio of synapses to neuropil greatly accelerates just before birth in both the macaque and the human and across a wide variety of cortical areas. In macaques, the peak of synaptic density across cortical areas is reached 2 to 4 months after birth. In humans, the curves are similar to those of macaques, with a marked perinatal increase in synaptic density that begins around birth and flattens postnatally across all cortical areas. It should be noted that synapse counts may, or may not, vary across different cortical regions. However, for methodological and technical reasons, the absolute values of synapse counts should be considered somewhat conditional, especially in human tissue. Moreover, we have attempted to normalize the data by plotting synapse numbers as a percentage of the total at puberty, which we defined as 12 years in human and 3 years in macaque. The "take home" message from the graph lies not in the absolute numbers but rather in the pattern of relative changes. The most interesting feature in both the macaque and the human data lies in the strikingly similar timing of acceleration and deceleration, not in the location of the exact peak.

In order to understand how synaptic numbers are changing, it is useful to place it in the context of brain growth, considering principally "neuropil," the component of cortical tissue including dendrites, axons, and synapses but not cell bodies of neurons or glia nor vasculature (i.e., the synaptic interface). In monkey cortex, the relative proportion of neuropil soars from initially insignificant values around PC 50 to very high values at PC 100, a period corresponding to PC 65 to PC 130 in humans, still well before birth. After that, the amount of neuropil remains constant at about 70% to 75% until about 1 year from birth, after which there is a

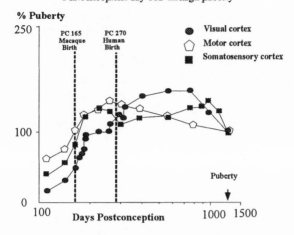

A   Macaque Synapse Production
Postconception day 112 through puberty

% Puberty

- ● Visual cortex
- ⬠ Motor cortex
- ■ Somatosensory cortex

PC 165 Macaque Birth
PC 270 Human Birth

Puberty

Days Postconception

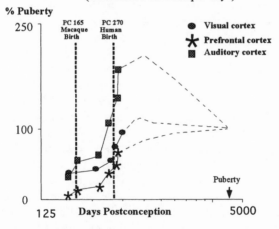

B   Human Synapse Production
Postconception day 192 through puberty
(normalized to macaque days)

% Puberty

- ● Visual cortex
- ✳ Prefrontal cortex
- ▦ Auditory cortex

PC 165 Macaque Birth
PC 270 Human Birth

Puberty

Days Postconception

Figure 1.4. Cortical synaptogenesis. A surge in the production of synapses in the developing cortex is coordinated with birth or eye opening (whichever occurs last)—timed to occur just at the verge of an onslaught of experience. The replotted synaptogenesis data from macaque (**A**) and human (**B**) cortex depict a rapid increase in the number of synapses coordinated across several cortical areas. If humans underwent an accelerated period of synaptogenesis at the maturational stage of macaques at birth, the synaptogenesis peaking would occur several weeks prior to the opportunity for most environmental stimuli. Synaptogenesis data obtained from Bourgeois, Goldman-Rakic, and Rakic (1994); Granger et al. (1995); Huttenlocher and Dabholkar (1997); Rakic et al. (1986); Zecevic, Bourgeois, and Rakic (1989); and Zecevic and Rakic (1991).

long slow decline to a value of about 50%, reached at some point past puberty. Meanwhile, the whole brain is getting bigger. In macaques and marmosets, the volume of visual cortex (with comparable increases in both depth and surface area) overshoots its adult size by about 45% at 6 months postnatal, then regresses to its adult volume. Overall brain volume increases from birth to adulthood by about a factor of two in monkeys and by a factor of almost four in humans. Because we know that the size of some components like primary visual cortex declines across the same period, the overall increase in brain size must be due to increases in the size of other cortical areas and in the number of glial cells, vasculature, and myelinated fibers in the brain.

What Causes the Synapse Surge?

Using visual cortex as a test case, Rakic and colleagues looked into the possibility that the marked synapse increase is actually *caused* by the barrage of experience that accompanies birth (Bourgeois & Rakic, 1996). However, when monkeys were deprived of visual input, the initial acceleration and peak of synaptogenesis in visual cortex were unchanged, though later events such as proportions, layering, and so forth, did change markedly. But this kind of deprivation experiment might be misleading, because the deprivation itself might induce a host of compensatory changes in other parts of the system. Yet in an experiment in which monkeys were delivered 3 weeks prematurely, so that external experience began much sooner than it would normally occur (Bourgeois, Jastreboff, & Rakic, 1989), there was no effect on the timing of synapse acceleration and peak—it occurred precisely when it should occur, based on the monkey's anticipated gestational birthdate, not the prematurely induced one. Secondary effects on types and distributions of synapses were also seen in this study, so certainly experience does matter. However, experience does not seem to be responsible for the burst in synaptogenesis.

Humans present an evolutionary experiment that is the opposite of the premature delivery manipulation, because we are actually born quite late with respect to many neural milestones (discussed below). Both birth and the accompanying surge of synaptogenesis occur much later in "neural time" in humans than they occur in the rhesus monkey. If humans underwent an accelerated period of synaptogenesis at the maturational stage corresponding to the stage when macaques show rapid synaptogenesis, it would occur several weeks prior to birth (see Figure 1.4). The human fetus would be in possession of a large reservoir of synaptic plasticity to simply contemplate the uterine wall! Timing of peak synaptogenesis to just precede the onset of experience is seen in other primates (Missler et al., 1993) and in animals such as rats (Blue & Parnavelas, 1983) where eye opening occurs after birth (which essentially marks a similar shift from a dark restricted environment into an onslaught of external experiences). Although less data are available for noncortical regions, a similarly timed burst and decline of synaptogenesis occurs in the striatum (Brand & Rakic, 1984). It should be noted that this peaking of synaptogenesis is the only instance we have found of a neural maturational event tied explicitly to birth rather than to the conserved intrinsic developmental timetable of the brain, which can be quite dissociated from birth (Clancy, Darlington, & Finlay, 2001).

One intriguing possibility for the source of the stimulus for the perinatal synapse surge is raised by work on mammalian parturition from Nathanielscz and colleagues. These recent studies have established that a signal from the fetus to the mother initiates the onset of labor (Nathanielsz, 1998). One could hypothesize that the same signal might trigger the synaptogenesis surge in the fetus itself.

As depicted in the graphs in Figure 1.4, the number of perinatal synapses are well in excess of the eventual adult number. It has become clear, however, that it would be a mistake to view early development as a "regressive" period. In both intermediately aged and mature nervous systems, additive and subtractive events co-occur and overlap (Quartz & Sejnowski, 1997).

MATURATIONAL GRADIENTS

Conventional hierarchical accounts of the development of human perception and behavior appeal to the successive maturation of midbrain versus cortex or the graded maturation of some parts of cortex versus other parts of cortex. Indeed, the hypothesis is often made that a part of the brain might "come online" at a particular point in development. But is there evidence for this?

Intrinsic Cortical Gradients

The isocortex has a gradient of neuron production and maturation that, as noted previously, is well conserved across all mammals. Bayer, Altman, and colleagues have produced detailed studies of the timing of neurogenesis in rodents (Altman & Bayer, 1979a, 1979b, 1988; Bayer et al., 1993), and we are able to apply the comparative mammalian model of Finlay and Darlington (1995) to predict a similar time sequence for humans. Neurogenesis begins at the front edge of the cortex where frontal cortex abuts inferotemporal cortex and proceeds back to primary visual cortex, framing a period of genesis that can last over 30 days in primates from front to back; in humans, this would lead us to expect a neurogenesis window of about 50 days in the first trimester extending from approximately PC 45 to PC 95. The limbic cingulate cortices also get an early start, with genesis beginning in humans about PC 45. The maturational edge possessed by frontal and limbic cortex may be expected to continue in various aspects of the intrinsic development of those parts of isocortex. For example, more mature neurons may begin to elaborate neuropil and extend local and long-range connections sooner. However, there is little direct association between the time of a neuron's genesis and when it makes its connections, as this also depends heavily on the maturational/trophic status of the regions it will connect to. Paradoxically, the frontal cortex (Fuster, 1997), often described as the last maturing cortical area, is in fact one of the first to be produced and thus quite "mature" in some features.

Imposed Thalamic Gradients

Each region of cortex receives thalamic input by maturity, but the order of thalamic development is different from the intrinsic cortical gradient. In general, the primary sensory nuclei in the thalamus, including the ventro-basal complex (somatosensory), parts of the medial geniculate body (auditory), and the LGN are generated first and establish their axonal connections to the cortex first. Various other nuclei (e.g., those projecting to motor and cingulate cortex) are intermediate in their timing, and the last to be produced are the nuclei that innervate the frontal, parietal, and part of the inferotemporal cortex. It is this thalamic order of neurogenesis that gives rise to the hierarchical notion of cortical development (e.g., "visual matures early; frontal matures late").

However, it is clear that different areas of the brain follow maturational gradients that do not match in order, and many temporal asynchronies are produced. In some areas, intracortical connections will be relatively more mature than thalamic connections (e.g., frontal cortex), and in others, the reverse will hold (e.g., primary visual cortex). This difference in developmental gradients might mean that frontal cortex, the area that bears so much weight in speculation about human evolution (e.g., Deacon, 1997), could be primed for higher-order associative function much earlier than previously thought. A direct comparison of the response properties of frontal versus visual neurons with regard to their responsiveness to thalamo-cortical and intracortical activation would be an interesting place to begin to explore the functional significance of this anatomical discrepancy.

UNEXPECTED MATURITY OF HUMANS AT BIRTH

There is another conventional developmental notion that should be reconsidered—the idea that neural tissue grows slowly in the human fetus, and consequently the human infant is born in a relatively altrical, or immature, state. This delayed and protracted human maturation is often presented as central to our unusual learning capacity. Clearly much neural development, including in the visual system, occurs postnatally, but is the human infant in fact neurally immature at birth? When we apply the comparative modeling approach to the timing of human neural events, we find instead that human neural development is relatively advanced at birth (Bates et al., 2002; Clancy, Darlington, & Finlay, 2000). This relative maturity makes intuitive sense (certainly to many parents), especially given recent empirical evidence that very young infants are capable of rapid and powerful forms of statistical learning, for example, the probabilistic relationship of syllables in speechlike streams or similar contingencies in visual events (Bates & Elman, 1996; Kirkham, Slemmer, & Johnson, 2001; Saffran, Aslin, & Newport, 1996).

In fact, months prior to parturition, human brains are at the neural maturational state of newborn macaques, primates that are conventionally considered advanced at birth. This human neural sophistication is perhaps best illustrated by fetal eye opening—the human fetus is capable of eye opening almost 3 months prior to birth (note: eye opening, which is difficult to observe in the human fetus, has been empirically determined to occur on PC day 182 of a 270-day gestation [Ashwell, Waite, & Marotte, 1996], although our model indicates it may actually occur about 2 weeks earlier). Why, then, is birth of the human infant delayed relative to brain maturation—and in fact delayed so late that the size of the human infant stretches the birth canal to its very limits?

Allometric analyses of primate data indicate that the human birth weight is above its predicted value, but contrary to conventional notions, the weight is not due to an enlarged brain. The weight is due to a disproportionately large size of the human fetus overall—the brain at birth is actually rather small relative to body size (reviewed in Leutenegger, 1982). It is somatic (nonneural) development that lags into the last months of human gestation (e.g., at 7 months gestation when neural tissue is comparatively developed, human lungs are not yet completely formed, the skin organ is not functioning properly, etc.).

The model translations suggest that despite the somatic immaturity of the human infant the human brain is relatively developed, perhaps even more developed than that of the recognized precocial nonhuman primates. The perinatal surge in synapse production (Figure 1.4), apparently postponed until the onslaught of environmental experience is imminent, may serve to "turn on" a relatively mature human infant brain. These suggestions are supported by recent research that indicates that the human infant rapidly acquires knowledge during the perinatal period, including some learning accomplished in utero (reviewed in Bates et al., 2002). It is even possible that the mismatch between the advanced neural and delayed somatic human maturational schedules is an important component of our learning capabilities, perhaps giving the human infant an enforced relatively nonactive period to observe and assimilate information prior to the extensive motor activity that will accompany later development. The oculomotor system is a relatively advanced volitional action system that can be used at birth to sample the optic array (Johnson & Johnson, 2001) and can provide a useful perception-action link, but without much physical peril.

SUMMARY

No single strategy holds any monopoly in visual system development. Genetics as well as internal and external activity combine in multiple, redundant, overlaid mechanisms and gradients that all contribute to an over-determined outcome. Virtually no evidence exists that the visual system, or any other neural area, "turns on" as a unit—most components of the visual system are responsive and plastic, and many change their functional profile as development occurs.

Although there is no evidence for a mosaic organization through which cortical divisions arise via discrete expression of single genes, visual cortex does seem to be a little "different." It has an overtly different structure in nonmammals, it scales differently from the rest of cortex, it is characterized by additional neurogenesis in primates, and it has some regionally specific molecular expression. One question of immediate and central interest is how species-specific recognition mechanisms, such as the recognition of faces and their properties, come to reside predictably in particular cortical areas, such as the inferotemporal cortex in primates (see Rodman, this volume).

The visual system as a whole is a complex and ancient sensory structure and one that has been vigorously studied for its contributions to our knowledge of both development and evolution. It is time to reconsider some conventional notions about such things as neural hierarchies and maturational schedules—just as the first genes that determine the properties of the eyes and brain are expressed in overlapping and nested fashion, so every subsequent aspect of structure and function shows overlapping and piecemeal development. Distinct in our vertebrate lineage, the developing human brain combines a surprising maturity at the time of birth, which could be viewed as readiness for experience, coupled with an unusually long time to assimilate that experience.

REFERENCES

Altman, J., & Bayer, S.A. (1979a). Development of the diencephalon in the rat. IV. Quantitative study of the time of origin of neurons and the internuclear chronological gradients in the thalamus. *Journal of Comparative Neurology, 188*, 455–471.

Altman, J., & Bayer, S.A. (1979b). Development of the diencephalon in the rat. VI. Reevaluation of the embryonic development of the thalamus on the basis of thymidine-radiographic datings. *Journal of Comparative Neurology, 188*, 501–524.

Altman, J., & Bayer, S.A. (1988). Development of the rat thalamus: II. Time and site of origin and settling pattern of neurons derived from the anterior lobule of the thalamic neuroepithelium. *Journal of Comparative Neurology, 275,* 378–405.

Angevine, J.B., & Sidman, R.L. (1961). Autoradiographic study of cell migration during histogenesis of cerebral cortex in the mouse. *Nature, 192,* 766–768.

Ashwell, K.W.S., Waite, P.M.E., & Marotte, L. (1996). Ontogeny of the projection tracts and commissural fibres in the forebrain of the tammar wallaby (*Macropus eugenii*): Timing in comparison with other mammals. *Brain Behavior and Evoution, 47,* 8–22.

Aslin, R.N. (1993). Perception of visual direction in human infants. In C.E. Granrud (Ed.), *Visual perception and cognition in infancy* (pp. 91–119). Hillsdale, NJ: Erlbaum.

Bates, E., & Elman, J. (1996). Learning rediscovered [comment]. *Science, 274,* 1849–1850.

Bates, E., Thal, D., Finlay, B., & Clancy, B. (2002). Early language development and its neural correlates. In F. Boller & J. Grafman (Series Eds.) & S.J. Segalowitz & I. Rapin (Vol. Eds.), *Handbook of Neuropsychology, Vol. 8: Child Neurology* (2nd ed., pp. 109–176). Amsterdam: Elsevier Science B.V.

Bayer, S.A., Altman, J., Russo, R.J., & Zhang, X. (1993). Timetables of neurogenesis in the human brain based on experimentally determined patterns in the rat. *Neurotoxicology, 14,* 83–144.

Bloom, F.E, & Lazerson, A. (1988). *Brain, mind and behavior* (2nd ed.). New York: Freeman.

Blue, M.E., & Parnavelas, J.G. (1983). The formation and maturation of synapses in the visual cortex of the rat. I. Qualitative analysis. *Journal of Neurocytology, 12,* 599–616.

Bodnarenko, S.R., Jeyarasasingam, G., & Chalupa, L.M. (1995). Development and regulation of dendritic stratification in retinal ganglion cells by glutamate-mediated afferent activity. *Journal of Neuroscience, 15,* 7037–7045.

Bourgeois, J.P., Goldman-Rakic, P.S., & Rakic, P. (1994). Synaptogenesis in the prefrontal cortex of rhesus monkeys. *Cerebral Cortex, 4,* 78–96.

Bourgeois, J.P., Jastreboff, P.J., & Rakic, P. (1989). Synaptogenesis in visual cortex of normal and preterm monkeys: Evidence for intrinsic regulation of synaptic overproduction. *Proceedings of the National Academy of Sciences (USA), 86,* 4297–4301.

Bourgeois, J.P., & Rakic, P. (1993). Changes of synaptic density in the primary visual cortex of the macaque monkey from fetal to adult stage. *Journal of Neuroscience, 13,* 2801–2820.

Bourgeois, J.P., & Rakic, P. (1996). Synaptogenesis in the occipital cortex of macaque monkey devoid of retinal input from early embryonic stages. *European Journal of Neuroscience, 8,* 942–950.

Brand, S., & Rakic, P. (1984). Cytodifferentiation and synaptogenesis in the neostriatum of fetal and neonatal rhesus monkeys. *Anatomy and Embryology, 169,* 21–34.

Bulfone, A., Smiga, S.M., Shimamura, K., Peterson, A., Puelles, L., & Rubenstein, J.L. (1995). T-brain-1: A homolog of Brachyury whose expression defines molecularly distinct domains within the cerebral cortex. *Neuron, 15,* 63–78.

Burkhalter, A. (1993). Development of forward and feedback connections between areas V1 and V2 of human visual cortex. *Cerebral Cortex, 3,* 476–487.

Butler, A.B., & Hodos, W. (1996). *Comparative vertebrate neuroanatomy: Evolution and adaptation.* New York: Wiley-Liss.

Callaerts, P., Halder, G., & Gehring, W.J. (1997). Pax-6 in development and evolution. *Annual Review of Neurosciences, 20,* 483–532.

Cepko, C.L. (1999). The roles of intrinsic and extrinsic cues and bHLH genes in the determination of retinal cell fates. *Current Opinion in Neurobiology, 9,* 37–46.

Cepko, C.L., Austin, C.P., Yang, X.J., & Alexiades, M. (1996). Cell fate determination in the vertebrate retina. *Proceedings of the National Academy of Sciences (USA), 93,* 589–595.

Chapman, B., Stryker, M.P., & Bonhoeffer, T. (1996). Development of orientation preference maps in ferret primary visual cortex. *Journal of Neuroscience, 16,* 6443–6453.

Cheng, H.J., Nakamoto, M., Bergemann, A.D., & Flanagan, J.G. (1995). Complementary gradients in expression and binding of ELF-1 and Mek4 in development of the topographic retinotectal projection map. *Cell, 82,* 371–381.

Clancy, B., Darlington, R.B., & Finlay, B.L. (2000). The course of human events: Predicting the timing of primate neural development. *Developmental Science, 3,* 57–66.

Clancy, B., Darlington, R.B., & Finlay, B.L. (2001). Translating developmental time across mammalian species. *Neuroscience, 105,* 7–17.

Cook, G., Tannahill, D., & Keynes, R. (1998). Axon guidance to and from choice points. *Current Opinion in Neurobiology, 8,* 64–72.

Coulombre, A.J., & Coulombre, J.L. (1956). The role of intraocular pressure in the development of the chick eye: I. Control of eye size. *Journal of Experimental Zoology, 133,* 211–225.

Crowley, J.C., & Katz, L.C. (1999). Development of ocular dominance columns in the absence of retinal input. *Nature Neuroscience, 2,* 1125–1130.

Crowley, J.C., & Katz, L.C. (2000). Early development of ocular dominance columns. *Science, 290,* 1321–1324.

Cudeiro, J., & Rivadulla, C. (1999). Sight and insight—on the physiological role of nitric oxide in the visual system. *Trends in Neuroscience, 22,* 109–116.

Curcio, C.A., & Hendrickson, A.E. (1992). Organization and development of the primate photoreceptor mosaic. *Progress in Retinal Research, 10,* 89–120.

Darlington, R.B., Dunlop, S.A., & Finlay, B.L. (1999). Neural development in metatherian and eutherian mammals: Variation and constraint. *Journal of Comparative Neurology, 411,* 359–368.

Deacon, T. (1997). *The symbolic species: The co-evolution of language and the brain.* New York: Norton.

Dehay, C., Giroud, P., Berland, M., Smart, I., & Kennedy, H. (1993). Modulation of the cell cycle contributes to the parcellation of the primate visual cortex. *Nature, 366,* 464–466.

Donoghue, M.J., & Rakic, P. (1999). Molecular gradients and compartments in the embryonic primate cerebral cortex. *Cerebral Cortex, 9,* 586–600.

Drescher, U., Kremoser, C., Handwerker, C., Loschinger, J., Noda, M., & Bonhoeffer, F. (1995). In vitro guidance of retinal ganglion cell axons by RAGS, a 25 kDa tectal protein related to ligands for Eph receptor tyrosine kinases. *Cell, 82,* 359–370.

Dunlop, S.A., Tee, I.B.G., Lund, R.D., & Beazley, L.D. (1997). Development of primary visual projections occurs entirely postnatally in the fat-tailed dunnart, a marsupial mouse, Sminthopsis crassicaudata. *Journal of Comparative Neurology, 384,* 26–40.

Easter, S.S., & Nicola, G.N. (1996). Development of vision in the zebrafish (Danio rerio). *Developmental Biology, 180,* 646–663.

Erskine, L., Williams, S.E., Brose, K., Kidd, T., Rachel, R.A., Goodman, C.S., Tessier-Lavigne, M., & Mason, C.A. (2000). Retinal ganglion cell axon guidance in the mouse optic chiasm: Expression and function of Robos and Slits. *Journal of Neuroscience, 20,* 4975–4982.

Felleman, D.J., & Van Essen, D.C. (1991). Distributed hierarchical processing in the primate cerebral cortex. *Cerebral Cortex, 1,* 1–47.

Fernald, R.D. (2000). Evolution of eyes. *Current Opinion in Neurobiology, 10,* 444–450.

Finlay, B.L. (1992). Cell death and the creation of regional differences in neuronal numbers. *Journal of Neurobiology, 23,* 1159–1171.

Finlay, B.L., & Darlington, R.B. (1995). Linked regularities in the development and evolution of mammalian brains. *Science, 268,* 1578–1584.

Finney, E.M., & Shatz, C.J. (1998). Establishment of patterned thalamocortical connections does not require nitric oxide synthase. *Journal of Neuroscience, 18,* 8826–8838.

Fitzpatrick, D. (2000). Seeing beyond the receptive field in primary visual cortex. *Current Opinion in Neurobiology, 10,* 438–443.

Flanagan, J.G., & Vanderhaeghen, P. (1998). The ephrins and Eph receptors in neural development. *Annual Review of Neuroscience, 21,* 309–345.

Franco, E.C.S., Finlay, B.L., Silveira, L.C.L., Yamada, Y.C., & Crowley, J.C. (2001). Conservation of absolute foveal area in New World primates: A constraint on eye size and conformation. *Brain, Behavior and Evolution, 56,* 276–286.

Frantz, G.D., Bohner, A.P., Akers, R.M., & McConnell, S.K. (1994). Regulation of the POU domain gene SCIP during cerebral cortical development. *Journal of Neuroscience, 14,* 472–485.

Frantz, G.D., Weimann, J.M., Levin, M.E., & McConnell, S.K. (1994). Otx1 and Otx2 define layers and regions in developing cerebral cortex and cerebellum. *Journal of Neuroscience, 14,* 5725–5740.

Fraser, S.E., & Perkel, D.H. (1990). Competitive and positional cues in the patterning of nerve connections. *Journal of Neurobiology, 21,* 51–72.

Fujita, S. (1963). The matrix cell cytogenesis in the developing nervous system. *Journal of Comparative Neurology, 120,* 37–42.

Fuster, J.M. (1997). *The prefrontal cortex* (3rd ed.). New York: Raven Press.

Gao, P.P., Yue, Y., Zhang, J.H., Cerretti, D.P., Levitt, P., & Zhou, R.P. (1998). Regulation of thalamic neurite outgrowth by the Eph ligand ephrin-A5: Implications in the development of thalamocortical projections. *Proceedings of the National Academy of Sciences (USA), 95,* 5329–5334.

Gao, P.P., Zhang, J.H., Yokoyama, M., Racey, B., Dreyfus, C.F., Black, I.B., & Zhou, R. (1996). Regulation of topographic projection in the brain: Elf-1 in the hippocamposeptal system. *Proceedings of the National Academy of Sciences (USA), 93,* 11161–11166.

Gao, W.J., & Pallas, S.L. (1999). Cross-modal reorganization of horizontal connectivity in auditory cortex without altering thalamocortical projections. *Journal of Neuroscience, 19,* 7940–7950.

Gilbert, C.D., Das, A., Ito, M., Kapadia, M., & Westheimer, G. (1996). Spatial integration and cortical dynamics. *Proceedings of the National Academy of Sciences (USA), 93,* 615–622.

Granger, B., Tekaia, F., Le Sourd, A.M., Rakic, P., & Bourgeois, J.P. (1995). Tempo of neurogenesis and synaptogenesis in the primate cingulate mesocortex: Comparison with the neocortex. *Journal of Comparative Neurology, 360,* 363–376.

Greenough, W.T. (1984). Structural correlates of information storage in the mammalian brain: A review and hypothesis. *Trends in Neurosciences, 7,* 229–233.

Gunhan-Agar, E., Kahn, D., & Chalupa, L.M. (2000). Segregation of on and off bipolar cell axonal arbors in the absence of retinal ganglion cells. *Journal of Neuroscience, 20,* 306–314.

Hendrickson, A. (1994). Primate foveal development: A microcosm of current questions in neurobiology. *Investigative Ophthalmology and Visual Sciences, 35,* 3129–3132.

Hendrickson, A., & Drucker, D. (1992). The development of parafoveal and mid-peripheral human retina. *Behavioral Brain Research, 49,* 21–31.

Hensch, T.K., & Stryker, M.P. (1996). Ocular dominance plasticity under metabotropic glutamate receptor blockade. *Science, 272,* 554–557.

Honig, L.S., Herrmann, K., & Shatz, C.J. (1996). Developmental changes revealed by immunohistochemical markers in human cerebral cortex. *Cerebral Cortex, 6,* 794–806.

Howland, H.C. (1983). Infant eyes: Optics and accommodation. *Current Eye Research, 2,* 217–224.

Howland, H.C., & Sayles, N. (1985). Photokeratometric and photorefractive measurements of astigmatism in infants and young children. *Vision Research, 25,* 73–81.

Hubel, D.H., & Wiesel, T.N. (1962). Receptive fields, binocular interaction and functional architecture in the cat's visual cortex. *Journal of Physiology, 160,* 106–154.

Hubel, D.H., & Wiesel, T.N. (1965). Binocular interaction in striate cortex of kittens reared with artificial squint. *Journal of Neurophysiology, 28,* 1041–1059.

Huttenlocher, P.R., & Dabholkar, A.S. (1997). Regional differences in synaptogenesis in human cerebral cortex. *Journal of Comparative Neurology, 387,* 167–178.

Huttenlocher, P.R., de Courten, C., Garey, L.J., & Van der Loos, H. (1982). Synaptogenesis in human visual cortex—evidence for synapse elimination during normal development. *Neuroscience Letters, 33,* 247–252.

Innocenti, G.M. (1991). The development of projections from cerebral cortex. *Progress in Sensory Physiology, 12,* 65–114.

Johnson, S.P., & Johnson, K.L. (2001). Early perception-action coupling: Eye movements and the development of object perception. *Infant Behavior and Development, 23,* 461–483.

Karlstrom, R.O., Trowe, T., & Bonhoeffer, F. (1997). Genetic analysis of axon guidance and mapping in the zebrafish. *Trends in Neurosciences, 20,* 3–8.

Karlstrom, R.O., Trowe, T., Klostermann, S., Baier, H., Brand, M., Crawford, A.D., Grunewald, B., Haffter, P., Hoffmann, H., Meyer, S.U., Muller, B.K., Richter, S., van Eeden, F.J.M., Nusslein Volhard, C., & Bonhoeffer, F. (1996). Zebrafish mutations affecting retinotectal axon pathfinding. *Development, 123,* 427–438.

Katz, L.C., & Shatz, C.J. (1996). Synaptic activity and the construction of cortical circuits. *Science, 274,* 1133–1138.

Kelling, S.T., Sengelaub, D.R., Wikler, K.C., & Finlay, B.L. (1989). Differential elasticity of the growing retina and the development of the area centralis. *Visual Neuroscience, 2,* 117–120.

Kirkham, N.Z., Slemmer, J.A., & Johnson, S.P. (2001). Statistical learning in infancy: A domain general learning mechanism. *Manuscript submitted for publication.*

Knudsen, E.I. (1994). Feature article: Supervised learning in the brain. *Journal of Neuroscience, 14,* 3985–3997.

LaVail, M.M., Rapaport, D.H., & Rakic, P. (1991). Cytogenesis in the monkey retina. *Journal of Comparative Neurology, 309,* 86–114.

Leutenegger, W. (1982). Encephalization and obstetrics in primates with particular reference to human evolution. In E. Armstrong & D. Falk (Eds.), *Primate brain evolution: Methods and concepts* (pp. 85–97). New York: Plenum.

LeVay, S., Wiesel, T.N., & Hubel, D.H. (1980). The development of ocular dominance columns in normal and visually deprived monkeys. *Journal of Comparative Neurology, 191,* 1–51.

Lidow, M.S., & Rakic, P. (1995). Neurotransmitter receptors in the proliferative zones of the developing primate occipital lobe. *Journal of Comparative Neurology, 360,* 393–402.

Mackarehtschian, K., Lau, C.K., Caras, I., & McConnell, S.K. (1999). Regional differences in the developing cerebral cortex revealed by ephrin-A5 expression. *Cerebral Cortex, 9,* 601–610.

Marin-Padilla, M. (1978). Dual origin of the mammalian neocortex and evolution of the cortical plate. *Anatomy and Embryology, 152,* 109–126.

Maslim, J., Webster, M., & Stone, J. (1986). Stages in the structural differentiation of retinal ganglion cells. *Journal of Comparative Neurology, 254,* 382–402.

Miles, F.A., & Wallman, J. (1990). Local ocular compensation for imposed local refractive error. *Vision Research, 30,* 339–349.

Miller, B., Chou, L., & Finlay, B.L. (1993). The early development of thalamocortical and corticothalamic projections. *Journal of Comparative Neurology, 335,* 16–41.

Miller, K.D., & Stryker, M.P. (1990). The development of ocular dominance columns: Mechanisms and models. In S.J. Hanson & C.R. Olson (Eds.), *Connectionist modeling and brain functions, the developing interface* (pp. 255–350). Cambridge, MA: MIT Press.

Misslar, M., et al. (1993). Prenatal and postnatal development of the primary visual cortex of the common marmoset. 1. A changing space for synaptogenesis. *Journal of Comparative Neurology, 333,* 41–52.

Molnar, Z., et al. (1998). Mechanisms underlying the early establishment of thalamocortical connections in the rat. *Journal of Neoroscience, 18,* 5723–5745.

Naegele, J.R., Jhaveri, S., & Schneider, G.E. (1988). Sharpening of topographical projections and maturation of geniculocortical axon arbors in the hamster. *Journal of Comparative Neurology, 281,* 1–12.

Nakagawa, Y., Johnson, J.E., & O'Leary, D.D. (1999). Graded and areal expression patterns of regulatory genes and cadherins in embryonic neocortex independent of thalamocortical input. *Journal of Neuroscience, 19,* 10877–10885.

Nathanielsz, P.W. (1998). Comparative studies on the initiation of labor. *European Journal of Obstetrics, Gynecology and Reproductive Biology, 78,* 127–132.

Nathans, J. (1999). The evolution and physiology of human color vision: Insights from molecular genetic studies of visual pigments. *Neuron, 24,* 299–312.

Neuman, T., Keen, A., Zuber, M.X., Kristjansson, G.I., Gruss, P., & Nornes, H.O. (1993). Neuronal expression of regulatory helix-loop-helix factor Id2 gene in mouse. *Developmental Biology, 160,* 186–195.

Northcutt, R.G., & Kaas, J.H. (1995). The emergence and evolution of mammalian neocortex. *Trends in Neurosciences, 18,* 373–379.

Nothias, F., Fishell, G., & Ruiz i Altaba, A. (1998). Cooperation of intrinsic and extrinsic signals in the elaboration of regional identity in the posterior cerebral cortex. *Current Biology, 8,* 459–462.

O'Kusky, J., & Colonnier, M. (1982). Postnatal changes in the number of neurons and synapses in the visual cortex (area 17) of the macaque monkey: A stereological analysis in normal and monocularly deprived animals. *Journal of Comparative Neurology, 210,* 291–306.

O'Leary, D.D., et al. (1994). Specification of neocortical areas and thalamocortical connections. *Annual Review of Neuroscience, 17,* 419–439.

O'Leary, D.D.M. (1989). Do cortical areas emerge from a protocortex? *Trends in Neurosciences, 12,* 400–406.

Olshausen, B.A., & Field, D.J. (1996). Emergence of simple-cell receptive field properties by learning a sparse code for natural images. *Nature, 381,* 607–609.

O'Rourke, N.A., Dailey, M.E., Smith, S.J., & McConnell, S.K. (1992). Diverse migratory pathways in the developing cerebral cortex. *Science, 258,* 299–302.

Pallas, S.L., Littman, T., & Moore, D.R. (1999). Cross-modal reorganization of callosal connectivity without altering thalamocortical projections. *Proceedings of the National Academy of Sciences (USA), 96,* 8751–8756.

Pallas, S.L., Roe, A.W., & Sur, M. (1990). Visual projection induced into the auditory pathway of ferrets. I. Novel inputs to primary auditory cortex (AI) from the LP/Pulvinar complex and the topography of the MGN/AI projection. *Journal of Comparative Neurology, 298,* 50–68.

Pettigrew, J.D., & Konishi, M. (1976). Neurons selective for orientation and binocular disparity in the visual Wulst of the barn owl (*Tyto alba*). *Science, 193,* 675–678.

Polley, E.H., Zimmerman, R.P., & Fortney, R.L. (1989). Neurogenesis and maturation of cell morphology in the development of the mammalian retina. In

B.L. Finlay & D.R. Sengelaub (Eds.), *Development of the vertebrate retina* (pp. 3–29). New York: Plenum.

Provis, J.M., & Penfold, P.L. (1988). Cell death and the elimination of retinal axons during development. *Progress in Neurobiology, 31,* 331–347.

Provis, J.M., van Driel, D., Billson, F.A., & Russell, P. (1985a). Development of the human retina: Patterns of cell distribution and redistribution in the ganglion cell layer. *Journal of Comparative Neurology, 233,* 429–451.

Provis, J.M., van Driel, D., Billson, F.A., & Russell, P. (1985b). Human fetal optic nerve: Overproduction and elimination of retinal axons during development. *Journal of Comparative Neurology, 238,* 92–100.

Quartz, S.R., & Sejnowski, T.J. (1997). The neural basis of cognitive development: A constructivist manifesto. *Behavioral Brain Science, 20,* 537.

Quiring, R., Walldorf, U., Kloter, U., & Gehring, W.J. (1994). Homology of the *eyeless* gene of *Drosophila* to the *Small eye* gene in mice and *Aniridia* in humans. *Science, 265,* 785–788.

Rakic, P. (1972). Mode of cell migration to the superficial layers of fetal monkey neocortex. *Journal of Comparative Neurology, 145,* 61–83.

Rakic, P. (1974). Neurons in rhesus monkey visual cortex: Systematic relation between time of origin and eventual disposition. *Science, 183,* 425–427.

Rakic, P. (1976). Prenatal genesis of connections subserving ocular dominance in the rhesus monkey. *Nature, 261,* 467–471.

Rakic, P. (1981). Development of visual centers in the primate brain depends on binocular competition before birth. *Science, 214,* 928–931.

Rakic, P. (1988). Specification of cerebral cortical areas. *Science, 241,* 170.

Rakic, P., Bourgeois, J.P., Eckenhoff, M.F., Zecevic, N., & Goldman-Rakic, P.S. (1986). Concurrent overproduction of synapses in diverse regions of the primate cerebral cortex. *Science, 232,* 232–235.

Rapaport, D.H., & Stone, J. (1982). The site of commencement of maturation in mammalian retina: Observations in the cat. *Developmental Brain Research, 5,* 273–279.

Reichenbach, A., Eberhardt, W., Scheibe, R., Deich, C., Seifert, B., Reichelt, W., Dahnert, K., & Rodenbeck, M. (1991). Development of the rabbit retina IV. Tissue tensility and elasticity in dependence on topographic specializations. *Experimental Eye Research, 53,* 241–251.

Reichenbach, A., Schnitzer, J., Reichelt, E., Osborne, N.N., Fritzsche, B., Puls, A., Richter, U., Friedrich, A., Knothe, A.K., Schober, W., & Timmermann, U. (1993). Development of the rabbit retina: III. Differential retinal growth, and density of projection neurons and interneurons. *Visual Neuroscience, 10,* 479–498.

Robinson, S.R. (1991). Development of the mammalian retina. In B. Dreher & S.R. Robinson (Eds.), *Neuroanatomy of the visual pathways and their development* (Vol. 3, pp. 69–128). London: Macmillan.

Robinson, S.R., & Dreher, B. (1990). The visual pathway of eutherian mammals and marsupials develop according to a common timetable. *Brain, Behavior and Evolution, 36,* 177–195.

Roe, A.W., Pallas, S.L., Kwon, Y.H., & Sur, M. (1992). Visual projections routed to the auditory pathway in ferrets: Receptive field of neurons in primary auditory cortex. *Journal of Neuroscience, 12,* 3651–3665.

Rubenstein, J.L., Anderson, S., Shi, L., Miyashita-Lin, E., Bulfone, A., & Hevner, R. (1999). Genetic control of cortical regionalization and connectivity. Cerebral Cortex, 9, 524–532.

Saffran, J.R., Aslin, R.N., & Newport, E.L. (1996). Statistical learning by 8-month-old infants. Science, 274, 1926–1928.

Sauer, F.C. (1935). Mitosis in the neural tube. Journal of Comparative Neurology, 62, 377–405.

Schaeffel, F., & Howland, H.C. (1991). Properties of the feedback loops controlling eye growth and refractive state in the chicken. Vision Research, 31, 717–734.

Sengelaub, D.R., Dolan, R.P., & Finlay, B.L. (1986). Cell generation, death and retinal growth in the development of the hamster retinal ganglion cell layer. Journal of Comparative Neurology, 246, 527–543.

Sengelaub, D.R., & Finlay, B.L. (1981). Early removal of one eye reduces normally occurring cell death in the remaining eye. Science, 213, 573–574.

Shatz, C.J. (1990). Competitive interactions between retinal ganglion cells during prenatal development. Journal of Neurobiology, 21, 197–211.

Shatz, C.J., Chun, J.J.M., & Luskin, M.B. (1988). The role of the subplate in the development of the mammalian telencephalon. In A. Peters & E.G. Jones (Eds.), The cerebral cortex (Vol. 7, pp. 35–58). New York: Plenum.

Shatz, C.J., & Sretavan, D.W. (1986). Interactions between ganglion cells during the development of the mammalian visual system. Annual Review of Neuroscience, 9, 171–207.

Sperry, R.W. (1963). Chemoaffinity in the orderly growth of nerve fiber patterns and their connections. Proceedings of the National Academy of Sciences (USA), 50, 703–710.

Stein, B.E. (1984). Development of the superior colliculus. Annual Review of Neuroscience, 7, 95–125.

Stryker, M.P., & Harris, W.A. (1986). Binocular impulse blockade prevents the formation of ocular dominance columns in cat visual cortex. Journal of Neuroscience, 6, 2117–2131.

Sur, M., Pallas, S.L., & Roe, A.W. (1990). Cross-modal plasticity in cortical development: Differentiation and specification of sensory neocortex. Trends in Neurosciences, 13, 227–233.

Troilo, D. (1992). Neonatal eye growth and emmetropization: A literature review. Eye, 6, 154–160.

Troilo, D., Gottlieb, M.D., & Wallman, J. (1987). Visual deprivation causes myopia in chicks with optic nerve section. Current Eye Research, 6, 993–999.

Udin, S.B., & Fawcett, J.W. (1988). The formation of topographic maps. Annual Review of Neuroscience, 11, 289–328.

Van Essen, D.C., Newsome, W.T., & Maunsell, J.H. (1984). The visual field representation in striate cortex of the macaque monkey: Asymmetries, anisotropies, and individual variability. Vision Research, 24, 429–448.

von Melchner, L., Pallas, S.L., & Sur, M. (2000). Visual behaviour mediated by retinal projections directed to the auditory pathway. Nature, 404, 871–876.

Wallman, J. (1992). Retinal control of eye growth and refraction. Progress in Retinal Research, 12, 47–63.

Walsh, C., & Cepko, C.L. (1988). Clonally related cortical cells show several migration patterns. *Science, 241*, 1342–1345.

Weliky, M., Kandler, K., Fitzpatrick, D., & Katz, L.C. (1995). Patterns of excitation and inhibition evoked by horizontal connections in visual cortex share a common relationship to orientation columns. *Neuron, 15*, 541–552.

Wiesel, T.N., & Hubel, D.H. (1974). Ordered arrangement of orientation columns in monkeys lacking visual experience. *Journal of Comparative Neurology, 158*, 307–318.

Wong, R.O. (1999). Retinal waves and visual system development. *Annual Review of Neuroscience, 22*, 29–47.

Wong, R.O.L., Hermann, K., & Shatz, C.J. (1991). Remodeling of retinal ganglion cell dendrites in the absence of action potential activity. *Journal of Neurobiology, 22*, 685–697.

Wong, R.O.L., Meister, M., & Shatz, C.J. (1993). Transient period of correlated bursting activity during development of the mammalian retina. *Neuron, 11*, 923–938.

Woo, T.U., Beale, J.M., & Finlay, B.L. (1991). Dual fate of subplate neurons in a rodent. *Cerebral Cortex, 1*, 433–443.

Wu, H.H., Williams, C.V., & Mcloon, S.C. (1994). Involvement of nitric oxide in the elimination of a transient retinotectal projection in development. *Science, 265*, 1593–1596.

Yakovlev, P., & Lecours, A. (1967). The myelinogenetic cycle of regional maturation of the brain. In A. Minkowski (Ed.), *Regional development of the brain in early life* (pp. 107–137). Philadelphia: Davis.

Zecevic, N., Bourgeois, J.P., & Rakic, P. (1989). Changes in synaptic density in motor cortex of rhesus monkey during fetal and postnatal life. *Developmental Brain Research, 50*, 11–32.

Zecevic, N., & Rakic, P. (1991). Synaptogenesis in monkey somatosensory cortex. *Cerebral Cortex, 1*, 510–523.

Chapter 2

Critical Periods in the Visual System

Nigel W. Daw

ABSTRACT

As the visual system develops, it goes through three stages: an initial period of development, a period during which it will degenerate if not normally stimulated, and a period over which it can recover from any degeneration. These periods may be different from each other; that is, the period over which degeneration can occur may last longer than the initial period of development, and the period over which recovery may occur may last longer still. These three periods are evaluated for a number of visual properties, namely, grating acuity, Snellen acuity, vernier acuity, binocular function, stereopsis, monocular optokinetic nystagmus, monocular visually evoked response for a moving stimulus, suppression, myopia, and contrast sensitivity. The periods of development and the critical periods for degeneration and recovery vary significantly from each other and with the visual property studied.

INTRODUCTION

A critical period in the visual system is a period during which some property of the system can be changed. In their pioneering experiments, Wiesel and Hubel (1963b) used it to describe the period during which the ocular dominance of cells in the visual cortex of cats can be changed by monocular deprivation, in other words, the period during which ocular dominance can be disrupted. This was clearly different from the initial period of development of ocular dominance, and authors have become increasingly aware that this is true of other properties. Considering acuity, Wick et al. (1992)

talk about the critical period for development and the plastic period for treatment. There is also the period during which a property can recover after it has been disrupted, and investigators have become increasingly aware that these are also not necessarily identical. Hardman Lea, Loades, and Rubinstein (1989) talk about the sensitive period for development of amblyopia and the sensitive period for its treatment.

Thus we have to distinguish three periods: the initial period for development of a property, the critical period for disruption of the property, and the critical period for recovery of the property after it has been disrupted. For some properties these may be the same, but for others, they are clearly not the same. The prime purpose of this chapter will be to discuss where there are similar time courses and where the time courses are different. In most people's minds the terms *critical period* and *sensitive period* are probably interchangeable. I will use the term *critical period* and talk about the initial period of development and the critical periods for disruption and recovery.

Critical periods have been studied in the visual system more extensively than anywhere else in the brain. The concept of the critical period is well known for other functions. For example, it becomes more difficult to learn a new language with the appropriate pronunciation after puberty. The advantage of the visual system is that there are a number of different functions that can be studied, and most of them can be measured, even in infants. Thus the visual system is the system of choice for a comparative and detailed study of critical periods.

The crucial visual factor in humans is, How well can one see, as measured by acuity? Poor vision (amblyopia) can result from a variety of conditions such as strabismus (one eye turned inward or outward) and anisometropia (one eye out of focus). Measurements of acuity show that this develops in normal children to adult levels in 3 to 5 years. However, acuity can be disrupted by strabismus or anisometropia until 7 or 8 years of age. After it has been disrupted, acuity can be improved by effective therapy in teenagers and sometimes even in adults with maintained therapy. This supports the point that the period for disruption of a property lasts longer than the period of initial development, and the period during which recovery is possible lasts longer still.

Experiments with animals also show that there are a variety of critical periods and that this depends on the part of the visual system being studied. Monocular deprivation has little effect on the retina, a very small effect on the lateral geniculate nucleus, and a major effect on primary visual cortex. Within primary visual cortex, the critical period for the effect on cells in layer IV ends earlier than the critical period for cells in layers outside IV. Furthermore, the critical period for direction of movement ends earlier than the critical period for monocular deprivation. Moreover, rearing an animal in the dark delays both the onset and the end of the critical period for monocular deprivation.

Thus, one cannot talk about the critical period as a single entity. One has to talk about the critical period for a particular function in a particular part of the nervous system after a particular history of visual exposure with a particular kind of visual deprivation. This chapter will discuss the evidence for these variations in the critical period and what general hypotheses may be drawn from the evidence.

GENERAL PRINCIPLES FROM EXPERIMENTS WITH ANIMALS

The System Is Plastic between Eye Opening and Puberty

The manipulation that has been carried out most often in animals, and is easiest to use for a comparison between species, is monocular deprivation. The eyelids of one eye are sutured shut for a period of time. Recordings are then made in the visual cortex, and a number of cells are assayed for whether they are dominated by the left eye or the right eye or both, to give an ocular dominance histogram. Ocular dominance may also be measured with the visually evoked potential (VEP).

In the cat, the critical period for monocular deprivation lasts from 3 weeks to 8 months of age (Daw et al., 1992; Jones, Spear, & Tong, 1984; Olson & Freeman, 1980). The eyes open at 3 to 12 days of age, and puberty occurs at 6 months of age. In the rat, the critical period lasts from before 3 to about 7 weeks of age (Fagiolini et al., 1994; Guire, Lickey, & Gordon, 1999). The eyes open at 10 to 12 days, and puberty occurs at 8 to 12 weeks, later for males than females. For mice, the critical period is before 18 to more than 35 days of age (Gordon & Stryker, 1996), with eye opening at 10 to 12 days and puberty at 6 to 8 weeks. Macaque monkeys have their eyes open at birth, with a critical period lasting from close to birth to nearly 1 year of age. Puberty is at 3 to 3½ years for males and 2 to 3 years for females. Humans also have their eyes open at birth, with a critical period for unilateral cataract lasting from 6 to 8 weeks of age to 10 years of age (Birch et al., 1998; Vaegan & Taylor, 1979).

It is often difficult to judge the start of the critical period, because experiments with infants can be very difficult and so can physiological recordings in young animals. Similarly, the end of the critical period depends on the severity of the deprivation, as described in the next section, and the technique used, for example, single unit recording versus visually evoked potentials. Thus the comparisons are difficult to make. Nevertheless, the generalization that the critical period starts soon after eye opening and ends around puberty seems to be true. The one exception seems to be the macaque, where current evidence shows that the critical period ends at about 1 to 2 years of age, and puberty occurs some time after that.

One consequence of this generalization is that the end of the critical period could vary with gender in species where puberty varies with gender, such as rat and macaque monkey. Experiments to test a direct relationship between the end of the critical period and levels of steroids that increase around puberty have been either negative (Daw, Baysinger, & Parkinson, 1987) or equivocal (Daw et al., 1991). However, the relationship might be indirect, and the possibility of a relationship between gender and the end of the critical period in rats and macaques, where the difference in puberty between the two genders is most striking, has never been tested.

Within the critical period the susceptibility increases to a peak during which the system is extremely sensitive, then declines. At the peak, 1 to 2 days of deprivation can have an effect in species like mice and cat, and 1 week can have an effect in others like macaque and human. The peak sensitivity is at 4 to 6 weeks in cat, around 4 weeks in rats and mice, around 6 weeks in macaque, and around 6 months in human, although it is not very well defined in the last two species.

More Severe Deprivations Have a Larger Effect

Numerous studies, starting with the first papers by Wiesel and Hubel (1963b) on cats and LeVay, Wiesel, and Hubel (1980) on macaque monkeys, have shown that the extent of the ocular dominance shift from monocular deprivation depends on both the length of deprivation and the time at which it is applied. During the most sensitive part of the critical period in the cat, 1 day of deprivation has a slight effect, 2½ to 3½ days has a large effect, and after 6 to 10 days of deprivation, nearly all cells in the cortex are totally dominated by the eye that remained open (Hubel & Wiesel, 1970; Olson & Freeman, 1975).

The first experiment that tested the effect of a constant period of monocular deprivation at various ages was done in the cat (Olson & Freeman, 1980). They used approximately 10 days of deprivation and showed a small ocular dominance shift for deprivation between 8 and 19 days of age, a substantial one with deprivation between 18 and 27 days of age, and significant shifts up to deprivation between 109 and 120 days of age when it was again very small. The conclusion was that the critical period lasted from 3 weeks to 3½ months of age. Subsequent experiments with 1 month (Jones, Spear, & Tong, 1984) and 3 months of deprivation (Daw et al., 1992) show that these longer periods of deprivation are effective at 9 months of age. Thus the end and the length of the critical period both depend on how long the deprivation lasts (Figure 2.1).

Deprivations more severe than suturing the eyelids shut can have an effect even in the adult (Gilbert & Wiesel, 1992). If large lesions are

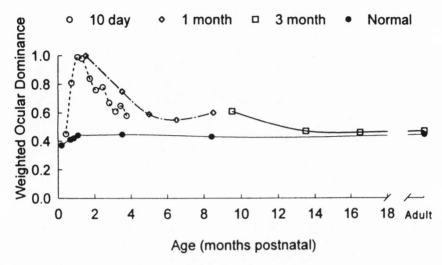

Figure 2.1. Critical period for ocular dominance changes from monocular deprivation in the cat. Weighted ocular dominance ranges from 0, when all cells are driven solely by the contralateral eye, to 1, when all cells are driven solely by the ipsilateral eye, and is 0.43 in normal animals, because there is a slight dominance by the contralateral eye. The contralateral eye is closed to produce shifts toward dominance by the ipsilateral eye. Points for 10 days of deprivation from Olson and Freeman (1980); for 1 month from Jones, Spear, and Tong (1984); for 3 months from Daw et al. (1992). Reprinted with permission from *Investigative Ophthalmology and Visual Science*, Daw (1994).

made in the retinas of both eyes, so that the cortex has no input in this part of the field of view, cells in the cortex representing the area of the lesion will start responding to areas in the retina outside the lesion. There is a short-term physiological change, and also a long-term anatomical change, through sprouting of lateral connections within the cortex (Darian-Smith & Gilbert, 1994). The physiological change can be produced with an artificial scotoma as well as a lesion (Pettet & Gilbert, 1992).

Higher Levels of the System Develop Later and Are More Plastic

Processing of signals in the visual system goes from retina to lateral geniculate nucleus to primary visual cortex to secondary visual cortex, then to visual areas in the temporal lobe for processing of form and color and to parietal areas for processing of location in space (Van Essen, Anderson, & Felleman, 1992). Development at these different levels has been compared using acuity for a black and white grating, with both physiological and behavioral measurements made in the macaque monkey. Grating acuity develops as a result of changes in both photoreceptors and visual cortex. The change in photoreceptors accounts for a factor of five in the improvement in acuity between newborn and adult. It is due to the photoreceptors becoming longer, which gives them more light-gathering power, and closer together (Banks & Bennett, 1988). This process is complete by about 6 months of age in the macaque, and the resolution for cells in the lateral geniculate nucleus reaches maturity at about the same time (Jacobs & Blakemore, 1988). The capabilities of the cortical cells continue to develop after this time (Figure 2.2). Thus development of grating acuity, measured in the cortex and by behavior, develops for a longer period of time than in the retina and lateral geniculate nucleus.

Visual deprivation also has larger effects in the cortex than in retina and lateral geniculate nucleus. Monocular deprivation has very little effect in the retina (Sherman & Stone, 1973; Wiesel & Hubel, 1963b) on any of the cell types found there (Cleland et al., 1980). There is also little effect on the physiological properties of cells in the lateral geniculate nucleus (Derrington & Hawken, 1981; Shapley & So, 1980; Wiesel & Hubel, 1963a). Cells in the lateral geniculate nucleus driven by the deprived eye are smaller (Wiesel & Hubel, 1963a), but this almost certainly occurs because they support reduced endings in the cortex, particularly in the part of the field of view that is binocular where competition between the two eyes occurs (Guillery & Stelzner, 1970).

The most noticeable effects of monocular deprivation occur in primary visual cortex, where cells are completely dominated by the open eye, and most cannot be driven at all by the closed eye after long periods of deprivation. This is true particularly of cells in extragranular layers (layers II, III, V, and VI), which are the output layers of the cortex. Some cells in the input layer, layer IV, can still be driven by the deprived eye (Shatz & Stryker, 1978). With deprivations late in the critical period, the ocular dominance of cells in layers II, III, V, and VI is altered, whereas the ocular dominance of cells in layer IV is not (Daw et al., 1992; Mower et al., 1985). Thus the critical period for the input layer ends earlier than the critical period for the output layers.

The critical period for secondary visual cortex (area 18) is the same as the critical period for primary visual cortex in the cat (Jones, Spear, & Tong, 1984), but this may be because the lateral geniculate nucleus projects to areas 17 and 18 in parallel in this species. A careful comparison of critical periods in areas 17 and 18 has not been made in the macaque monkey where area 18 receives input from area 17 but not from the lateral geniculate nucleus. Plasticity in inferotemporal cortex, which is implicated in many object recognition tasks, continues for some period of time after primary visual cortex is no longer mutable (Rodman, 1994).

There are problems in comparing plasticity at different levels of the visual system. One has to use an appropriate manipulation. Monocular depriva-

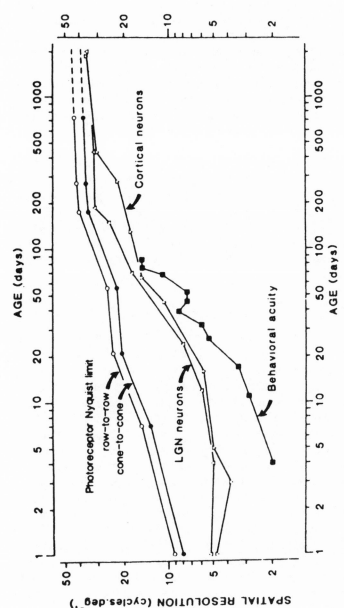

Figure 2.2. Development of acuity in the monkey measured in behavioral experiments, compared to the capabilities of neurons in the lateral geniculate nucleus and cortex, and the theoretical limit of acuity (Nyquist limit) based on the spacing of photoreceptors. Reprinted with kind permission from Jacobs, D.S., & Blakemore, C. (1988). Factors limiting the postnatal development of visual acuity in the monkey. *Vision Research, 28,* 947–958. Copyright 1988, Elsevier Science, Ltd., The Boulevard, Langford Lane, Kidlington OX5 1GB, UK.

tion is a powerful manipulation for primary visual cortex, because that is the first level at which signals from the two eyes converge onto a single neuron. The effects of competition between the two eyes for synaptic space on visual cortex neurons results in the dramatic ocular dominance shifts seen there. After a cell in primary visual cortex has become monocular, this property may simply be carried on to higher levels of the system. Moreover, monocular deprivation may not be such a powerful manipulation at lower levels of the system, where no competition is involved. However, other manipulations that may be more appropriate for the retina also give no plasticity. The rabbit retina contains a large percentage of ganglion cells that are directionally selective, responding to upward, leftward, downward, or rightward movement in approximately equal numbers. Rearing rabbits in an environment that continually moves in one direction does not change the percentage of cells responding to movement in that direction (Daw & Wyatt, 1974). This occurs either because the retina is not plastic or because the rabbit is not plastic, since a similar experiment in the cat cortex gives positive results (Daw & Wyatt, 1976). Generally speaking, the retina can be affected by chemical manipulations before birth (Bodnarenko, Jeyarasasingam, & Chalupa, 1995) but does not appear to be affected by sensory manipulations after birth.

Different Properties Have Different Critical Periods

The first experiment comparing critical periods for different properties was done with ocular dominance and direction selectivity in the cat visual cortex. Kittens were reared in a drum moving continually in one direction; then the direction was switched to the reverse direction, and the cortex was assayed for the percentage of cells preferring the direction seen first compared to the percentage preferring the direction seen second (Daw & Wyatt, 1976). The results were compared to data on ocular dominance where one eye was open first, then closed, and the other eye opened (Blakemore & van Sluyters, 1974). With ocular dominance, the eye opened second dominated for switches before 7 weeks of age, and the eye open first dominated for switches after that. With direction, the direction seen second dominated for switches before 4 weeks, and the direction seen first dominated for switches after that, implying that the critical period for direction selectivity ends earlier than the critical period for ocular dominance (Figure 2.3). Interestingly, when one eye was open until 5 weeks of age looking at a drum moving in one direction, then both eyes and direction were switched, the majority of cells preferred the direction seen first and the eye open second (Daw, Berman, & Ariel, 1978), as expected for critical periods ending at different times. The general point is supported by the observation that orientation selectivity becomes fixed in place before ocular dominance in ferrets (Chapman & Stryker, 1993; Issa et al., 1999).

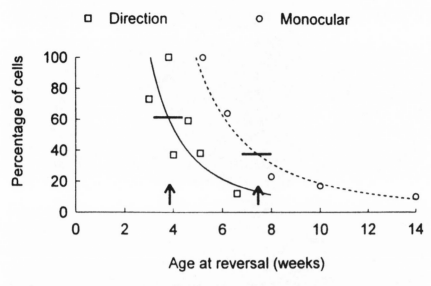

Figure 2.3. Comparison of critical periods for direction-selective and ocular dominance changes. Animals were reared in one condition (right eye open, or environment moving right) and then switched to the opposite (left eye open or movement left) at an age that varied from animal to animal. Points plot the percentage of cells preferring the direction seen second, or the eye open second. The curve for direction-selective changes passes through the normal ratio (60%) before 4 weeks of age, and the curve for ocular dominance changes passes through the normal ratio (43%) after 7 weeks of age. Points from Blakemore and van Sluyters (1974) and Daw and Wyatt (1976). Reprinted with permission from *Investigative Ophthalmology and Visual Science*, Daw (1994).

To fit this result in with the previous generalization that critical periods end earlier at lower levels of the system, one has to argue that directional selectivity is created at a lower level than ocular dominance. This is partly true in the cat. Many cells in layer IV are directionally selective, and many are also monocular. Thus direction selectivity is a property created at the input level of primary visual cortex, at least in the cat where these experiments were conducted, whereas binocularity is a property created primarily at higher levels of the system.

Another example of different critical periods for different properties occurs in layer IV of primary visual cortex in the macaque monkey. There are two parallel pathways for processing of different properties within the geniculostriate projections in the macaque. Form and color are processed in the P pathway, which projects to the parvocellular layers of the lateral geniculate nucleus and layer IVC in primary visual cortex. Movement is processed in the M pathway, which projects to the magnocellular layers of the lateral geniculate nucleus and layer IVC in primary visual cortex. Mo-

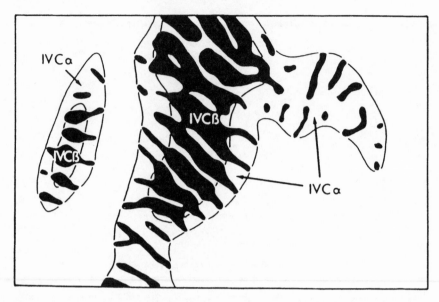

Figure 2.4. Effect of reverse suture at 3 weeks of age on labeling pattern in the right cortex from amino acids injected into the eye and transported to the cortex to label endings from that eye. Right eye sutured first, then opened and left eye sutured. Right eye was injected. Right eye endings (black area) dominated in layer IVC ß because this layer was still plastic at 3 weeks of age; left eye endings (white area) dominated in layer IVC a, because the critical period for this layer was over at 3 weeks of age. Reprinted with permission from LeVay, S., Wiesel, T.N., & Hubel, D.H. (1980). The development of ocular dominance columns in normal and visually deprived monkeys. *Journal of Comparative Neurology, 191*, 1–51. Copyright 1980, John Wiley & Sons, Inc.

nocular deprivation leads to a reduction in the extent of the geniculocortical endings in the visual cortex. In animals where one eye is open until 3 weeks of age, then closed and the other eye opened, layer IVC α is dominated by the endings from the eye open first, while layer IVC β is dominated by the endings from the eye opened second (LeVay, Wiesel, & Hubel, 1980; Figure 2.4). Thus the critical period for the magnocellular endings comes to a close before the critical period for the parvocellular endings. Connections for movement get wired into place, while connections for form and color are still plastic.

A further example comes from experiments with monocular deprivation in the macaque monkey (Harwerth et al., 1986). Monocular deprivation can affect a variety of behavioral measures, such as sensitivity to light in the dark-adapted state, sensitivity to increments of light in the light-adapted state, sensitivity to contrast at high spatial frequencies, and binocular summation. Dark-adapted sensitivity is affected by monocular deprivation before 3 months of age, increment sensitivity before 6 months, contrast sensitivity at high spatial frequencies before 18 months, and binocular summation before 24 months (Figure 2.5). This sequence of effects also fits in with the generalization that properties dealt with at a higher level of the system have critical periods that end later.

The Critical Period Depends on the Previous Visual History of the Animal

It is now well established that rearing an animal in the dark affects the critical period. Monocular deprivation changes the ocular dominance in dark-reared animals at several months of age, when there is little effect in light-reared animals of the same age (Cynader & Mitchell, 1980). Early in the critical period, monocular deprivation has a larger effect on light-reared animals than dark-reared animals (Beaver, Ji, & Daw, 2002; Mower, 1991). Thus rearing in the dark delays both the start and the end of the critical period. This leads to the interesting result that dark-reared cats are less plastic than light-reared cats at 5 to 6 weeks of age, equally plastic at 8 to 9 weeks, and more plastic at 12 to 20 weeks (Figure 2.6). This result can be used to distinguish factors that are related to plasticity, as opposed to factors that simply increase or decrease with age during the development of the visual cortex (Chen, Cooper, & Mower, 2000; Mower & Kaplan, 1999; Reid et al., 1996).

The Periods of Development, Disruption, and Reversal May Be Different

There are several examples of these differences coming out of experiments with animals. Looking at anatomical changes, the geniculocortical endings in layer IV of the visual cortex are initially overlapping and come to be segregated into separate bands of left and right eye endings. This is assayed by transport of substances injected into the eye and carried through the lateral geniculate nucleus to the terminals in the visual cortex. This process of ocular dominance segregation is complete in the macaque monkey by 6 to 8 weeks of age (LeVay, Wiesel, & Hubel, 1980) or earlier (Horton & Hocking, 1996). Nevertheless, the pattern of ocular dominance can be affected by monocular deprivation up to 10 to 12 weeks of age (Horton & Hocking, 1997). Moreover, geniculocortical endings that have been induced to retract by monocular deprivation can be made to expand again by opening the initially closed eye and closing the initially open eye (Swindale, Vital-Durand, & Blakemore, 1981). Recent experiments in the ferret show that the segregation of ocular dominance columns in the cortex initially occurs between P 15 and P 20, while monocular deprivation between P 40 and P 65 can modify these columns, supporting the distinction

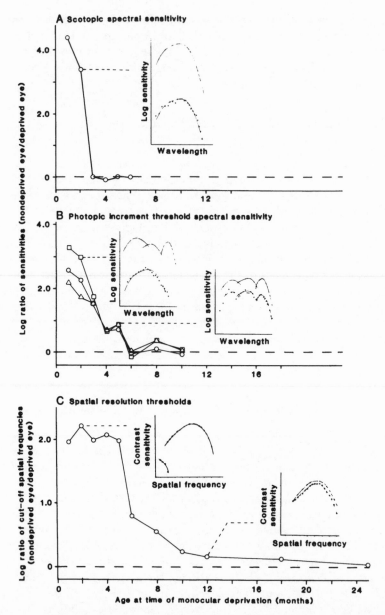

Figure 2.5. Different critical periods for different functions in the macaque monkey. (**A**) Comparison of the dark-adapted (scotopic) spectral sensitivity in the two eyes, for deprivations starting at various ages. (**B**) Comparison of the light-adapted (photopic) spectral sensitivity in the two eyes. (**C**) Comparison of contrast sensitivity curves in the two eyes. Reprinted with permission from Harwerth, R.S., Smith, E.L., Duncan, G.C., Crawford, M.J. & von Noorden, G.R. (1986). Multiple sensitive periods in the development of the primate visual system. *Science, 232,* 235–238. Copyright 1986, American Association for the Advancement of Science.

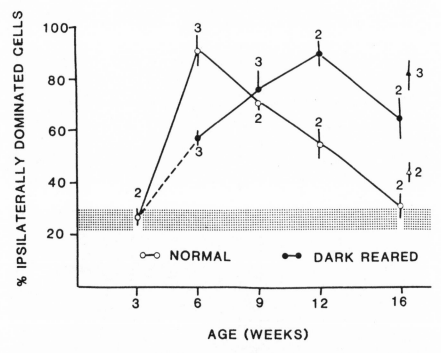

Figure 2.6. Dark-reared cats are less plastic than normal at 6 weeks of age, equally plastic at 9 weeks of age, and more plastic at 12 to 16 weeks of age. Percentage of ipsilaterally dominated cells is plotted after 2 days of monocular deprivation at these ages. Shaded region indicates the percentage in normal adult cats. At 16 weeks, data from cats who experienced prolonged deprivation are also plotted. Numbers indicate the number of cats. Reprinted with kind permission from Mower, G.D. (1991). The effect of dark rearing on the time course of the critical period in cat visual cortex. *Developmental Brain Research, 58*, 151–158. Copyright 1991, Elsevier Science, Ltd., The Boulevard, Langford Lane, Kidlington OX5 1GB, UK.

between the period of initial development and the period of plasticity (Crowley & Katz, 2000).

A more clear-cut example comes from observation of the ocular dominance histograms assembled from recording cells in all layers of primary visual cortex. In normal animals, the histogram contains a large percentage of binocular cells and is dominated slightly by the contralateral eye at all ages. It changes as the geniculocortical afferents change, becoming slightly less binocular and slightly less dominated by the contralateral eye (Albus & Wolf, 1984; Hubel & Wiesel, 1970). By 6 weeks of age, in both cats and macaque monkeys, the histogram is indistinguishable from that recorded in adults. Nevertheless, monocular deprivation has a dramatic influence on the histogram for many months after this (Figure 2.7).

In terms of behavioral responses, the acuity of kittens develops to

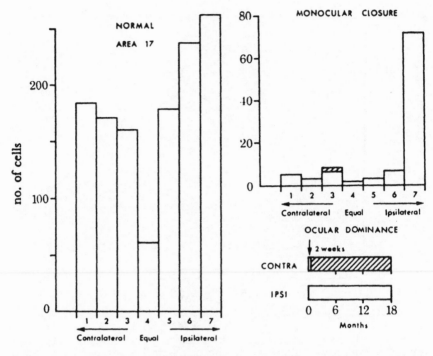

Figure 2.7. Ocular dominance histograms in normal and monocularly deprived monkeys. A sample of cells is recorded from the visual cortex. Each cell is characterized according to whether it is driven solely by the contralateral eye (group 1), solely by the ipsilateral eye (group 7), equally by both eyes (group 4), or somewhere in between (groups 2, 3, 5, and 6). The histogram on the left was based on 1,256 cells recorded from visual cortex in juvenile and adult monkeys. The histogram on the right was obtained from a monkey with the right eye closed from 2 weeks to 18 months and recordings then made from the left hemisphere. Reprinted with permission from Hubel, D.H., Wiesel, T.N., & LeVay, S. (1977). Plasticity of ocular dominance columns in monkey striate cortex. *Philosophical Transactions of the Royal Society of London, Series B, 278,* 377–409.

maturity at 3 months of age (Giffin & Mitchell, 1978). Both reductions in acuity after deprivation by occlusion of one eye and increases in acuity when the occluded eye is opened and the other eye is occluded (reverse occlusion) can be obtained up to 1 year of age (Mitchell, 1988, 1991). In some cases, increases were also seen in the previously occluded eye without reductions in acuity in the previously open eye, but this point was not stringently tested because the purpose of the experiments was to obtain recovery, not cause amblyopia (Mitchell, 1991).

The point that the effect of a deprivation can be reversed for some time after the critical period for the creation of the deficit has ended comes out most clearly in relation to strabismus in humans. The comparable experiments in macaque monkeys or cats have yet not been done. The experiments that have been done will be discussed below, after the human data.

DEVELOPMENT OF ACUITY IN HUMANS

Acuity is commonly measured in the eye practitioner's office with a series of lines of letters of decreasing size. This is called Snellen acuity. For children who cannot read, the letters can be replaced by a series of Es, pointing up, down, right, or left. The child is asked to state which direction the "fingers" point to. It can also be measured with a grating of black and white lines, the task being to detect the orientation of the lines of the grating (grating acuity). Numerous other stimuli have been employed with varying results (Fern & Manny, 1986). The reaction can be tested by a verbal answer, measurement of the visually evoked potential (VEP), or the forced-choice preferential looking (FPL) technique. In the last technique (FPL), used most often with infants, two stimuli are placed side by side on a screen. An observer behind the screen, who does not know what the stimuli are, is forced to state whether the infant is looking to the right or to the left. Infants tend to look more often at an interesting stimulus, for example, a grating with detectable lines, rather than a uniform gray square of the same luminance, so this test gives an indication of whether or not the infant can see the lines.

Results from the various methods vary slightly, but the overall conclusion is the same: Grating acuity develops from 10% of the adult value near birth to close to the adult value, which is 30 cycles per degree, by 3 to 5 years (Figure 2.8). Most of this improvement occurs in the first 6 to 8 months (Dobson & Teller, 1978; Norcia & Tyler, 1985), and there is a small further improvement between 8 months and 3 to 5 years of age (Sireteanu, 2000).

It is of interest to determine, for reasons described in detail below, whether Snellen acuity and grating acuity develop over the same period of time. Snellen acuity involves an additional factor called crowding. Letters in a line are less distinguishable than letters seen by themselves, because letters on either side of the letter being observed can interfere with its visibility. This has been described inter alia as crowding (Irvine, 1948), separation difficulty (Stuart & Burian, 1962), and contour interaction (Flom, Weymouth, & Kahneman, 1963) and depends on the spacing of the letters. It is due to neural interactions, rather than optical interference in the formation of the image on the retina.

Experience in the clinic shows that it is important to test acuity for letters in a line as well as single letters or gratings (von Noorden, 1990). Acuity with letters in surrounding contours shows continued development after 5 years of age (Simons, 1983). Crowding occurs at all ages but is significantly

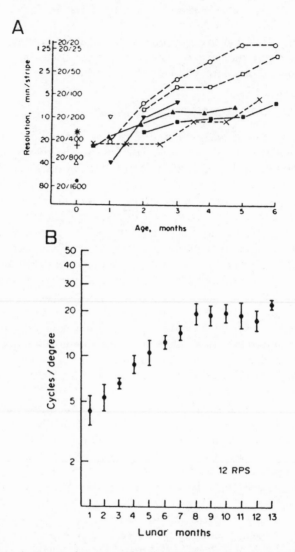

Figure 2.8. Improvement of acuity with age. (A) Compendium of results from different authors, using different techniques. Reprinted with kind permission from Dobson, V., & Teller, D.Y. (1978). Visual acuity in human infants: A review and comparison of behavioral and electrophysiological techniques. *Vision Research, 18,* 1469–1483. Copyright 1978, Elsevier Science, Ltd., The Boulevard, Langford Lane, Kidlington OX5 1GB, UK. (B) Measurements using the "sweep" technique. Reprinted with kind permission from Norcia, A.M., & Tyler, C.W. (1985). Spatial frequency sweep VEP: Visual acuity during the first year of life. *Vision Research, 25,* 1399–1408. Copyright 1985, Elsevier Science, Ltd., The Boulevard, Langford Lane, Kidlington OX5 1GB, UK. (C) A comparison of data from three studies of older children. Reprinted with permission from Sireteanu, R. (2000). Development of the visual system in the human infant. In A.F. Kalverboer & A. Gramsberger (eds.), *Handbook on brain and behaviour in human development* (pp. 629–652). London: Kluwer.

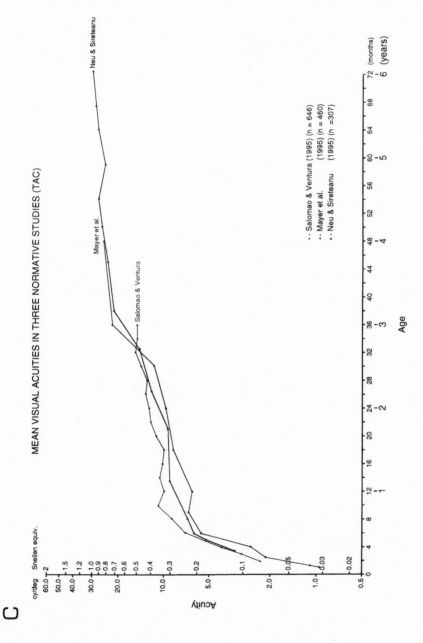

MEAN VISUAL ACUITIES IN THREE NORMATIVE STUDIES (TAC)

Neu & Sireteanu

Mayer et al.

Salomao & Ventura

·- Salomao & Ventura (1995) (n = 646)
·- Mayer et al.   (1995) (n = 460)
·- Neu & Sireteanu   (1995) (n =307)

Age

Acuity

cy/deg   Snellen equiv.

59

greater in 3- to 4-year-old children than in 5- to 7-year-old children or adults (Atkinson et al., 1988). When the spacing between letters is 17.2 minutes of arc, most normal children with correct refraction can see a line of letters as well as single letters at the age of 7, but when the spacing is 2.6 minutes of arc, many 9- to 11-year-old children do not see the letters in a line as well as single letters (Hohmann & Haase, 1982). All of this suggests that the crowding effect develops, or rather diminishes, for several years after grating acuity has reached adult levels.

DISRUPTION OF ACUITY

Acuity can be degraded by any optical or motor problem that leads to a poor image on the retina or a lack of coordination between the images that fall on the left and right retinas.

By Stimulus Deprivation

The most severe disruption of acuity occurs with stimulus deprivation. This can be caused by cataract, when the cataract is so dense that no clear image reaches the retina; traumatic injury; ptosis; lid hemangioma; vitreous hemorrhage; and operations that require patching the eye continuously for a week or more.

Patients with spontaneous and traumatic cataract provide detailed information on the critical period for stimulus deprivation in humans (Vaegan & Taylor, 1979). It lasts from a few weeks after birth (Gair & Adams, 1999) to 10 years of age (Figure 2.9). Susceptibility declines with age: For example, patient SH deprived for about a year at age 1 year was completely blind; patient LF deprived for about the same period from 4 to 5 years of age had acuity reduced to $\frac{1}{10}$ normal; and patient AN deprived for the same period from 8 to 9 years had normal acuity. Longer periods of deprivation have a greater effect, as shown by comparing patient SD, who was deprived for 6 months at 3 years of age and had acuity $\frac{1}{20}$ normal at the end, with patients SR and AB, who were deprived for 3 years and had acuity of $\frac{1}{160}$ normal. Similar results have been obtained by other investigators (von Noorden, 1981). All of this agrees with the general principles coming out of experiments with animals.

Bilateral cataract has less severe consequences than unilateral cataract. The comparison is most easily made in patients who have cataract from birth, since cases of bilateral cataract with dense cataracts in both eyes starting and treated at the same time rarely occur after this (Maurer & Lewis, 1993). After treatment, acuity in cases of bilateral cataract reaches somewhere between 20/30 and 20/200 in most cases (Figure 2.10B). Acuity in cases of unilateral cataract rarely gets better than 20/200, and reaches this value only when the patient follows the patching procedure well (Figure

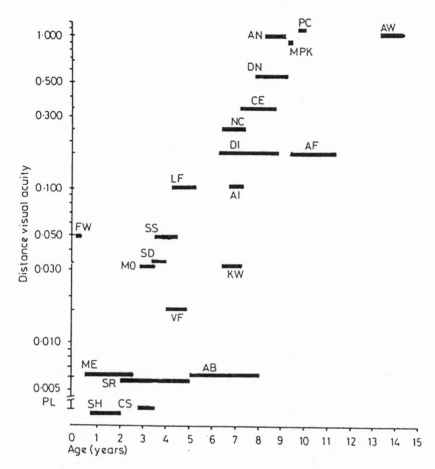

Figure 2.9. Cases of unilateral cataract in man in which the beginning and end of deprivation are well defined. Heavy horizontal bars span the period of deprivation and are set at the level of the first visual acuity score obtained after adequate correction after taking out the cataract. Reprinted with permission from Vaegan, M., & Taylor, D. (1979). Critical period for deprivation amblyopia in children. *Transactions of the Ophthalmological Society (UK)*, 99, 432–439.

2.10A). Interestingly, the duration of the deprivation does not make a large difference in cases of bilateral cataract, and compliance with patching is much more important than duration of deprivation in cases of unilateral cataract.

The difference between unilateral and bilateral congenital cataracts is only apparent when treatment is started after 2 months of age (Birch et al., 1998). With treatment started before 6 to 8 weeks of age, there is very little difference. Thus the effects of competition between the two eyes does not make itself felt until after 2 months of age. The competition could

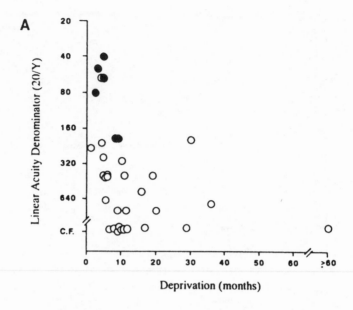

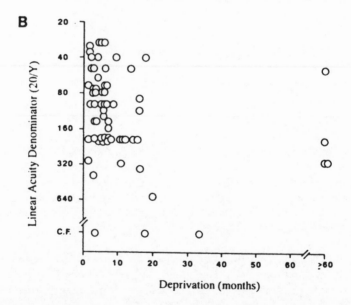

Figure 2.10. (A) Linear letter acuity as a function of the duration of deprivation. In some cases the good eye was patched 40 to 50% of the waking time (○), and in some cases it was not (●). (B) Children treated for bilateral congenital cataracts. From Maurer, D., & Lewis, T.L. (1993). Visual outcomes after infantile cataract. In K. Simons (ed.), *Early visual development: Normal and abnormal* (pp. 459–484). Copyright © 1993 by Oxford University Press, Inc. Reprinted with permission.

be due to a reduction in the connections from the deprived eye to the visual cortex or to suppression of the signals from the deprived eye by signals from the good eye, or both. Whatever the mechanism, it does not develop in the first 2 months of life.

An interesting comparison of similar deprivations at different ages is provided by surgery for eyelids that turn inward (Awaya, Sugawara, & Miyake, 1979). This is usually binocular, so surgery is done on one eye, then the other. Each eye has to be patched for one week after the surgery. As far as a study of critical periods is concerned, the procedure is complicated because strabismus often results from the operation. Thus the deprivation involves stimulus deprivation followed by a less well defined period of strabismus. In all cases, it is the eye closed second that becomes amblyopic. Good recovery of acuity is obtained if the operation is performed after 18 months of age. Before this time, there is poor recovery in 50 to 70% of the cases. Thus the critical period for short-term occlusion is over by 18 months of age. However, the interpretation is uncertain because of the unknown period of strabismus occurring after the short-term occlusion.

By Anisometropia

The critical period for disruption of acuity by anisometropia is much less well defined (Hardman Lea, Loades, & Rubinstein, 1989). Cases rarely occur where anisometropia starts after birth, the starting date is known, it is not treated for a sufficient period of time, and amblyopia results. The onset is almost always below the age of 5, and it does not lead to amblyopia unless it is persistent for 3 years or more (Abrahamsson, Andersson, & Sjostrand, 1990; von Noorden, 1990). There is not a significant correlation between the age at which treatment is started and the initial acuity before treatment (Hardman Lea, Loades, & Rubinstein, 1989).

Useful information could be obtained from animals, comparing the critical period for anisometropia with the critical period for monocular deprivation. Experiments in cats (Eggers & Blakemore, 1978) and macaque monkeys (Hendrickson et al., 1987; Kiorpes et al., 1987; Movshon et al., 1987) have studied the long-term effects of anisometropia, and the behavioral effects are very similar to those in humans. Unfortunately, nobody has looked at the effect of a constant period of anisometropia starting at different ages in any animal model.

By Strabismus

Testing for degradation of acuity by strabismus requires a prospective study. Such a study has been done by Dobson and Sebris (1989) on infants with or at risk for esotropia. There was no significant difference in grating acuity between esotropic and normal infants at 6, 9, 12, 18, or 24 months of age. There was a significant difference at 30 and 36 months of age, by which time most subjects had had a surgical procedure for eye alignment (could the degradation of acuity be a result of surgery rather than esotropia?!).

The clinical experience is that amblyopia from strabismus does not develop after 6 to 8 years of age (von Noorden, 1990). Keech and Kutsche (1995) investigated the age after which visual deprivation does not produce amblyopia, in a series of patients that included 17 with strabismus, 27 with corneal lacerations, 31 with cataract, and 7 others. None of them had amblyopia if the visual deprivation started after 73 months of age. Unfortunately, the data do not give the length of deprivation for each individual patient, as in Figure 2.9. Quite possibly they might have seen some reduction in acuity for a deprivation lasting 2 years at a later age, as for patient AF in Figure 2.9.

Most people would consider that monocular deprivation is the most severe form of deprivation, with strabismus and anisometropia both being milder. The data from Vaegan and Taylor (1979) show a critical period lasting to 10 years of age for monocular deprivation. The critical period for disruption of acuity by strabismus and anisometropia almost certainly ends earlier than this, making the general clinical estimate of 6 to 8 years reasonable.

RECOVERY FROM DISRUPTION OF ACUITY

Whereas acuity is not disrupted by stimulus deprivation, strabismus, or anisometropia after the age of 10, recovery can be obtained after this age with appropriate therapy. In reviewing the literature on this subject, one has to pay more attention to the successes than the failures. The therapy can be very time-consuming for patient, parent, and eye care practitioner (Greenwald & Parks, 1989). The nonamblyopic eye must be patched to bring up the acuity in the amblyopic eye, before eye muscle surgery in the case of strabismus, but not so much that acuity in the nonamblyopic eye is reduced (Odom, Hoyt, & Marg, 1982). Exercises may be required to get the eyes to move together, particularly after strabismus surgery. Use of the amblyopic eye in visual tasks helps the improvement. Continual monitoring is required to assess progress. Failure can easily be due to lack of persistence in the therapy, rather than lack of capability in the visual system of the patient (Simmers & Gray, 1999).

A review of the literature shows that considerable improvement is possible after 7 years of age (Birnbaum, Koslowe, & Sanet, 1977). Indeed, using an improvement of 4 lines on the acuity chart as the criterion, success was more than 50% for children in the 7- to 10-year and 11- to 15-year groups and dropped to 40% in the over 15-year group. Lack of compliance may be one of the reasons for failure in older groups of children (Oliver et al., 1986). In anisometropic amblyopes, large improvements can be obtained at all ages with full refractive correction, added lenses or prisms to improve alignment of the visual axes, 2 to 5 hours per day of patching, and active vision therapy (Wick et al., 1992). The vision therapy included visual stimulation during patching, binocular antisuppression therapy, and stimulation of vergence eye movements. With these treatments, results in older patients were much better than with refractive correction and patching alone (Figure 2.11), although improvements were obtained in previous studies with less extensive therapy in teenagers (Meyer, Mizrahi, & Perlman, 1991; Sen, 1982).

A study of 407 strabismic children treated by patching suggested that some recovery can be obtained up 12 years of age (Epelbaum et al., 1993). Acuity in the patched eye was reduced temporarily over the same age range, suggesting that the critical period for induction of amblyopia by stimulus deprivation is coextensive with the critical period for recovery of amblyopia from strabismus (Figure 2.12).

Recovery after strabismus is more complicated than recovery after anisometropia. Acuity may be degraded by several factors: because vision in the foveal area is reduced; because the patient fixates with an area outside the fovea where acuity is limited by the coarser connections between photoreceptors and visual cortex; by suppression of vision in the amblyopic eye by signals from the nonamblyopic eye; and by masking when the non-amblyopic and amblyopic eyes view different scenes (Freeman, Nguyen, & Jolly, 1996). Most studies do not distinguish these factors, which may have different critical periods. One of the few that did distinguish them included 14 patients from 13 to 54 years old but did not follow the various components during treatment and recovery (Figure 2.13). There did not seem to be any correlation between age and the magnitude of any of the components.

What happens with Snellen acuity in strabismus is interesting. Grating acuity and Snellen acuity are degraded in proportion to each other in anisometropes, but Snellen acuity is degraded more than grating acuity in strabismics (Levi & Klein, 1982). This is partly due to eccentric fixation in the strabismics. During treatment, grating acuity improves faster than Snellen acuity (Pasino & Cordella, 1959; Stuart & Burian, 1962). The authors describe this as an increase in separation difficulty during treatment. The explanation needs further study, with careful attention to changes in the point of fixation during recovery.

A number of cases have been recorded where acuity is improved in the amblyopic eye after loss of function in the nonamblyopic eye. A review of the literature, including loss of function from vascular causes, glaucoma, tumors, macular degeneration, and retinal detachment, showed significant improvements (Vereecken & Brabant, 1984). Patients who get macular degeneration in their nonamblyopic eye can also have dramatic and sustained

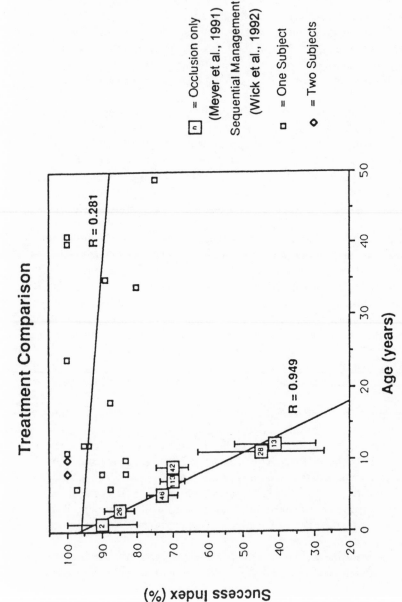

Figure 2.11. Comparison of success in anisometropic amblyopes treated with occlusion only (Meyer, Mizrahi, & Perlman, 1991) and those treated with full refractive correction, prisms, or lenses to improve alignment, and therapy as well (Wick et al., 1992). Success index is defined as initial acuity – final acuity / initial acuity – test distance × 100. Reprinted with permission from Wick, B., Wingard, M., Cotter, S., & Scheiman, M. (1992). Anisometropic amblyopia: Is the patient ever too old to treat? *Optometry and Vision Science, 69,* 866–878.

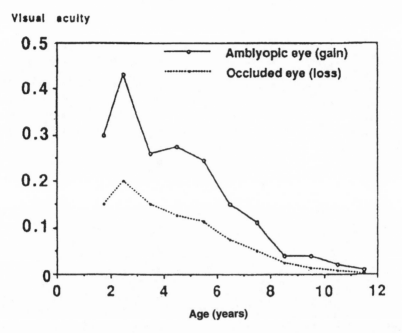

Figure 2.12. Comparison between the gain in acuity (expressed in decimal unities) of the amblyopic eye and the loss in acuity of the occluded eye, measured at the end of the occlusion, as a function of the age of initiation of the therapy in strabismic children. Reprinted with permission from Epelbaum, M., Milleret, C., Buisseret, P., & Dufier, J.L. (1993). The sensitive period for strabismic amblyopia in humans. *Ophthalmology, 100,* 323–327.

improvements in the amblyopic eye (El Mallah, Chakravarthy, & Hart, 2000; Tierney, 1989). Even elderly patients with cataract can find large improvements in acuity in their amblyopic eye, which can be maintained after the cataract is removed, and the vision is restored in that eye (Wilson, 1992). The assumption is that the degradation in the nonamblyopic eye leads to a removal of suppression of the amblyopic eye. All of these cases reinforce the point that recovery can be obtained over a long period of time.

VERNIER ACUITY

Vernier acuity is the ability to detect a lateral break in a line, rather than the gaps in or between lines (Figure 2.14). It is approximately 10 times better than grating acuity: Lines closer than 50 seconds of arc are at the limit of detection in the adult, compared to lateral displacements of 5 to 6 seconds (Carkeet, Levi, & Manny, 1997). Consequently it is called hyperacuity. The discrimination is finer than the spacing of photoreceptors and

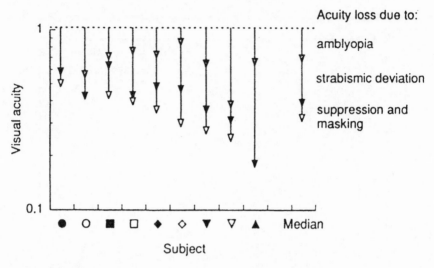

Figure 2.13. Components of acuity loss in nine strabismic eyes. The dashed line gives the mean acuity recorded in subjects with normal binocular vision. The length of each arrow gives the acuity loss due to the stated factor in a strabismic subject; arrows smaller than their arrowheads are not shown. Amblyopic loss was determined from the acuity during monocular viewing compared with that in normal subjects. The loss due to strabismic deviation was calculated, and the loss due to strabismic deviation, suppression, plus masking was found by comparing acuity during binocular viewing with that during monocular viewing. The loss due to suppression and masking was then found by subtraction. Median losses across subjects are also shown. Reprinted with kind permission from Freeman, A.W., Nguyen, V.A., & Jolly, N. (1996). Component of visual acuity loss in strabismus. *Vision Research, 36,* 765–774. Copyright 1988, Elsevier Science, Ltd., The Boulevard, Langford Lane, Kidlington OX5 1GB, UK.

is assumed to depend on cortical mechanisms (Levi, Klein, & Aitsebaomo, 1985).

Vernier acuity changes faster and develops for a longer period of time than grating acuity. Grating acuity reaches half its adult value at about 2 years of age, whereas Vernier acuity does not reach half its adult value until 5 to 8 years of age, when grating acuity is fully developed (Carkeet, Levi, & Manny, 1997). The relationship between the two is similar in different species using various methods but is distinctly nonlinear (Skoczenski & Norcia, 1999). It would appear that the cortical mechanisms responsible for the hyperacuity of Vernier acuity develop between 1 and 10 years of age (Levi & Carkeet, 1993).

In anisometropic amblyopes, vernier acuity, like Snellen acuity, is degraded in proportion to grating acuity (Levi & Klein, 1982). In strabismic amblyopes, vernier acuity, again like Snellen acuity, is degraded by a larger

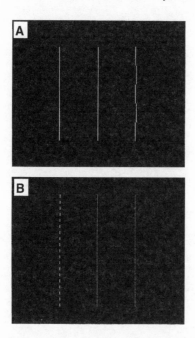

Figure 2.14. Three alternative, forced-choice stimuli for (A) Vernier acuity and (B) resolution.

factor than grating acuity (Figure 2.15). This is not due to eccentric fixation, because the stimulus was always large enough to cover the fovea. It is due to the degradation of positional information that is evident from many tests in strabismic amblyopes (Flom & Bedell, 1985; Hess & Holliday, 1992). This degradation of positional information affects lateral interactions to reduce Snellen acuity and vernier acuity similarly. The degradation of vernier acuity occurs independent of the age of onset of the strabismus, showing that strabismus and anisometropia affect the visual system in different ways (Birch & Swanson, 2000)—the difference is not due to onsets in the two types of deprivation occurring at different ages (Levi & Carkeet, 1993).

There is very little information on how the disruption of vernier acuity varies with age for strabismus or anisometropia. One paper on congenital unilateral cataract shows that best results are obtained if surgery is performed before 6 weeks of age (Birch & Stager, 1996). However, vernier acuity in adults with amblyopia can be improved by sustained practice at the task, by a factor of about two (Levi, Polat, & Hu, 1997). This shows that vernier acuity is plastic in the adult. There are other discriminations that can also be improved by practice in adults (see Levi, Polat, & Hu, 1997). Moreover, Vernier acuity can be improved by practice in normal people as well as in amblyopes, although the improvement is considerably

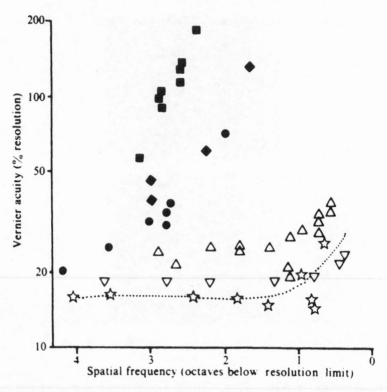

Figure 2.15. Vernier acuity tested with two gratings offset from each other, as a function of the fundamental frequency of the grating. Both the abscissa and the ordinate have been scaled to take account of each observer's grating resolution. Results from normal eyes are shown by the dotted line. Results from anisometropic amblyopes are shown by open symbols. Results from strabismic amblyopes shown by filled symbols. Vernier acuity, when scaled like this, is close to normal for anisometropic amblyopes and far from normal for strabismic amblyopes. Reprinted with permission from Levi, D.M., & Klein, S. (1982). Hyperacuity and amblyopia. *Nature, 298,* 268–270. Copyright 1982, MacMillan Magazines Limited.

smaller—on the order of 20 to 30% (Beard, Levi, & Reich, 1995). Thus one cannot say that the critical period for this function lasts longer than for normal people, only that amblyopes are more plastic than normal people.

BINOCULARITY

The development of binocular function is a coordinated sensory and motor process (Helveston, 1993). Acuity develops as the fovea develops, to provide a precise fixation point in the two eyes. At the same time, vergence eye movements become more precise, so that the same view of the world is conveyed to the same cells in the visual cortex (Mitkin & Orestova, 1988). This occurs at 4 to 5 months of age. Full convergence, as judged by the ability of an infant to follow a toy to within 12 centimeters of its face, appears between 2 and 4 months of age (Thorn et al., 1994). Stereoscopic depth perception depends on binocular fusion, and this also develops rapidly at 3 to 5 months of age (Held, Birch, & Gwiazda, 1980). Thus 3 to 5 months of age is the period for fine-tuning of both stereopsis and vergence to give good binocular function. Some authors such as Worth (1903) may have emphasized the sensory aspects, and others such as Chevasse (1939) the motor, but the real point is that the two develop together, and disruption of either one can lead to problems.

Binocular fusion can be tested in a number of different ways (von Noorden, 1990). One is to ask the subject to fixate on a white light with one eye and probe the visibility of a red light as it is moved around the field of view in the other eye. Another is to put glasses with lines scratched on the surface over the two eyes with the scratches for one eye perpendicular to the scratches for the other eye (Bagolini lenses). A gap in one set of striations shows suppression in that eye. Another is to look at four dots, one red, two green, and one white, through a red glass over one eye and a green glass over the other (Worth four dot test). A disappearance of one or more of the dots shows suppression. The test most often used for experiments with animals is a grating presented to one eye, and another grating, orthogonal to or displaced from the first, presented to the other eye. These stimuli test different aspects of binocular fusion and suppression, so the interpretation is complicated (Jampolsky, 1955). Moreover, since the receptive fields of cells in the peripheral part of the field of view are much larger than those in the fovea, one frequently finds fusion is present in the periphery and absent in the fovea (Parks, 1969; Sireteanu, Fronius, & Singer, 1981).

Binocularity depends on cells in the visual cortex receiving signals from corresponding points of the two retinas. This can be disrupted by strabismus, which makes most cells in the visual cortex monocular—that is, each cell is driven by the left eye or by the right eye but not by both (Crawford, Pesch, & von Noorden, 1996; Hubel & Wiesel, 1965). The critical period for this effect is the same as the critical period for ocular dominance shifts by monocular deprivation (Levitt & van Sluyters, 1982), which is not surprising because they both involve ocular dominance shifts at the same level of the system, primary visual cortex.

Binocular function can be tested in the human by a phenomenon called interocular transfer of the tilt aftereffect (Banks, Aslin, & Letson, 1975; Hohmann & Creutzfeldt, 1975). If one stares at slanted lines for a period of time, then looks at vertical lines, the vertical lines appear to be tilted in the opposite direction. The amount of tilt can be quantified. For measurement of interocular transfer, one stares at the slanted lines with one eye, then measures the aftereffect in that eye and compares it with the size of the aftereffect in the other eye. No aftereffect in the other eye implies that the cells in the visual cortex do not have binocular input. Modeling of the results from this test in early and late-onset strabismus patients suggests a critical period that starts at 3 to 6 months of age, peaks at 1 to 2 years of age, and declines over 2 to 8 years of age (Figure 2.16).

Binocular fusion, tested with FPL and checkerboards or random dot displays, develops rapidly between 2 and 6 months of age (Birch, Shimojo, & Held, 1985). It can also be tested by measuring the VEP response to a dynamic random dot correlogram (Eizenman et al., 1999). The authors tested esotropes before surgery (4.4 to 33 months of age) and compared the results to esotropes after surgery (13 to 102 months of age) and normal children. Five out of 13 had detectable responses in the first group, and 11 out of 13 in the second. In another study, von Noorden (1988) showed that binocular vision can be obtained in a number of cases with alignment after 2 or even 4 years of age, but stereopsis was rare. The results suggested that binocular fusion is more robust than stereopsis to abnormal visual experience and has a later critical period.

STEREOPSIS

Stereopsis is the ability to detect depth using disparity signals. Objects nearer than the fixation point fall on noncorresponding points of the two retinas with crossed disparity, and objects further than the fixation point fall on noncorresponding points of the two retinas with uncrossed disparity. There is coarse stereopsis, which drives vergence eye movements, and fine stereopsis, which detects the fine details of depth in the object being viewed and objects nearby, without necessarily leading to eye movements.

Stereopsis develops very rapidly between 3 and 5 months of age (Braddick et al., 1980; Fox et al., 1980; Held, Birch, & Gwiazda, 1980; Petrig et al., 1981). In any one individual, stereoacuity may go from more than 80 minutes of arc to less than 1 minute of arc in a period of less than a month (Held, Birch, & Gwiazda, 1980). There is further development of stereoacuity at a slower rate between 5 months and 5 years of age, with considerable variation between subjects and methods of testing (see Birch & Salomao, 1998; Ciner, Schanelklitsch, & Herzberg, 1996). One would like to suggest that the rapid development of stereoacuity at 3 to 5 months of age is related to the development of vergence eye movements around the same time, and involves coarse stereopsis, and that the later slower development of stereoacuity determines fine stereopsis involved with perception of depth rather than eye movements, but no experiments have tested this hypothesis in detail.

It is interesting that the rapid development of stereoacuity occurs at the

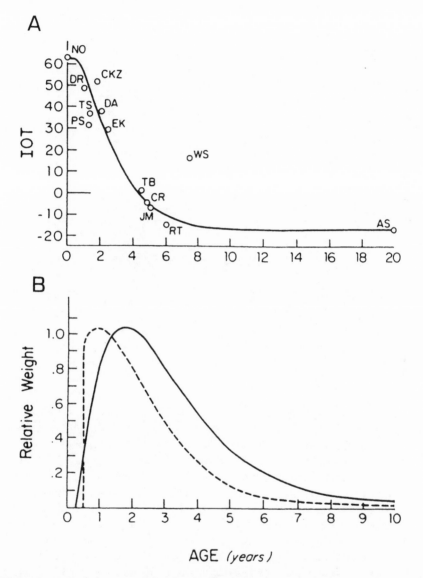

Figure 2.16. Sensitive period for the development of human binocular vision. (A) Interocular transfer of the tilt aftereffect for 13 congenital esotropes, plotted as a function of the age at which corrective surgery was done. Esotropes identified by their initials. (B) Weights given to binocular experience at various ages that provided the best fit measurements in (A) (—) and to measurements made from 12 late-onset esotropes (-----). Reprinted with permission from Banks, M.S., Aslin, R.N., & Letson, R.D. (1975). Sensitive period for the development of human binocular vision. *Science, 190,* 675–677. Copyright 1975, American Association for the Advancement of Science.

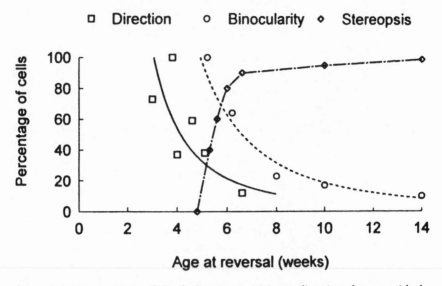

Figure 2.17. Comparison of the decline in sensitivity to direction changes with the increase in sensitivity to stereopsis, and the decline in sensitivity to ocular dominance changes in the cat. At 5 weeks of age, cells are not very susceptible to direction changes. Between 5 and 6 weeks of age, the ability to discriminate stereoscopic targets increases rapidly, while cells are still sensitive to ocular dominance changes. Reprinted with permission from *Investigative Ophthalmology and Visual Science*, Daw (1994).

same time as the segregation of geniculocortical afferents in layer IV of the visual cortex (Held, 1993). This is also the time at which binocular thresholds start to be summated (Birch & Swanson, 1992), and binocular stimuli that lead to binocular rivalry are avoided (Shimojo et al., 1986). Several aspects of binocular function change at the same time during this period.

A similar correspondence occurs in cats (LeVay, Stryker, & Shatz, 1978; Timney, 1981) where the critical periods for cellular properties in the visual cortex have been worked out. The time period for rapid development of stereoscopic acuity in the cat is 5 to 7 weeks of age (Timney, 1981). This occurs after connections for orientation and direction are largely set in place and while connections for ocular dominance in layers outside layer IV are still plastic (Figure 2.17). It would make no sense for a disparity-sensitive cell to have input for vertical lines from one eye and input for horizontal lines for the other. It seems likely that the system has arranged to have the critical period for orientation and direction selectivity end earlier than the critical period for ocular dominance to provide appropriate coordinated input for cells that determine stereopsis (Daw, 1994, 1995).

In infants with infantile esotropia, stereopsis develops to 4 months of age, then declines (Birch, 1993). After 6 months of age, only 20% have

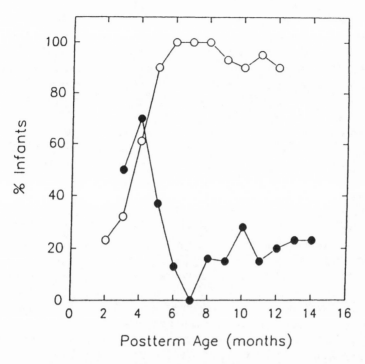

Figure 2.18. Percent of normal (○) and esotropic (●) infants who reached criterion (45 minutes of arc) for stereopsis. All esotropic infants were diagnosed by age 6 months, had no known neurological or neuromuscular disorders, and were tested at the initial visit prior to any treatment. Reprinted with permission from Stager, D.R., & Birch, E.E. (1986). Preferential-looking acuity and stereopsis in infantile esotropia. *Journal of Pediatric Ophthalmology and Strabismus, 23,* 160–165.

any stereopsis, when tested at the initial visit prior to treatment (Figure 2.18). The criterion was a disparity of 45 minutes of arc, representing a coarse level of stereopsis, and the graph shows the percentage of infants passing this test. Thus the results show a degradation of coarse stereopsis over the same period of time that development takes place. However, stereopsis can also be degraded after the initial period of development in cases, for example, of accommodative esotropia (Fawcett, Leffler, & Birch, 2000).

Some recovery can be obtained up to at least 2 years of age. When the results are tallied according to the time at which eye alignment is achieved, binocularity is seen in nearly all cases up to 2 years of age, and coarse stereopsis is found in over 40% of the cases. For those treated before 6 months of age, stereopsis is found in three quarters of the cases, while for those treated after 6 months of age, it is less than half (Birch, Fawcett, & Stager, 2000b). Taylor (1972) found that all of his patients (30/50) who were operated before 23 months of age and converted from a tropia to a phoria had stereopsis. Stereoscopic acuity after treatment varied from 40 to 400 arc seconds, and the stereoscopic acuity depended on the size of the area of suppression in the macula. Those with a suppression scotoma of 1 degree or less had acuities of 40 to 60 arc seconds. For alignment after 2 years of age, less than 50% have binocularity, and less than 30% have stereopsis (Ing, 1983).

Whether fine stereopsis can ever be achieved after strabismus is uncertain. In 1988 von Noorden stated, "The noteworthy isolated case of Parks (1984) notwithstanding, there is universal agreement between strabismologists that complete restoration of normal binocular vision with normal random dot stereopsis is unattainable in infantile esotropia." Since von Noorden's summary, Wright et al. (1994) have reported two patients who achieved stereo of 40 to 70 arc seconds, after surgery at 13 and 19 weeks of age, out of a group of seven. There are few other cases, because surgery at this age is controversial. It is difficult to achieve correct alignment, and some alignment might be achieved without the surgery, making the surgery unnecessary. In theory, early alignment should help if good stereopsis is desired, as well as good acuity (Helveston, 1993). However, *alignment* is the operative word. Early surgery is not enough if it does not lead to alignment. Unless practice evolves to where good alignment can be achieved and maintained by 4 months of age, the point will not be tested.

In summary, stereopsis can be degraded over a period after the initial period of development. Some recovery can also be obtained after this time, adequate to drive vergence eye movements and achieve binocular fusion. What happens in the case of fine stereopsis is largely unknown. Nobody knows whether fine stereopsis can be degraded in the period 6 months to 2 years of age, after coarse stereopsis is established, without affecting coarse stereopsis. All the evidence suggests that recovery of fine stereopsis once it has been disrupted is difficult at all ages, and almost impossible after the age of 2, which is before it finally finishes developing in normal people. Thus fine stereopsis may be an exception to the generalization above that the critical periods for development, degradation, and recovery are different. If anything, the critical period for recovery may end earlier than the critical period for development. However, the real answers can only be obtained from experiments with animals.

Experiments done so far with macaque monkeys help somewhat. Stereocauity in the macaque has a rapid period of initial development, as in human and cat, between 2 and 10 weeks of age (O'Dell & Boothe, 1997). Animals reared with prisms for 2 weeks to produce strabismus had a greater deficit when the rearing was started at 6 weeks of age than when it was started at 2 weeks of age (Kumagami et al., 2000). Both of these periods of deprivation were within the period of development of stereopsis, and it would clearly be of interest to extend the study to periods of deprivation starting after the period of development of stereopsis is complete. Further experiments are needed to clarify the questions that cannot be answered easily in humans.

MOVEMENT

There is an interesting asymmetry in movement perception and responses in infants. When placed in a drum rotating around them (Figure 2.19A) with one eye open, they follow the drum better for movement in the temporal-nasal direction than for movement in the nasotemporal direction. This asymmetry disappears between birth and 3 to 5 months of age (Atkinson, 1979; Naegele & Held, 1982; see Figure 2.19B). The symmetry does not develop in infantile esotropes (Schor & Levi, 1980), depending on the age of onset of the esotropia. In patients studied by Demer and von Noorden (1988), 58% of the patients with onset before 6 months showed asymmetry, 22% of those with onset at 6 to 12 months, 9% of those with onset at 12 to 24 months, and 5% of those with onset after 24 months. In patients studied by Bourron-Madignier et al. (1987), the numbers were 92% of those with onset under 6 months, 64% of those with onset at 6 to 12 months, 33% of those with onset at 12 to 24 months, and 23% of those with onset over 24 months. Whether the difference in the numbers is due to different techniques or different populations of patients is not clear, but it is clear that the symmetry in the monocular optokinetic nystagmus (OKN) can be disrupted for some time after it develops in normal infants (Figure 2.20).

There is also an asymmetry in the response to motion, assayed by VEPs. This is in the opposite direction from the OKN asymmetry—with VEPs, nasotemporal movement produces a better response (Mason et al., 2001). The motion VEP is not seen at 0.5 to 1 month of age, is asymmetric when it appears, and eventually becomes symmetric. The time course of this maturation is between 2 and 10 months of age in normal infants in one study (Birch, Fawcett, & Stager, 2000a), between 5 months and 2 years in another (Norcia, 1996), and between 6 and 15 weeks in a third (Mason et al., 2001). The asymmetry depends on cortical mechanisms and has a period of development that lasts longer than the period of development for OKN asymmetry, because different mechanisms are involved: The motion VEP is obviously a purely cortical response, whereas OKN has subcortical components (Hoffmann, Distler, & Markner, 1996). The development of symmetrical motion VEPs is related to the ability to fuse an image with the two foveas (bifoveal fusion) rather than the presence of stereoscopic vision (Fawcett & Birch, 2000). For infants with infantile esotropia, the asymmetry is within normal limits at 4 to 6 months of age and becomes abnormal at 7 to 9 months of age (Birch, Fawcett, & Stager, 2000a). Some 73% of infants with infantile esotropia show asymmetry in this response, com-

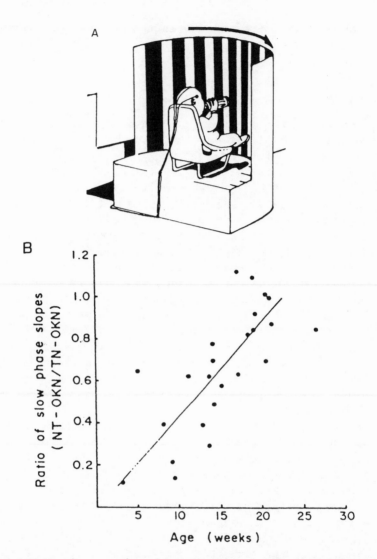

Figure 2.19. Development of optokinetic nystagmus in infants. (A) Infant faces a semicircular screen on which stripes are projected, continually moving in one direction. The ability of the infant to follow the stripes is measured. (B) Ratio of the slope of eye movement curves for nasalward compared to temporalward directions plotted against the age of the infant (in weeks). NT-OKN = slope of slow phase monocular OKN with nasal-temporal motion; TN-OKN = slope of slow phase monocular OKN with temporal-nasal motion. A linear regression line was fit to the data; $r = 0.60$, slope = 1.1. Data from 24 infants are shown. Reprinted with kind permission from Naegele, J.R., & Held, R. (1982) The postnatal development of monocular optokinetic nystagmus in infants. *Vision Research, 22,* 341–346. Copyright 1982, Elsevier Science, Ltd., The Boulevard, Langford Lane, Kidlington OX5 1GB, UK.

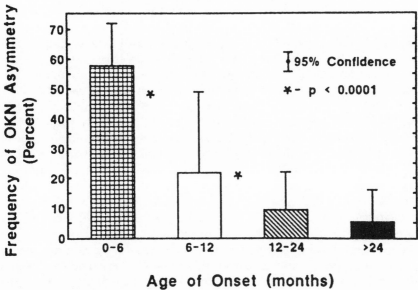

Figure 2.20. Histogram showing the prevalence of clinical monocular optokinetic nystagmus (OKN) asymmetry in esotropic patients with various ages of onset of strabismus. The asterisks indicate statistically significant differences in prevalence between adjacent columns, and the error bars indicate 95% confidence intervals for mean prevalence. Thus, there was a significantly greater prevalence of asymmetry in esotropic patients with onset before the age of 6 months than those with onset between 6 and 12 months, and these in turn had a significantly greater prevalence than those with later onset. Reprinted with permission from Demer, J.L., & von Noorden, G.K. (1988). Optokinetic asymmetry in esotropia. *Journal of Pediatric Ophthalmology and Strabismus, 25,* 286–292.

pared to 20% of infants with onset after 2 years (Hamer et al., 1993). The latter figure shows that motion VEPs, like monocular optokinetic nystagmus, can be disrupted by strabismus after the initial period of development is over. This general point is confirmed for OKN, perceptual, and motion VEP direction biases in a more recent summary of the data (Brosnahan et al., 1998).

The critical period for recovery is determined by looking at asymmetry as a function of age of alignment. Infants aligned at 11 to 18 months had asymmetry indices for motion VEPs that were significantly worse than those aligned by 10 months of age (Birch, Fawcett, & Stager, 2000a). Those aligned after 2 years of age had asymmetry significantly worse than those aligned before (Norcia, Hamer, & Jampolsky, 1995). Moreover, alternate occlusion therapy between 35 and 60 weeks of age can reduce the asymmetry significantly (Norcia, 1996). All these points show that the critical period for recovery also lasts longer than the initial period of development for infantile esotropia. Whether the critical period for recovery extends beyond the critical period for disruption needs further data, or further analysis of data that have already been collected, in order to settle the point.

The developmental time course for the perception of direction of movement, as well as orientation, is not well characterized. Newborns can discriminate the orientation of a stimulus if they are habituated to one orientation, then presented with a choice of two orientations side by side (Slater, Morison, & Somers, 1988). VEP responses to a grating jittering in one orientation, then the perpendicular orientation with three reversals of orientation per second, appear at 3 weeks of age, and responses to eight reversals per second appear at 6 weeks of age (Braddick, Wattam-Bell, & Atkinson, 1986). VEP responses to direction of movement at 5 degrees per second were first found at 74 days, and for 20 degrees per second at 90 days of age (Wattam-Bell, 1991). Unfortunately, no one has taken some specific measure of a movement response and measured it as a function of age. As far as degradation is concerned, the sensitive period for degradation of global motion sensitivity is very short: Patients who receive normal patterned input before visual deprivation by monocular or binocular cataract, even for as little as 4 to 8 months, perform normally on global movement tests (Ellemberg et al., 2002). Thus, the data are all consistent with the proposition that orientation and direction selectivity develop before ocular dominance is finally set into place, coming out of experiments with cats (Daw, 1994).

SUPPRESSION

There are several different kinds of suppression, which can be seen in normal people as well as people with amblyopia (Harrad, 1996). There is dichoptic masking, where a stimulus of higher contrast prevents the detection of a lower-contrast stimulus in the other eye (Abadi, 1976). This is probably most important in anisometropia and small-angle strabismus. There are disparity-specific suppression and fusional suppression, apparent, for example, when a portion of a far object is covered by a near object in one eye but not in the other. Finally, there is binocular rivalry, which probably operates primarily in large-angle strabismus. Suppression may vary with the part of the field of view: A frequent finding is suppression in the central part of the field of view with fusion in the periphery (Helveston & von Noorden, 1967; Jampolsky, 1951; Parks, 1969; Sireteanu, Fronius, & Singer, 1981). Different types of suppression may also operate in the same person in different parts of the field of view. Interestingly, there is a negative correlation between suppression and amblyopia, looking at gratings in the central 1.2 degree part of the field of view (Holopigian, Blake, & Greenwald, 1988). Suppression is most powerful in alternately fixating strabismics, intermediate in strabismic amblyopia, and weakest in anisometropic amblyopia. Thus the subject is very complicated (see Jampolsky, 1955; Travers, 1938).

The form of suppression that has received most attention from the developmental point of view is binocular rivalry, which is the form of suppression that is least important in strabismic suppression (Smith et al., 1985). Infants express preference for a nonrivalrous stimulus until about 3 to 4 months of age (Shimojo et al., 1986) when stereopsis develops. However, the VEP response is still immature at 5 to 15 months of age (Brown, Candy, & Norcia, 1999). The complete time course for development of binocular rivalry has not been studied. Other forms of suppression, such as dichoptic masking of a pattern of dots, appear to be similar in infants and adults (Odom & Harter, 1983) insofar as the question has been studied.

There is a form of dichoptic suppression that is known as crossorientation inhibition, with a grating presented to one eye and a perpendicular grating presented to the other. Measurements in infants suggest that this form of suppression develops between 6 and 8 months of age (Morrone & Burr, 1986). Sengpiel et al. (1994) have proposed that orientation inhibition is similar in normal and amblyopic people, occurring with all angles of relative orientation, and that the excitatory input is reduced in amblyopes so that the inhibition becomes predominant.

Dichoptic suppression may be measured in single cells by observing the binocular response to drifting sinewave gratings and comparing it to the monocular response (Kumagami et al., 2000). The percentage of cells showing suppression by this test in macaques declines with age. It is increased by strabismus from wearing prisms, more in animals deprived from 6 to 8 weeks of age than in animals deprived from 2 to 4 weeks of age (Figure 2.21). More data with older animals will be required to determine when the percentage of cells with suppression reaches adult levels and whether the changes induced by a 2-week period of strabismus are larger when the strabismus is imposed at a later time. What is known is that the percentage of cells with suppression is not changed in animals deprived from 6 to 8 weeks if the prisms are then removed and the animal reared normally for another several months (Smith et al., 1997). In this case, the period of recovery does not extend beyond the critical period for disruption.

In summary, all forms of suppression develop early, and all are found in adults as well as in normal and strabismic infants. The results suggest increases with age in binocular rivalry. In the case of dichoptic masking, the results are confusing and probably depend on the details of the procedures, which may or may not be comparable. Suppression in strabismic and anisometropic infants may develop just as it does in normal infants for stimuli that are not concordant in the two eyes. The primary mechanism may be that an image in focus in the nonamblyopic eye suppresses an image out

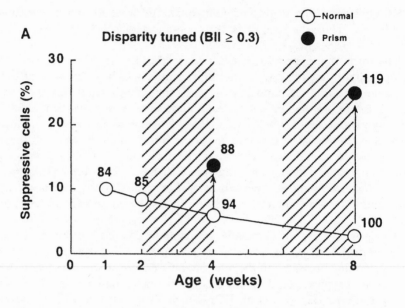

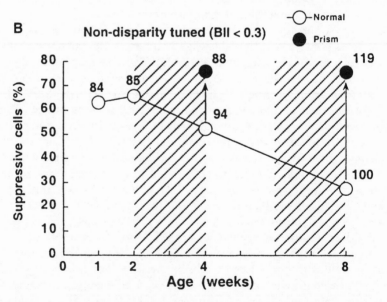

Figure 2.21. The proportions of binocularly suppressive units as a function of age for prism-reared and normal monkeys. (A) Disparity tuned units. (B) Non-disparity tuned units. Shaded areas indicate the prism effects on the respective response properties. Small numbers next to data points indicate the number of sample units. Reprinted with permission from *Investigative Ophthalmology and Visual Science*, Kumagami et al. (2000).

of focus in the amblyopic eye, just as afterimages are suppressed in normal vision (Daw, 1962).

MYOPIA

Myopia can occur through growth of the eyeball from too much near work. The mechanism involves local signals within the eyeball. Indeed, one part of the eyeball in birds can grow more than another part if images in one part of the field of view are focused at a different distance from the other (Wallman et al., 1987). Epidemiological studies would suggest that progression of myopia can continue until at least the college years, since the percentage of the population that is myopic increases from grade school to high school to college, at least in the studious countries of East Asia (Curtin, 1985).

Lengthening of the eyeball is also induced by suturing the eyelids of one eyelid shut, an observation that was a by-product of the original experiments on monocular deprivation (Wiesel & Raviola, 1977). This is now known as form deprivation myopia. Form deprivation induces myopia in marmosets after puberty, when growth of the eyeball is normally complete (Troilo, Nickla, & Wildsoet, 2000) and in "teenage" macaque monkeys (Smith et al., 1999). The system is most susceptible in tree shrews at 6 to 9 weeks of age, when the eyeball is almost adult in size, and is still susceptible at 10 to 12 weeks of age, when the eyeball is fully grown (Siegwart & Norton, 1998; Figure 2.22). The conclusion, in both humans and animals, is that myopia can be induced after the eyeball is mature. However, the eyeball cannot contract. Recovery is limited to the period of normal growth, during which it can stop growing and let growth of other components of the system such as the lens catch up. All of this is obviously an exception to the rule that the system is more plastic at higher levels of the system.

CONTRAST SENSITIVITY

Contrast sensitivity is measured with gratings of variable contrast. Lines of medium spatial frequency, about 2 cycles per degree, are most visible (Figure 2.23). Finer lines are less visible, until they are so close that they cannot be seen at all, which represents the limit of grating acuity. Wider lines are less visible because of lateral inhibitory interactions. The lowest contrast that can be seen, at the peak of the contrast sensitivity curve, has a contrast of about 0.5% of the background.

Contrast sensitivity develops over a wide range from birth (Atkinson, Braddick, & Moar, 1977). Five-week infants cannot distinguish a contrast of 20%, no matter what the spatial frequency. Infants at 8 weeks need 20%, and infants at 12 weeks need 10% (Figure 2.24). Contrast sen-

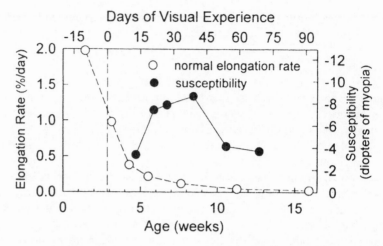

Figure 2.22. Axial elongation rate (○, scale on the left ordinate) and susceptibility to induced myopia (●, scale on the right ordinate) from form deprivation in tree shrews. Lower abscissa scale is age; the upper abscissa scale is days of visual experience. The elongation rate was calculated as the amount of daily elongation divided by the axial length at birth. Susceptibility is the difference between the control eye and deprived eye retinoscopy values in diopters. The vertical dashed line indicates natural eyelid opening. Reprinted with kind permission from Siegwart, J.T., & Norton, T.T. (1998). The susceptible period for deprivation-induced myopia in tree shrew. *Vision Research, 38*, 3505–3515. Copyright 1998, Elsevier Science, Ltd., The Boulevard, Langford Lane, Kidlington OX5 1GB, UK.

sitivity develops at low spatial frequency to an asymptote at 9 weeks of age and continues to develop at high spatial frequencies until grating acuity is fully developed (Norcia, Tyler, & Hamer, 1990). Contrast sensitivity at the peak of the curve reaches adult levels by 7 years of age by some procedures (Ellemberg et al., 1999) but not by others (Scharre et al., 1990).

Contrast sensitivity can be disrupted by strabismus (Hess, Campbell, & Greenhalgh, 1978), astigmatism (Mitchell & Wilkinson, 1974), myopia (Fiorentini & Maffei, 1976), and cataract (Tytla et al., 1988). Results on disruption and recovery of contrast sensitivity at high spatial frequencies generally follow results for grating acuity, since the two are closely related. We will therefore just discuss the results at low and middle spatial frequencies. The two main examples come from measurements in humans with cataract and macaque monkeys with strabismus.

Three children who had traumatic injury and cataract at 5.5, 8.9, and 9.3 years of age, for a period of at least 4½ months, had normal contrast sensitivity for low and middle spatial frequencies (Tytla et al., 1988), suggesting that it cannot be disrupted after 5 years of age. Children who had congenital cataract showed improvement after the cataract was removed

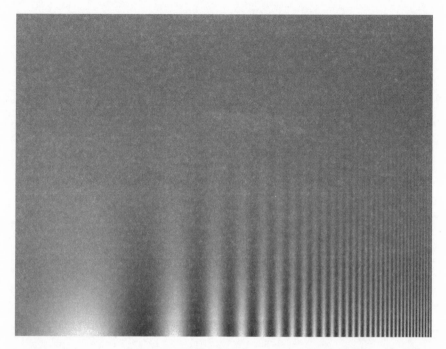

Figure 2.23. Grating of variable spatial frequency, and variable contrast. One can see that the stripes are most visible in the middle, less visible on the left edge, and invisible on the right edge. Photograph provided by John Robson.

up to 7 years of age at these spatial frequencies (Lewis et al., 2000). Thus the critical periods for development, disruption, and recovery all appear to be over by 7 years of age for these measurements, which are taken in the central part of the field of view. The critical period for sensitivity in the peripheral part of the field view may last longer (Bowering et al., 1993).

A number of naturally strabismic monkeys were studied by Kiorpes (1989). Peak sensitivity for contrast, as well as acuity, developed over the first 2 years, compared to development over the first year for normal macaques. This certainly suggests that the time period for disruption lasts longer than the initial period of development. One would also like to see what happens in macaques with strabismus created after 1 year of age to confirm the point.

In summary, peak sensitivity to contrast seems to have similar critical periods for development, disruption, and recovery in cataract but not in strabismus. When one thinks about it, the first result seems more reasonable than the second. Nobody knows whether peak sensitivity for contrast is entirely a retinal phenomenon or whether the cortex is also involved in some aspect of the discrimination. Most people would probably suggest

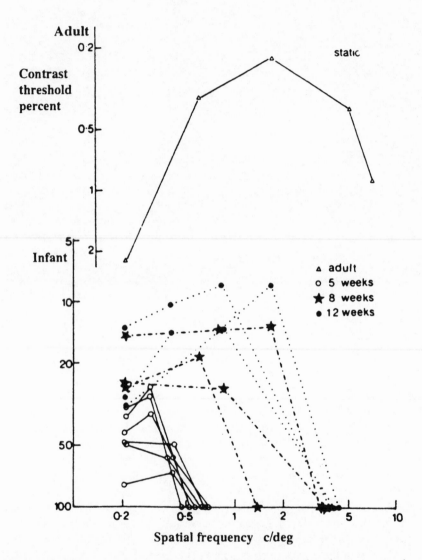

Figure 2.24. Contrast sensitivity curves at 5, 8, and 12 weeks of age compared to adult. Data obtained from individual subjects by VEP technique. Reprinted with kind permission from Atkinson, J., Braddick, O.J., & Moar, K. (1977). Development of contrast sensitivity over the first 3 months of life in the human infant. *Vision Research, 17,* 1037–1044. Copyright 1977, Elsevier Science, Ltd., The Boulevard, Langford Lane, Kidlington OX5 1GB, UK.

that it is primarily retinal, and the results of Harwerth et al. (1986) would support this. The results from Kiorpes (1989) are contradictory to this from the theoretical point of view and bring up the possibility that there might be a cortical component to the discrimination.

COMPARISON WITH CRITICAL PERIODS IN OTHER SYSTEMS

Critical periods have been investigated in considerably more detail in the visual system than in any other system. Where they have been investigated in other systems, the general principles seem to be the same. For example, musicians have an increased representation in both sensory and motor cortex, shown by functional magnetic source imaging. The dipole moments for piano tones are about 25% larger than dipole moments for pure tones in musicians, but there is no difference for control subjects (Pantev et al., 1998). The difference was found in musicians who started to practice before the age of 8 but not in those who started later. Moreover, the cortical representation of the left hand is found to be larger in violinists than in controls (Elbert et al., 1995). The size of this effect drops between 12 and 20 years of age. These results bring out two points: first, that the critical period in sensory cortex lasts to around puberty, in agreement with results from the visual system, and second, that the motor system is plastic for longer than the sensory system. The latter point has not been discussed in this chapter in relation to the visual system, but it is likely to be true. It is certainly true that visuomotor coordination is plastic in the adult (Held, 1965), but the location of this plasticity has not been determined—it could well be cerebellum rather than cortex. Nevertheless, auditory plasticity seems to be similar to visual plasticity.

There are other examples of critical periods that end around puberty (Doupe & Kuhl, 1999). For example, speech deteriorates markedly if deafness occurs prior to puberty (Plant & Hammarberg, 1983). Language can develop fully if acquired before puberty, and it is much more difficult to acquire a second language after puberty (Lennenberg, 1967). Speech can be learned after a left hemispherectomy up to puberty (Vargha-Khadem et al., 1997).

There are other examples of experience affecting subsequent plasticity. For example, English infants can discriminate both Hindi and Salish (native Canadian Indian) consonants at 6 to 8 months of age (Werker & Tees, 1984). This ability declines rapidly by 1 year of age. Hindi infants retain the ability to distinguish the Hindi consonants, and Salish infants retain the ability to distinguish the Salish consonants.

There are also clear examples of the period for recovery ending after the critical period for disruption. There is a map of space in the optic tectum of the barn owl that is similar for both auditory and visual input, since the owl does not move its eyes (Knudsen, 1982). The auditory map can be shifted by rearing barn owls with prisms over their eyes (Knudsen & Brainard, 1991). The shift was large for owls reared with prisms from 21 days of age, and small when the prism rearing was started at 102 days of age (Knudsen & Knudsen, 1990). However, when the prisms were removed at 182 days of age, recovery was rapid. The range of adjustment that older animals were capable of was expanded considerably by experience with prisms at an early age (Knudsen, 1998). These experiments also show that prior experience can change later capabilities for plasticity.

SUMMARY OF CURRENT KNOWLEDGE

This description and analysis of critical periods can be summarized in Figure 2.25 and Table 2.1—the figure showing the periods over which different properties develop, and the table showing whether the critical period for disruption of a property lasts longer than the initial period of development and whether the critical period for recovery also lasts longer.

Acuity develops between birth and 3 to 5 years of age; vernier acuity between a few months and 10 years of age; binocularity between 2 and 6 months of age; stereopsis between 3 and 5 months of age and more slowly after that; monocular OKN between birth and 3 to 5 months of age; motion VEP between 2 months and 2 years of age; and contrast sensitivity between birth and 7 years of age (Figure 2.25). The period of development for suppression is unknown. The time course for the development of these various visual functions definitely supports the point that functions dealt with at lower levels of the system develop earlier.

Disruption of acuity can certainly occur after acuity has first developed in cases of stimulus deprivation (Figure 2.9). How far this is true in cases of strabismus and anisometropia is unclear. There are few tabulations of the clinical data, and a variety of measures of acuity are used. Thus many comparisons are like apples and oranges. Binocularity can be disrupted over several years, with a critical period similar to that for acuity. Stereopsis is disrupted by strabismus over the same period as it is developing, and also afterward. Monocular OKN and the motion VEP can both be disrupted after the period of development is over. Myopia can certainly be induced after the eyeball is fully grown. There is not a lot of information on disruption of vernier acuity and changes in suppressive effects as a function of age of onset of the deprivation.

Recovery of acuity can certainly occur for anisometropia long after the period of disruption has passed, and for strabismus in cases where the nonamblyopic eye loses function. With stimulus deprivation, there is not a lot of recovery later on. Vernier acuity can be improved in the adult, in normal as well as deprived people, but the improvement is much larger in deprived people. Recovery of stereopsis is difficult after 2 years of age,

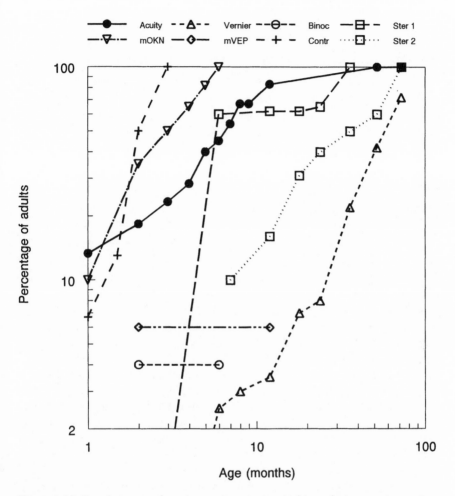

Figure 2.25. Development of grating acuity, stereopsis, binocularity, vernier acuity, monocular OKN, motion VEP, and contrast sensitivity as a function of age. Grating acuity measurements from Dobson and Teller (1978), Norcia and Tyler (1985) and Neu and Sireteanu (1995). Stereopsis measurements from Birch, Gwiazda, and Held (1982), and Birch and Hale (1996) for projected patterns and line stereograms (stereo 1), and from Birch and Salomao (1998) and Ciner, Schanelkitsch, and Herzberg (1996) for random dot stereocards (stereo 2). Vernier acuity averaged from Carkeet, Levi, and Manny (1997), Gwiazda, Bauer, and Held (1989), and Zanker et al. (1992). Monocular OKN from Naegele and Held (1982). Contrast sensitivity from Norcia, Tyler, and Hamer (1990). There are few numerical values for binocularity or motion VEPs, so the horizontal line simply shows the period over which these develop.

Table 2.1
Critical Periods for Disruption and Recovery of Various Properties

Property	Is CP for Disruption Later?	Is CP for Recovery Later?
Acuity	maybe	yes
Vernier acuity	?	yes
Binocularity	yes	?
Stereopsis	yes	no
Monocular OKN	yes	yes
Motion VEP	yes	yes
Suppression	?	?
Myopia	yes	?
Contrast sensitivity	no	no

which is still within the period of development of fine stereopsis, although coarse stereopsis is probably fully developed by then. There is recovery for both monocular OKN and motion VEPs, when they have been disrupted, after the initial period of development.

All of this emphasizes the point that we started off with: One has to define the visual property, the previous visual history, and the type of visual deprivation when discussing a critical period. Strabismus and anisometropia change the critical period in humans just as rearing in the dark does in animals. Disruption differs for strabismus, anisometropia, and stimulus deprivation, and so does recovery. These three types of deprivation have different effects on different properties. Not all the critical periods have been worked out because of limitations in the data available from humans and the difficulty and tediousness of the experiments required to find the answer from animals. However, the general rule that the critical period for disruption of a property lasts longer than the initial period of development, and that recovery can be obtained at a time when disruption no longer occurs, seems to be true for most properties with the exception of contrast sensitivity.

PROMINENT GAPS IN CURRENT KNOWLEDGE

The most serious gap in our current knowledge is information on development of the crowding phenomenon and on Snellen acuity. It is clear that this is not complete until after grating acuity is developed. Strabismus affects Snellen acuity and vernier acuity much more than grating acuity.

Looking at Figure 2.25, it is clear that Vernier acuity develops more rapidly and at a later time than grating acuity, and one might expect that the curve for Snellen acuity would lie somewhere between the two curves for grating and vernier acuity, but nobody knows exactly where. One needs to adopt a specific spacing of letters or specific distance for surrounding symbols to give constancy in the results. Part of the reason that so much attention has been paid to the development of grating acuity, and comparatively little to the development of crowding and Snellen acuity, is that it is much easier to standardize and test the former.

The question is of importance in practical terms because of the use that we make of reading and the need to see fine detail in objects. It is also of importance in theoretical terms within the framework of this chapter. Vaegan and Taylor (1979) showed clearly that stimulus deprivation will disrupt acuity at 10 years of age. They used grating acuity in their younger children and Snellen acuity in their older ones. It seems that the disruption of Snellen acuity in child AF, the latest serious disruption found in their series, is beyond the period of development of Snellen acuity with even the closest spacing of letters. However, without the evidence for development in normal children, one does not conclusively know if this is the case.

A second serious gap concerns the development of coarse versus fine stereopsis. These have not been distinguished in developmental studies, nor have linear and nonlinear stereopsis. The two curves for the development of stereopsis in Figure 2.25 show two very different time courses. These curves are distinguished by the use of different stimuli—line stereograms and projected patterns versus random dot stereocards—rather than by the distinctions of coarse and fine or linear and nonlinear stereopsis, but the fact that there are two such different curves suggests that there may be two different developmental processes. Again, there is a practical point: Stereopsis is used, on the one hand, to guide vergence movements and, on the other hand, to perceive shape and depth in objects. One needs to know if one of these processes can be disrupted at a certain age without the other being affected. There is also the theoretical point brought out above: It is clear that coarse stereopsis can be degraded by strabismus starting after the initial period of rapid development. Can fine stereopsis also be degraded by strabismus after stereoacuity has finally reached adult levels?

A third serious gap, as pointed out above, is the development of suppression mechanisms in normal children. Clearly suppression is an important phenomenon in normal vision, to avoid diplopia for a further object that is hidden in one eye but not the other by a nearer object. Data on this phenomenon are extremely thin. Given that suppression is a major component of poor vision in strabismus, one needs to know how suppression in strabismics varies from suppression in normal children. One cannot start to answer this question until one knows how suppression develops in normal children, using stimuli that relate to the real-world stimuli that produce suppression in both cases.

This is just a short list of questions for which we need the answers. Others will no doubt have their own list. It may be that the information is there sitting in the experience of some clinician who has not had the time to document it. One of my frustrations in writing this chapter has been to read statements that seem very likely to be true but cannot be used because the documentation and quantification are not there. I hope that the chapter has gone over the data within a slightly novel framework, which will encourage some new experiments as well as documentation of points known from clinical experience.

ACKNOWLEDGMENTS

I thank Eileen Birch and Donald Mitchell for comments on this chapter. The author's research is supported by PHS grant RO1 EY00053. The author is a Senior Scientific Investigator of Research to Prevent Blindness.

REFERENCES

Abadi, R.V. (1976). Induction masking: A study of some inhibitory interactions during dichoptic viewing. *Vision Research, 16,* 269–275.

Abrahamsson, M., Andersson, A.K., & Sjostrand, J. (1990). A longitudinal study of a population based sample of astigmatic children I. Refraction and amblyopia II. The changeability of anisometropia (Fabian). *Acta Ophthalmologica Copenhagen, 68,* 428–434.

Albus, K., & Wolf, W. (1984). Early postnatal development of neuronal function in the kitten's visual cortex: A laminar analysis. *Journal of Physiology, 348,* 153–185.

Atkinson, J. (1979). Development of optokinetic nystagmus in the human infant and monkey infant. In R.D. Freeman (Ed.), *Developmental neurobiology of vision* (pp. 277–287). New York: Plenum.

Atkinson, J., Anker, S., Evans, C., Hall, R., & Pimm-Smith, E. (1988). Visual acuity testing of young children with the Cambridge Crowding Cards at 3 m and 6 m. *Archives of Ophthalmology, 66,* 505–508.

Atkinson, J., Braddick, O.J., & Moar, K. (1977). Development of contrast sensitivity over the first 3 months of life in the human infant. *Vision Research, 17,* 1037–1044.

Awaya, S., Sugawara, M., & Miyake, S. (1979). Observations in patients with occlusion amblyopia. *Transactions of the Ophthalmological Society (UK), 99,* 447–454.

Banks, M.S., Aslin, R.N., & Letson, R.D. (1975). Sensitive period for the development of human binocular vision. *Science, 190,* 675–677.

Banks, M.S., & Bennett, P.J. (1988). Optical and photoreceptor immaturities limit the spatial and chromatic vision of human neonates. *Journal of the Optical Society of America A, 5,* 2059–2079.

Beard, B.L., Levi, D.M., & Reich, L.N. (1995). Perceptual learning in parafoveal vision. *Vision Research, 35,* 1679–1690.

Beaver, C.J., Ji, Q.H., & Daw, N.W. (2002). Layer differences in the effect of monocular deprivation in light- and dark-reared kittens during and after the critical period. *Visual Neuroscience, 18*, 811–820.

Birch, E.E. (1993). Stereopsis in infants and its developmental relation to visual acuity. In K. Simons (Ed.), *Early visual development, normal and abnormal* (pp. 224–236). New York: Oxford University Press.

Birch, E.E., Fawcett, S., & Stager, D.R. (2000a). Co-development of VEP motion response and binocular vision in normal infants and infantile esotropes. *Investigative Ophthalmology and Visual Science, 41*, 1719–1723.

Birch, E.E., Fawcett, S., & Stager, D.R. (2000b). Why does early sugical alignment improve stereoacuity outcomes in infantile esotropia? *Journal of American Association of Pediatric Ophthalmology and Strabismus, 4*, 10–14.

Birch, E.E., Gwiazda, J., & Held, R. (1982). Stereoacuity development for crossed and uncrossed disparities in human infants. *Vision Research, 22*, 507–513.

Birch, E.E., & Hale, L.A. (1996). Operant assessment of stereoacuity. *Clinical Vision Sciences, 4*, 295–300.

Birch, E.E., & Salomao, S. (1998). Infant random dot stereoacuity cards. *Journal of Pediatric Ophthalmology and Strabismus, 35*, 86–90.

Birch, E.E., Shimojo, S., & Held, R. (1985). Preferential-looking assessment of fusion and stereopsis in infants aged 1–6 months. *Investigative Ophthalmology, 26*, 366–370.

Birch, E.E., & Stager, D.R. (1996). The critical period for surgical treatment of dense congenital unilateral cataract. *Investigative Ophthalmology and Visual Science, 37*, 1532–1538.

Birch, E.E., Stager, D.R., Leffler, J., & Weakley, D.R. (1998). Early treatment of congenital unilateral cataract minimizes unequal competition. *Investigative Qphthalmology and Visual Science, 39*, 1560–1566.

Birch, E.E., & Swanson, W.H. (1992). Probability summation of acuity in the human infant. *Vision Research, 32*, 1999–2003.

Birch, E.E., & Swanson, W.H. (2000). Hyperacuity deficits in anisometropic and strabismic amblyopes with known ages of onset. *Vision Research, 40*, 1035–1040.

Birnbaum, M.H., Koslowe, K., & Sanet, R. (1977). Success in amblyopia therapy as a function of age: A literature survey. *American Journal of Optometry and Physiological Optics, 54*, 269–275.

Blakemore, C., & van Sluyters, R.C. (1974). Reversal of the physiological effects of monocular deprivation in kittens: Further evidence for a sensitive period. *Journal of Physiology, 237*, 195–216.

Bodnarenko, S.R., Jeyarasasingam, G., & Chalupa, L.M. (1995). Development and regulation of dendritic stratification in retinal ganglion cells by glutamate-mediated afferent activity. *Journal of Neuroscience, 15*, 7037–7045.

Bourron-Madignier, M., Ardoin, M.L., Cypres, C., et, al. (1987). Study of opto-kinetic nystagmus in children. In M. Lenk-Schaeffer (Ed.), *Transactions of the Sixth International Orthoptic Congress* (pp. 134–139). London: International Orthoptic Association.

Bowering, E.R., Maurer, D., Lewis, T.L., & Brent, H.P. (1993). Sensitivity in the nasal and temporal hemifields in children treated for cataract. *Investigative Ophthalmology and Visual Science, 34*, 3501–3509.

Braddick, O.J., Atkinson, J., Julesz, B., Kropfl, W., Bodis-Wollner, I., & Raab, E. (1980). Cortical binocularity in infants. *Nature, 288,* 363–365.

Braddick, O.J., Wattam-Bell, J., & Atkinson, J. (1986). Orientation-specific cortical responses develop in early infancy. *Nature, 320,* 617–619.

Brosnahan, D., Norcia, A.M., Schor, C., & Taylor, D.G. (1998). OKN, perceptual and VEP direction biases in strabismus. *Vision Research, 38,* 2833–2840.

Brown, R.J., Candy, T.R., & Norcia, A.M. (1999). Development of rivalry and dichoptic masking in human infants. *Investigative Ophthalmology and Visual Science, 40,* 3324–3333.

Carkeet, A., Levi, D.M., & Manny, R.E. (1997). Development of Vernier acuity in childhood. *Optometry and Vision Science, 74,* 741–750.

Chapman, B., & Stryker, M.P. (1993). Development of orientation selectivity in ferret visual cortex and effects of deprivation. *Journal of Neuroscience, 13,* 5251–5262.

Chen, L., Cooper, N.G.F., & Mower, G.D. (2000). Developmental changes in the expression of NMDA receptor subunits (NR1, NR2A, NR2B) in the cat visual cortex and the effects of dark rearing. *Molecular Brain Research, 78,* 196–200.

Chevasse, F.B. (1939). *Worth's squint or the binocular reflexes and the treatment of strabismus* (7th ed., p. 519). London: Baillier, Tindall and Cox.

Ciner, E.B., Schanelklitsch, E., & Herzberg, C. (1996). Stereoacuity development— 6 months to 5 years—a new tool for testing and screening. *Optometry and Vision Science, 73,* 43–48.

Cleland, B.G., Mitchell, D.E., Crewther, S.G., & Crewther, D.P. (1980). Visual resolution of retinal ganglion cells in monocularly deprived cats. *Brain Research, 192,* 261–266.

Crawford, M.J., Pesch, T.W., & von Noorden, G.K. (1996). Excitatory binocular neurons are lost following prismatic binocular dissociation in infant monkeys. *Behavioral Brain Research, 79,* 227–232.

Crowley, J.C., & Katz, L.C. (2000). Early development of ocular dominance columns. *Science, 290,* 1321–1325.

Curtin, B.J. (1985). *The myopias: Basic science and clinical management.* Philadelphia: Harper & Row.

Cynader, M.S., & Mitchell, D.E. (1980). Prolonged sensitivity to monocular deprivation in dark-reared cats. *Journal of Neurophysiology, 43,* 1026–1040.

Darian-Smith, C., & Gilbert, C.D. (1994). Axonal sprouting accompanies functional reorganization in adult cat striate cortex. *Nature, 368,* 737–740.

Daw, N.W. (1962). Why after-images are not seen in normal circumstances. *Nature, 196,* 1143–1145.

Daw, N.W. (1994). Mechanisms of plasticity in the visual cortex. *Investigative Ophthalmology and Visual Science, 35,* 4168–4179.

Daw, N.W. (1995). *Visual development.* New York: Plenum.

Daw, N.W., Baysinger, K.J., & Parkinson, D. (1987). Increased levels of testosterone have little effect on visual cortical plasticity in the kitten. *Journal of Neurobiology, 18,* 141–154.

Daw, N.W., Berman, N.J., & Ariel, M. (1978). Interaction of critical periods in the visual cortex of kittens. *Science, 199,* 565–567.

Daw, N.W., Fox, K.D., Sato, H., & Czepita, D. (1992). Critical period for monocular deprivation in the cat visual cortex. *Journal of Neurophysiology, 67,* 197–202.

Daw, N.W., Sato, H., Fox, K.D., Carmichael, T., & Gingerich, R. (1991). Cortisol reduces plasticity in the kitten visual cortex. *Journal of Neurobiology, 22,* 158–168.

Daw, N.W., & Wyatt, H.J. (1974). Raising rabbits in a moving visual environment: An attempt to modify directional sensitivity in the retina. *Journal of Physiology, 240,* 309–330.

Daw, N.W., & Wyatt, H.J. (1976). Kittens reared in a unidirectional environment: Evidence for a critical period. *Journal of Physiology, 257,* 155–170.

Demer, J.L., & von Noorden, G.K. (1988). Optokinetic asymmetry in esotropia. *Journal of Pediatric Ophthalmology and Strabismus, 25,* 286–292.

Derrington, A.M., & Hawken, M.J. (1981). Spatial and temporal properties of cat geniculate neurons after prolonged deprivation. *Journal of Physiology, 316,* 1–10.

Dobson, V., & Sebris, S.L. (1989). Longitudinal study of acuity and stereopsis in infants with or at-risk for esotropia. *Investigative Ophthalmology, 30,* 1146–1158.

Dobson, V., & Teller, D.Y. (1978). Visual acuity in human infants: A review and comparison of behavioral and electrophysiological studies. *Vision Research, 18,* 1469–1483.

Doupe, A.J., & Kuhl, P.K. (1999). Birdsong and human speech: Common themes and mechanisms. *Annual Review of Neuroscience, 22,* 567–631.

Eggers, H.M., & Blakemore, C. (1978). Physiological basis of anisometropic amblyopia. *Science, 201,* 264–266.

Eizenman, M., Westfall, C.A., Geer, I., Smith, K., Chatterjee, S., Panton, C.M., Kraft, S.P., & Skarf, B. (1999). Electrophysiological evidence of cortical fusion in children with early-onset esotopia. *Investigative Ophthalmology and Visual Science, 40,* 354–362.

Elbert, T., Pantev, C., Wienbruch, C., Rockstroh, B., & Taub, E. (1995). Increased cortical representation of the fingers of the left hand in string players. *Science, 270,* 305–307.

Ellemberg, D., Lewis, T.L., Liu, C.H., & Maurer, D. (1999). Development of spatial and temporal vision during childhood. *Vision Research, 39,* 2325–2333.

Ellemberg, D., Lewis, T.L., Maurer, D., Brar, S., & Brent, H.P. (2002). Better perception of global motion after monocular than after binocular deprivation. *Vision Research, 42,* 167–179.

El Mallah, M.K., Chakravarthy, U., & Hart, P.M. (2000). Amblyopia: Is visual loss permanent? *British Journal of Ophthalmology, 84,* 952–956.

Epelbaum, M., Milleret, C., Buisseret, P., & Dufier, J.L. (1993). The sensitive period for strabismic amblyopia in humans. *Ophthalmology, 100,* 323–327.

Fagiolini, M., Pizzorusso, T., Berardi, N., Domenici, L., & Maffei, L. (1994). Functional postnatal development of the rat primary visual cortex and the role of visual experience: Dark rearing and monocular deprivation. *Vision Research, 34,* 709–720.

Fawcett, S., & Birch, E.E. (2000). Motion VEPs, stereopsis, and bifoveal fusion in children with strabismus. *Investigative Ophthalmology and Visual Science, 41,* 411–416.

Fawcett, S., Leffler, J., & Birch, E.E. (2000). Factors influencing stereoacuity in accommodative esotropia. *Journal of the American Association of Pediatric Ophthalmology and Strabismus, 4*, 15–20.

Fern, K.D., & Manny, R.E. (1986). Visual acuity of the preschool child: A review. *American Journal of Optometry and Physiological Optics, 63*, 319–345.

Fiorentini, A., & Maffei, L. (1976). Spatial contrast sensitivity of myopic subjects. *Vision Research, 16*, 437–438.

Flom, M.C., & Bedell, H.E. (1985). Identifying amblyopia using associated conditions, acuity, and nonacuity features. *American Journal of Optometry and Physiological Optics, 62*, 153–160.

Flom, M.C., Weymouth, F.W., & Kahneman, D. (1963). Visual resolution and contour interaction. *Journal of the Optical Society of America A, 53*, 1026–1032.

Fox, R., Aslin, R.N., Shea, S.L., & Dumais, S.T. (1980). Stereopsis in human infants. *Science, 207*, 323–324.

Freeman, A.W., Nguyen, V.A., & Jolly, N. (1996). Component of visual acuity loss in strabismus. *Vision Research, 36*, 765–774.

Gair, E.J., & Adams, G.G.W. (1999). Normal visual development after unilateral complete ptosis at birth. *Journal of the American Association of Pediatric Ophthalmology and Strabismus, 3*, 58–59.

Giffin, F., & Mitchell, D.E. (1978). The rate of recovery of vision after early monocular deprivation in kittens. *Journal of Physiology, 274*, 511–537.

Gilbert, C.D., & Wiesel, T.N. (1992). Receptive field dynamics in adult primary visual cortex. *Nature, 356*, 150–152.

Gordon, J.A., & Stryker, M.P. (1996). Experience-dependent plasticity of binocular reponses in the primary visual cortex of the mouse. *Journal of Neuroscience, 16*, 3274–3286.

Greenwald, M.J., & Parks, M.M. (1989). Treatment of amblyopia. In T.D. Duane (Ed.), *Clinical ophthalmology* (pp. 1–9). Hagerstown, MD: Harper and Row.

Guillery, R.W., & Stelzner, D.J. (1970). The differential effects of unilateral eye closure on the monocular and binocular segments of the dorsal lateral geniculate nucleus in the cat. *Journal of Comparative Neurology, 139*, 413–422.

Guire, E.S., Lickey, M.E., & Gordon, B. (1999). Critical period for the monocular deprivation effect in rats: Assessment with sweep visually evoked potentials. *Journal of Neurophysiology, 81*, 121–128.

Gwiazda, J., Bauer, J., & Held, R. (1989). From visual acuity to hyperacuity: A 10-year update. *Canadian Journal of Psychology, 43*, 109–120.

Hamer, R.D., Norcia, A.M., Orel-Bixler, D., & Hoyt, C.S. (1993). Motion VEPs in late-onset esotropia. *Clinical Vision Sciences, 8*, 55–62.

Hardman Lea, S.J., Loades, J., & Rubinstein, M.P. (1989). The sensitive period for anisometropic amblyopia. *Eye, 3*, 783–790.

Harrad, R. (1996). Psychophysics of suppression. *Eye, 10*, 270–273.

Harwerth, R.S., Smith, E.L., Duncan, G.C., Crawford, M.J., & von Noorden, G.K. (1986). Multiple sensitive periods in the development of the primate visual system. *Science, 237*, 235–238.

Held, R. (1965). Plasticity in sensory-motor systems. *Scientific American, 213*, 84–94.

Held, R. (1993). Two stages in the development of binocular vision and eye alignment. In K. Simons (Ed.), *Early visual development: Normal and abnormal* (pp. 250–257). New York: Oxford University Press.

Held, R., Birch, E.E., & Gwiazda, J. (1980). Stereoacuity of human infants. *Proceedings of the National Academy of Sciences (USA), 77*, 5572–5574.

Helveston, E.M. (1993). The origins of congenital esotropia. *Journal of Pediatric Ophthalmology and Strabismus, 30*, 215–232.

Helveston, E.M., & von Noorden, G.K. (1967). Microtropia. *Archives of Ophthalmology, 78*, 272–281.

Hendrickson, A.E., Movshon, J.A., Eggers, H.M., Gizzi, M.S., Boothe, R.G., & Kiorpes, L. (1987). Effects of early unilateral blur on the macaque's visual system. II. Anatomical observations. *Journal of Neuroscience, 7*, 1327–1339.

Hess, R.F., Campbell, F.W., & Greenhalgh, T. (1978). On the nature of the neural abnormality in human amblyopia: Neural aberrations and neural sensitivity loss. *Pfluger's Archives gesamte Physiologie, 377*, 201–207.

Hess, R.F., & Holliday, I.E. (1992). The spatial localization deficit in amblyopia. *Vision Research, 32*, 1319–1339.

Hoffmann, K.P., Distler, C., & Markner, C. (1996). Optokinetic nystagmus in cats with congenital strabismus. *Journal of Neurophysiology, 75*, 1495–1502.

Hohmann, A., & Creutzfeldt, O.D. (1975). Squint and the development of binocularity in humans. *Nature, 254*, 613–614.

Hohmann, A., & Haase, W. (1982). Development of visual line acuity in humans. *Ophthalmic Research, 14*, 107–112.

Holopigian, K., Blake, R., & Greenwald, M.J. (1988). Clinical suppression and amblyopia. *Investigative Ophthalmology and Visual Science, 29*, 444–451.

Horton, J.C., & Hocking, D.R. (1996). An adult-like pattern of ocular dominance columns in striate cortex of newborn monkeys prior to visual experience. *Journal of Neuroscience, 16*, 1791–1807.

Horton, J.C., & Hocking, D.R. (1997). Timing of the critical period for plasticity of ocular dominance columns in macaque striate cortex. *Journal of Neuroscience, 17*, 3684–3709.

Hubel, D.H., & Wiesel, T.N. (1965). Binocular interaction in striate cortex of kittens reared with artificial squint. *Journal of Neurophysiology, 28*, 1041–1059.

Hubel, D.H., & Wiesel, T.N. (1970). The period of susceptibility to the physiological effects of unilateral eye closure in kittens. *Journal of Physiology, 206*, 419–436.

Hubel, D.H., Wiesel, T.N., & LeVay, S. (1977). Plasticity of ocular dominance columns in monkey striate cortex. *Philosophical Transactions of the Royal Society of London, Series B, 278*, 377–409.

Ing, M.R. (1983). Early surgical alignment for congenital esotropia. *Ophthalmology, 90*, 132–135.

Irvine, S.R. (1948). Amblyopia ex anopsia. Observations on retinal inhibition, scotoma, projection, light difference discrimination and visual acuity. *Transactions of the American Ophthalmological Society, 66*, 527–575.

Issa, N.P., Trachtenberg, J.L., Chapman, B., Zahs, K.R., & Stryker, M.P. (1999).

The critical period for ocular dominance plasticity in the ferret's visual cortex. *Journal of Neuroscience, 19,* 6965–6978.

Jacobs, D.S., & Blakemore, C. (1988). Factors limiting the postnatal development of visual acuity in the monkey. *Vision Research, 28,* 947–958.

Jampolsky, A. (1951). Retinal correspondence in patients with small degree strabismus. *Archives of Ophthalmology, 45,* 18–26.

Jampolsky, A. (1955). Characteristics of suppression in strabismus. *Archives of Ophthalmology, 54,* 683–696.

Jones, K.R., Spear, P.D., & Tong, L. (1984). Critical periods for effects on monocular deprivation: Differences between striate and extrastriate cortex. *Journal of Neuroscience, 4,* 2543–2552.

Keech, R.V., & Kutsche, P.J. (1995). Upper age limit for the development of amblyopia. *Journal of Pediatric Ophthalmology and Strabismus, 32,* 89–93.

Kiorpes, L. (1989). The development of spatial resolution and contrast sensitivity in naturally strabismic monkeys. *Clinical Vision Sciences, 4,* 279–293.

Kiorpes, L., Boothe, R.G., Hendrickson, A.E., Movshon, J.A., Eggers, H.M., & Gizzi, M.S. (1987). Effects of early unilateral blur on the macaque's visual system I. Behavioural observations. *Journal of Neuroscience, 7,* 1318–1326.

Knudsen, E.I. (1982). Auditory and visual maps of space in the optic tectum of the barn owl. *Journal of Neuroscience, 2,* 1177–1194.

Knudsen, E.I. (1998). Capacity for plasticity in the adult owl auditory system expanded by juvenile experience. *Science, 279,* 1531–1533.

Knudsen, E.I., & Brainard, M.S. (1991). Visual instruction of the neural map of auditory space in the developing optic tectum. *Science, 253,* 85–87.

Knudsen, E.I., & Knudsen, P.F. (1990). Sensitive and critical periods for visual calibration of sound localization by barn owls. *Journal of Neuroscience, 10,* 222–232.

Kumagami, T., Zhang, B., Smith, E.L., & Chino, Y.M. (2000). Effect of onset age of strabismus on the binocular responses of neurons in the monkey visual cortex. *Investigative Ophthalmology and Visual Science, 41,* 948–954.

Lenneberg, E. (1967). *Biological foundations of language.* New York: Wiley.

LeVay, S., Stryker, M.P., & Shatz, C.J. (1978). Ocular dominance columns and their development in layer IV of the cat's visual cortex: A quantitative study. *Journal of Comparative Neurology, 179,* 223–244.

LeVay, S., Wiesel, T.N., & Hubel, D.H. (1980). The development of ocular dominance columns in normal and visually deprived monkeys. *Journal of Comparative Neurology, 191,* 1–51.

Levi, D.M., & Carkeet, A. (1993). Amblyopia: A consequence of abnormal visual development. In K. Simons (Ed.), *Early visual development: Normal and abnormal* (pp. 391–408). New York: Oxford University Press.

Levi, D.M., & Klein, S. (1982). Hyperacuity and amblyopia. *Nature, 298,* 268–270.

Levi, D.M., Klein, S.A., & Aitsebaomo, A.P. (1985). Vernier acuity, crowding and cortical magnification. *Vision Research, 25,* 963–977.

Levi, D.M., Polat, U., & Hu, Y.S. (1997). Improvement in vernier acuity in adults with amblyopia. *Investigative Ophthalmology and Visual Science, 38,* 1492–1510.

Levitt, F.B., & van Sluyters, R.C. (1982). The sensitive period for strabismus in the kitten. *Developmental Brain Research, 3,* 323–327.

Lewis, T.L., Ellemberg, D., Maurer, D., & Brent, H.P. (2000). Changes in spatial vision during middle childhood in patients treated for congenital cataract. *Vision Research, 39,* 3480–3489.

Mason, A.J.S., Braddick, O.J., Wattam-Bell, J., & Atkinson, J. (2001). Directional motion asymmetry in infant VEPs—which direction? *Vision Research, 41,* 201–211.

Maurer, D., & Lewis, T.L. (1993). Visual outcomes after infantile cataract. In K. Simons (Ed.), *Early visual development: Normal and abnormal* (pp. 454–484). New York: Oxford University Press.

Mayer, D.L., Beiser, A.S., Warner, A.F., Pratt, E.M., Raye, K.N., & Lang, J.M. (1995). Monocular acuity norms for the Teller acuity cards between ages of one month and four years. *Investigative Ophthalmology and Visual Science, 36,* 671–685.

Meyer, E., Mizrahi, E., & Perlman, I. (1991). Amblyopia success index: A new method of quantitative assessment of treatment efficiency; application in a study of 473 anisometropic amblyopic patients. *Binocular Vision Quarterly, 6,* 83–90.

Mitchell, D.E. (1988). The extent of visual recovery from early monocular or binocular visual deprivation in kittens. *Journal of Physiology, 395,* 639–660.

Mitchell, D.E. (1991). The long-term effectiveness of different regimens of occlusion on recovery from early monocular deprivation in kittens. *Philosophical Transaction of the Royal Society, Series B, 333,* 51–79.

Mitchell, D.E., & Wilkinson, F.E. (1974). The effect of early astigmatism on the visual resolution of gratings. *Journal of Physiology, 243,* 739–756.

Mitkin, A., & Orestova, E. (1988). Development of binocular vision in early ontogenesis. *Psychologische Beiträge, 30,* 65–74.

Morrone, M.C., & Burr, D.C. (1986). Evidence for the existence and development of visual inhibition in humans. *Nature, 321,* 235–237.

Movshon, J.A., Eggers, H.M., Gizzi, M.S., Hendrickson, A.E., & Kiorpes, L. (1987). Effects of early unilateral blur on the macaque's visual system. III. Physiological observations. *Journal of Neuroscience, 7,* 1340–1351.

Mower, G.D. (1991). The effect of dark rearing on the time course of the critical period in cat visual cortex. *Developmental Brain Research, 58,* 151–158.

Mower, G.D., Caplan, C.J., Christen, W.G., & Duffy, F.H. (1985). Dark rearing prolongs physiological but not anatomical plasticity of the cat visual cortex. *Journal of Comparative Neurology, 235,* 448–466.

Mower, G.D., & Kaplan, I.V. (1999). Fos expression during the critical period in visual cortex: Differences between normal and dark reared cats. *Molecular Brain Research, 64,* 264–269.

Naegele, J.R., & Held, R. (1982). The postnatal development of monocular optokinetic nystagmus in infants. *Vision Research, 22,* 341–346.

Neu, B., & Sireteanu, R. (1995). Monocular acuity in preschool children: Assessment with the Teller and Keeler acuity cards in comparison to the C-test. *Strabismus, 5,* 185–201.

Norcia, A.M. (1996). Abnormal motion processing and binocularity: Infantile esotropia as a model system for effects of early interruptions of binocularity. *Eye, 10,* 259–265.

Norcia, A.M., Hamer, R.D., & Jampolsky, A. (1995). Plasticity of human motion processing mechanisms following surgery for infantile esotropia. *Vision Research, 35,* 3279–3296.

Norcia, A.M., & Tyler, C.W. (1985). Spatial frequency sweep VEP: Visual acuity during the first year of life. *Vision Research, 25,* 1399–1408.

Norcia, A.M., Tyler, C.W., & Hamer, R.D. (1990). Development of contrast sensitivity in the human infant. *Vision Research, 30,* 1475–1486.

O'Dell, C., & Boothe, R.G. (1997). The development of stereoacuity in infant rhesus monkeys. *Vision Research, 37,* 2675–2684.

Odom, J.V., & Harter, M.R. (1983). Interocular suppression in adults and infants using anaglyphic stimuli: Visually evoked potential measures. *Electroencephalography and Clinical Neurophysiology, 56,* 232–243.

Odom, J.V., Hoyt, C.S., & Marg, E. (1982). Eye patching and visual evoked potential acuity in children four months to eight years old. *American Journal of Optometry and Physiological Optics, 59,* 706–717.

Oliver, M., Neumann, R., Chaimovitch, Y., Gotesman, N., & Shimshoni, M. (1986). Compliance and results of treatment for amblyopia in children more than 8 years old. *American Journal of Ophthalmology, 102,* 340–345.

Olson, C.R., & Freeman, R.D. (1975). Progressive changes in kitten striate cortex during monocular vision. *Journal of Neurophysiology, 38,* 26–32.

Olson, C.R., & Freeman, R.D. (1980). Profile of the sensitive period for monocular deprivation in kittens. *Experimental Brain Research, 39,* 17–21.

Pantev, C., Osstenveld, R., Engellen, A., Ross, B., Roberts, L.E., & Hoke, M. (1998). Increased auditory cortical representation in musicians. *Nature, 392,* 811–814.

Parks, M.M. (1969). The monofixation syndrome. *Transactions of the American Ophthalmological Society, 67,* 609–657.

Parks, M.M. (1984). Congenital esotropia with a bifixation result: Report of a case. *Documenta Ophthalmologica, 58,* 109–114.

Pasino, L., & Cordella, M. (1959). Il comportamento della difficoltà di separazione durante il trattamento dell'ambliopia strabica. *Istituto di clinica oculistica dell'università di Sassari, 25,* 111–115.

Petrig, B., Julesz, B., Kropfl, W., Baumgartner, G., & Anliker, M. (1981). Development of stereopsis and cortical binocularity in human infants: Electrophysiological evidence. *Science, 213,* 1402–1405.

Pettet, M.W., & Gilbert, C.D. (1992). Dynamic changes in receptive-field size in cat primary visual cortex. *Proceedings of the National Academy of Sciences (USA), 89,* 8366–8370.

Plant, G., & Hammarberg, B. (1983). Acoustic and perceptual analysis of the speech of the deafened. *Speech Transmission Laboratory Quarterly Progress and Status Report, 2–3,* 85–107.

Reid, S.M., Daw, N.W., Gregory, D.S., & Flavin, H.J. (1996). cAMP levels increased by activation of metabotropic glutamate receptors correlate with visual plasticity. *Journal of Neuroscience, 16,* 7619–7626.

Rodman, H.R. (1994). Development of inferior temporal cortex in the monkey. *Cerebral Cortex, 5,* 484–498.

Salomao, S.R., & Ventura, D.F. (1995). Large sample population for visual acuities obtained with Vistech-Teller cards. *Investigative Ophthalmology and Visual Science, 36,* 657–670.

Scharre, J.E., Cotter, S., Block, S.S., & Kelly, S.A. (1990). Normative contrast sensitivity data for young children. *Optometry and Vision Science, 67,* 826–832.

Schor, C., & Levi, D.M. (1980). Disturbances of small-field horizontal and vertical optokinetic nystagmus in amblyopia. *Investigative Ophthalmology, 19,* 668–683.

Sen, D.K. (1982). Results of treatment of anisohypermetropic amblyopia without strabismus. *British Journal of Ophthalmology, 66,* 680–684.

Sengpiel, F., Blakemore, C., Kind, P.C., & Harrad, R. (1994). Interocular suppression in the visual cortex of strabismic cats. *Journal of Neuroscience, 14,* 6855–6871.

Shapley, R.M., & So, Y.T. (1980). Is there an effect of monocular deprivation on the proportion of X and Y cells in the cat lateral geniculate nucleus? *Experimental Brain Research, 39,* 41–48.

Shatz, C.J., & Stryker, M.P. (1978). Ocular dominance in layer IV of the cat's visual cortex and the effects of monocular deprivation. *Journal of Physiology, 281,* 267–283.

Sherman, S.M., & Stone, J. (1973). Physiological normality of the retina in visually deprived cats. *Brain Research, 60,* 224–230.

Shimojo, S., Bauer, J., O'Connell, K.M., & Held, R. (1986). Pre-stereoptic binocular vision in infants. *Vision Research, 26,* 501–510.

Siegwart, J.T., & Norton, T.T. (1998). The susceptible period for deprivation-induced myopia in tree shrew. *Vision Research, 38,* 3505–3515.

Simmers, A.J., & Gray, L.S. (1999). Improvement of visual function in an adult amblyope. *Optometry and Vision Science, 76,* 82–87.

Simons, K. (1983). Visual acuity norms in young children. *Survey of Ophthalmology, 28,* 84–92.

Sireteanu, R. (2000). Development of the visual system in the human infant. In A.F. Kalverboer & A. Gramsbergen (Eds.), *Handbook on brain and behavior in human development* (pp. 629–652). London: Kluwer.

Sireteanu, R., Fronius, M., & Singer, W. (1981). Binocular interaction in the peripheral visual field of humans with strabismic and anisometropic amblyopia. *Vision Research, 21,* 1065–1074.

Skoczenski, A.M., & Norcia, A.M. (1999). Development of vernier acuity and grating acuity in human infants. *Investigative Ophthalmology and Visual Science, 40,* 2411–2417.

Slater, A.M., Morison, V., & Somers, M. (1988). Orientation discrimination and cortical function in the human newborn. *Perception, 17,* 597–602.

Smith, E.L., Bradley, D.V., Fernandes, A., & Boothe, R.G. (1999). Form deprivation myopia in adolescent monkeys. *Optometry and Vision Science, 76,* 428–432.

Smith, E.L., Chino, Y.M., Cheng, H., Crawford, M.J., & Harwerth, R.S. (1997). Residual binocular interactions in the striate cortex of monkeys reared with abnormal binocular vision. *Journal of Neurophysiology, 78,* 1353–1362.

Smith, E.L., Levi, D.M., Manny, R.E., Harwerth, R.S., & White, J.M. (1985). The relationship between binocular rivalry and strabismic suppression. *Investigative Ophthalmology and Visual Science, 26,* 80–87.

Stager, D.R., & Birch, E.E. (1986). Preferential-looking acuity and stereopsis in infantile esotropia. *Journal of Pediatric Ophthalmology and Strabismus, 23,* 160–165.

Stuart, J.A., & Burian, H.M. (1962). A study of separation difficulty. *American Journal of Ophthalmology, 53,* 471–477.

Swindale, N.V., Vital-Durand, F., & Blakemore, C. (1981). Recovery from monocular deprivation in the monkey. III. Reversal of anatomical effects in the visual cortex. *Proceedings of the Royal Society, Series B, 213,* 435–450.

Taylor, D.M. (1972). Is congenital esotropia functionally curable? *Transactions of the American Ophthalmological Society, 70,* 529–576.

Thorn, F., Gwiazda, J., Cruz, A., Bauer, J., & Held, R. (1994). The develoment of eye alignment, sensory binocularity and convergence in young infants. *Investigative Ophthalmology, 35,* 544–553.

Tierney, D.W. (1989). Vision recovery in amblyopia after contralateral subretinal hemorrhage. *Journal of the American Optometric Association, 60,* 281–283.

Timney, B.N. (1981). Development of binocular depth perception in kittens. *Investigative Ophthalmology, 21,* 493–496.

Travers, T. (1938). Suppression of vision in squint and its association with retinal correspondence and amblyopia. *British Journal of Ophthalmology, 22,* 577–604.

Troilo, D., Nickla, D., & Wildsoet, C. (2000). Form deprivation myopia in mature common marmosets (*Callithrix jacchus*). *Investigative Ophthalmology and Visual Science, 41,* 2043–2049.

Tytla, M.E., Maurer, D., Lewis, T.L., & Brent, H.P. (1988). Contrast sensitivity in children treated for congenital cataract. *Clinical Vision Sciences, 2,* 251–264.

Vaegan, M., & Taylor, D. (1979). Critical period for deprivation amblyopia in children. *Transactions of the Ophthalmological Society (UK), 99,* 432–439.

Van Essen, D.C., Anderson, C.H., & Felleman, D.J. (1992). Information processing in the primate visual system: An integrated systems perspective. *Science, 255,* 419–423.

Vargha-Khadem, F., Carr, L.J., Isaacs, E., Brett, E., Adams, C., & Mishkin, M. (1997). Onset of speech after a left hemispherectomy in a nine-year old boy. *Brain, 120,* 159–182.

Vereecken, E.P., & Brabant, P. (1984). Prognosis for vision in amblyopia after loss of the good eye. *Archives of Ophthalmology, 102,* 220–224.

von Noorden, G.K. (1981). New clinical aspects of stimulus deprivation amblyopia. *American Journal of Ophthalmology, 92,* 416–421.

von Noorden, G.K. (1988). A reassessment of infantile esotropia. *American Journal of Ophthalmology, 105,* 1–10.

von Noorden, G.K. (1990). *Binocular vision and ocular motility.* St Louis: Mosby.

Wallman, J., Gottlieb, M.D., Rajaram, V., & Fugate-Wentzek, L. (1987). Local retinal regions control local eye growth in chicks. *Science, 237,* 73–77.

Wattam-Bell, J. (1991). Development of motion-specific cortical responses in infancy. *Vision Research, 31,* 287–297.

Werker, J.F., & Tees, R.C. (1984). Cross-language speech perception: Evidence for perceptual reorganization during the first year of life. *Infant Behavior and Development, 7,* 49–63.

Wick, B., Wingard, M., Cotter, S., & Scheiman, M. (1992). Anisometropic amblyopia: Is the patient ever too old to treat? *Optometry and Vision Science, 69,* 866–878.

Wiesel, T.N., & Hubel, D.H. (1963a). Effects of visual deprivation on morphology and physiology of cells in the cat's lateral geniculate body. *Journal of Neurophysiology, 26,* 978–993.

Wiesel, T.N., & Hubel, D.H. (1963b). Single cell responses in striate cortex of kittens deprived of vision in one eye. *Journal of Neurophysiology, 26,* 1003–1017.

Wiesel, T.N., & Raviola, E. (1977). Myopia and eye enlargement after neonatal lid fusion in monkeys. *Nature, 266,* 66–68.

Wilson, M.E. (1992). Adult amblyopia reversed by contralateral cataract formation. *Journal of Pediatric Ophthalmology and Strabismus, 29,* 100–102.

Worth, C. (1903). *Squint. Its causes, pathology and treatment.* Philadelphia: Blakiston.

Wright, K.W., Edelman, P.M., McVey, J.H., Terry, A.P., & Lin, M. (1994). High-grade stereo acuity after early surgery for congenital esotropia. *Archives of Ophthalmology, 112,* 913–919.

Zanker, J., Mohn, G., Weber, U., Zeitler-Driess, K., & Fahle, M. (1992). The development of vernier acuity in human infants. *Vision Research, 32,* 1557–1564.

Chapter 3

Development of Temporal Lobe Circuits for Object Recognition: Data and Theoretical Perspectives from Nonhuman Primates

Hillary R. Rodman

ABSTRACT

In humans, relatively little is known about the normal structural and physiological development of the temporal neocortex circuits underlying object recognition. In addition, relatively little has been done to develop theoretical accounts for understanding perceptual/behavioral changes that aim at biological plausibility at the level of offering specific candidate mechanisms. In this chapter, I review data obtained from studies in macaque monkeys and suggest that the longtime course of behavioral development of object perception and recognition in primates is paralleled by a built-in developmental delay in some of the neural plasticity that characterizes temporal lobe function in the adult. These data and arguments are then used as the basis for a conceptual framework that postulates rudimentary early neural capacity, a very long maturational time course, and specific signals that may be used in the generation of *relatively dedicated circuitry* underlying complex object perception. Finally, I identify some important predictions of the framework and domains of future inquiry that, based on both the framework and a comparison of the human and monkey literature, stand out as fruitful areas of concentration.

INTRODUCTION

Development of Object Recognition: The Problem and Ways to Approach It

How does one come to know what has never been seen before? For human and nonhuman primates alike, the recognition of significant objects in the environment is a skill crucial to survival, social success, and general well-being. For diurnal primates, the capacity for object identification is heavily dependent upon the exquisite processes of vision to which large portions of the brain contribute. However, determining what is and what is not a significant object is both a complex process and one that cannot, by definition, be fully organized prior to birth. Even if one postulates "innate"[1] detectors for such stimulus classes as faces, facial expressions, and specific foodstuffs, some learning is required to detect and predict when and where these and other important stimuli will occur and in what combination. For example, recognition of *particular* conspecifics cannot be preprogrammed and requires both stimulus input and contextual information.

These are not novel insights but rather reflect a growing consensus that visual object recognition capacities may be present in rudimentary form early in life but in any case only gradually mature completely (e.g., Carey, 1992; M. Johnson, 1994; Rodman & Nace, 1997). The mechanisms by which the system goes from ground zero at birth to the sophisticated performance of the adult have, however, only begun to be elucidated. In the most general sense—for myriad cognitive domains as well as vision—what does the hardware first show up with, what exactly are the signals provided by experience, and most critically, *how* does the process of change take place in terms of neural circuits?

Two very general approaches may be identified to this rather daunting set of questions. One strategy is to mathematically model the self-organization of complex circuits or systems underlying specific and diverse functions (see Grossberg, this volume), such as orientation discrimination (Kuroiwa et al., 2000; Swindale, 1992), discrimination of tonality (Tillmann, Bharucha, & Bigand, 2000), problems in language learning (Plunkett & Marchman, 1993), and object recognition itself (Mareschal & Johnson, 2002). A second strategy is to use observations taken at a variety of levels of analysis to generate hypotheses about what evolution has provided in terms of inherent biases and organizing mechanisms, as well as the mechanisms by which signals from the environment reorganize circuitry in temporary or long-lasting fashion. One influential example of this approach has been the work of Mark Johnson and colleagues (e.g., M. Johnson, 1990, 2000; Johnson & Vecera, 1993), who have drawn on a combination of behavioral and neurobiological considerations to generate and evolve an integrated view (see also "Toward a Biologically Plausible Framework" below). Ideally, such views are used in turn to inform mathematical models, and vice versa.

In this chapter, I will first review what we know, in primates, about the development of temporal lobe circuits underlying object recognition, in the context of both neuroscience and behavioral/perceptual development. I will then briefly discuss some earlier theoretical contributions and present a new integrated model for understanding the ontogeny of object recognition, both in terms of capacity and substrate. Having done so, I will look again at some aspects of the neurobiological data that are especially relevant to the framework and its assumptions and make some predictions. It should be noted that although some of our hypotheses propose changes intrinsic to temporal cortex, I do not claim that *all* predicted or likely age-dependent changes are purely intrinsic to temporal cortex. However, I propose that it is the signals that derive from temporal lobe regions that are what the developing animal has to *work with* in learning about the visual world, and these signals are what our efforts are focused on understanding. Finally, I will identify domains of future inquiry that, based on both the theoretical framework and the comparison of the human and monkey literature, stand out as needed areas of focus.

The Role of the Temporal Lobe

In both monkeys and humans, the neural pathways for object recognition depend heavily on a largely ventral and medial subset of extrastriate cortical territories in the temporal lobes. This so-called *ventral stream* consists, in adult monkeys, of a well-studied set of areas assumed to have some functional and structural independence as separate, distinct regions (Figure 3.1). Going from posterior to anterior within this domain as a whole, successively encountered areas show increasing degrees of retinotopic organization, larger visual receptive field size, more specific "trigger features" for eliciting neuronal responses for at least subpopulations of cells, and more evidence of memory- and eye movement–related modulation of the visual responses that occur (reviewed in Gross et al., 1993). The original proposal for a division between ventral stream processing of physical object attributes and dorsal stream processing of object location (Ungerleider & Mishkin, 1982) has since been broadened to highlight, in particular, the role of dorsal regions in using object attributes for visuomotor guidance (Goodale & Milner, 1992; see also Gilmore, this volume). In addition, discussion of the "two cortical visual systems" has increasingly emphasized the extensive crosstalk between the two streams, their functional interdependence, their extension into relatively segregated regions of the frontal lobes, and their partially overlapping but distinguishable connections with subcortical regions associated with memory and motor control.

Research clearly indicates, however, a primary role for ventral stream regions in object recognition, as well as neural correlates of how that role is made possible. Within the ventral stream of monkeys, the so-called *inferior temporal cortex (IT)* and related nearby regions play a crucial role in extracting the invariant aspects that characterize individual objects. In adult monkeys, damage to this tissue leads to deficits in discriminating between and reacting appropriately to objects on the basis of visual texture, overall shape, color, and internal arrangement of detail (Gross, 1973; Weis-

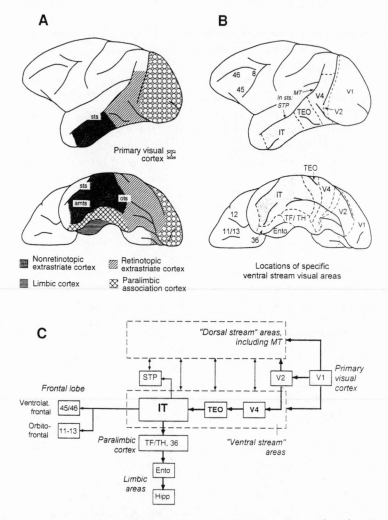

Figure 3.1. Location and interconnections of cortical regions referred to in this chapter, illustrated with respect to the macaque monkey brain. Although the story is still evolving, it appears that most or all of the regions specified here have identifiable homologs in humans. (**A**) Different classes of cortical areas shown on a side view (*top*) and bottom view (*bottom*) of a representative brain. Different types of shading are used to differentiate areas that have a significant degree of topographic organization (retinotopy) from territory (mainly IT for purposes of this chapter) in which receptive fields, typically large, are not organized into a systematic representation or map. Paralimbic and limbic cortical regions contributing to the object recognition process are also shown. (**B**) Approximate location and borders of widely recognized "ventral stream" extrastriate cortical areas. (**C**) Main feedforward pathways in the ventral cortical pathway for object recognition. Not all existing pathways are shown; most illustrated connections are reciprocal. Abbreviations: amts = anterior medial temporal sulcus; ento = entorhinal cortex; hipp = hippocampus; ots = occipitotemporal sulcus; sts = superior temporal sulcus. See text for other terms.

krantz & Saunders, 1984). In humans, damage to homologous ventral temporal cortex likewise produces impairments in object perception and recognition, that is, visual agnosia (reviewed in Farah, 1990). At the neural level, small but well-studied populations of cells in adult monkey temporal cortex respond to sometimes amazingly complex conjunctions of features, such as the prototypical arrangements of features in the primate face (Desimone, 1991; Rodman, 1999). Even more striking are findings demonstrating that these cells shift their properties with experience, a proposed cellular correlate of learning (e.g., Kobatake, Wang, & Tanaka, 1998; Miller, Li, & Desimane, 1991; Miyashita, 2000). Recent imaging work in humans illustrates comparable phenomena at the systems level, that is, shifts in activation patterns associated with experience of novel visual objects (Gauthier et al., 1999), although the specifics of processing stages and areas involved remain to be worked out.

DEVELOPMENT OF TEMPORAL CIRCUITS: EVIDENCE FROM NEUROSCIENCE

Although a substantial body of data has accrued on functional development of object recognition, far less is known about the development of its neural substrates, especially those beyond the preliminary stages of visual processing (Rodman & Moore, 1997). In the following sections, I will briefly summarize what neuroscience has taught us about the status of the object processing hardware in infancy, using a nonhuman primate model.

Structural Development of the Underpinnings of Object Recognition

A first question is that of when cortical circuits are physically in place. In primates, the vast majority, if not all[2], of the pool of available neurons is presumed to be in place in their target regions by birth. Generation and subsequent winnowing of synaptic connections continue furiously, however, in the early postnatal period (Goldman-Rakic, Bourgeois, & Rakic, 1997; Huttenlocher & Dabholkar, 1997; Rakic et al., 1986). While the presence of suitable connectivity of a brain region is not synonymous with the presence of mature function, it is a necessary precondition to it. Thus, the degree to which the wiring of the immature brain deviates from the wiring of the adult's is a potentially valuable source of information about functional capacity. There is relatively little work on the structural maturation of the primate temporal lobe relative to our knowledge of "primary" areas, but the existing data suggest some important principles.

Connectivity of Inferior Temporal Areas

Virtually all that is known about the development of cellular communication within inferior temporal areas relates to inter-areal connectivity;

unlike for V1 (e.g., Callaway, 1998, and references therein), virtually nothing has been published to date on local circuit development in this portion of the brain. In adult monkeys, the highest level of the object processing hierarchy (anterior inferior temporal cortex) receives convergent visual input from posterior temporal and occipital areas V4, TEO, and posterior inferior temporal cortex, as well as projections from parahippocampal areas, "dorsal stream" regions, and feedback pathways from the frontal lobe. In order to determine whether similar inputs are in place early in life, we injected anatomical tracers into anterior IT in infant animals ranging from 2 to 18 weeks of age as well as adults (Rodman, 1994; Rodman & Consuelos, 1994; Rodman & Nace, 1997). Mapping out the ensuing patterns of retrograde labeling revealed that anterior IT receives input from essentially the same set of ipsilateral ventral visual areas as does IT in the adult monkey. No "exuberant" connectivity was found with visual areas (such as V2) that do not provide input to anterior IT in adults. Notably, in contrast to the more posterior retinotopic area TEO (and some of the extrastriate areas of cats), area IT does *not* receive transient inputs directly from the lateral geniculate nucleus early in life, although, as in adults, it is heavily innervated by afferents from the pulvinar (Sorenson & Rodman, 1996).

Thus, the main patterns of inputs providing purely visual drive to IT are in place at an early age and do not appear to include transient connections from regions that do not contribute in adulthood. Moreover, other connections from primarily visual regions of the temporal lobes, notably parahippocampal cortex, the temporal pole, and the superior temporal polysensory area, also appear adultlike early in life. A different conclusion emerges, however, when one considers sources of inputs from "high-order" areas that are not primarily visual in function, connections from the contralateral hemisphere, feedback connections from the frontal lobe, and outputs from IT.

Insular cortex. Our injections revealed a substantial number of labeled cells within the cortex of the ipsilateral insula in seven of eight of the infant cases but in none of the four adults tested. Typically, a dense patch of label was found in the so-called granular insula, with a smaller number of cells scattered more ventrally in the dysgranular region. The insula is a site of converging projections from multiple sensory systems (Mesulam & Mufson, 1982); in our own recordings (driving electrodes through this region to reach IT from a vertical approach), both visual and somatosensory responses were frequently encountered in this portion of the insula in both infant and adult monkeys. Thus, enhanced inputs from the insula may allow IT of the infant a privileged source of information about sensory processing in other modalities, in addition to the strong inputs from the more dominantly visual area STP and the temporal pole that are also seen in adults.

Contralateral and frontal inputs. Connections with the opposite hemisphere and with frontal cortex generally were more widespread in infants than in adults and most so in the youngest monkeys. Figure 3.2 illustrates, in a "flat-map" format, the overall patterns of retrogradely labeled cells in the frontal lobes of each hemisphere in a 2-week-old monkey injected with the retrograde tracer CTB. Many of the specific frontal cortex architectonic zones that gave rise to IT projections (namely, areas 11, 12, 13, 45, and lateral 46) were the same in infant and adult monkeys. However, in infants 7 weeks or younger, but not older infants or adults, labeling was found *bilaterally* in these regions. Inputs from frontal cortex to IT in the youngest infants also originated in a more extensive zone of frontal cortex than in older animals, involving a substantial portion of the lower bank of the principal sulcus and a portion of area 10. Notably, this extended zone also included regions primarily associated with motor function, namely, the frontal eye fields (area 8) and ventral premotor cortex (area 6). In addition, a variable and often bilateral projection back to IT from the anterior cingulate cortex (area 24) was seen in the infants but not in the adults. Finally, the laminar organization of projections from the contralateral temporal lobe differed in infants and adults, with a component from deep layers of cortex only in the infants (Rodman & Consuelos, 1994). These patterns suggest that infant IT also has preferential access, relative to adults, to signals originating in the opposite hemisphere and frontal lobes. Additional implications of early "exuberant" connectivity are discussed later.

Subcortical connections and outputs from IT. In addition to more widespread inputs from anterior and contralateral cortical regions, infant IT also provides more widespread outputs to perirhinal and parahippocampal cortices, which feed into the medial temporal lobe memory system (Rodman & Consuelos, 1994; Webster, Ungerleider, & Bachevalier, 1991a). Expanded projection territories in the superior colliculus, thalamus, and caudate nucleus are also found in infants relative to adults (Webster, Ungerleider, & Bachevalier, 1995), suggesting, perhaps, a less precise relationship to the inherent topography of these areas.

Myelination

In primates, it has long been recognized that cortical "association" or "higher-order" areas myelinate only very slowly (Flechsig, 1901; Yakovlev & LeCours, 1967), with some frontal regions remaining very myelin sparse even in adulthood (Preuss & Goldman-Rakic, 1991). Although the postnatal deposition of myelin on axons does not constitute a simple metric of circuit formation or synaptic viability (Goldman-Rakic, Bourgeois, & Rakic, 1997), a number of workers have noted or proposed a correlation between myelination and the appearance of function (e.g., Konner, 1991; Paus et al., 1999; Van der Knaap et al., 1991). Moreover, it has been

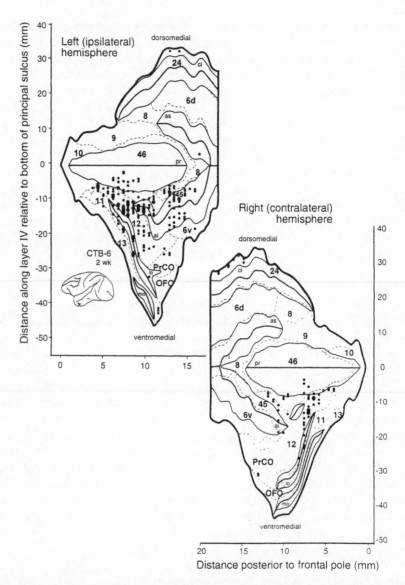

Figure 3.2. Pattern of cell labeling in frontal lobe after injections of CTB tracer into the inferior temporal cortex in a 2-week-old macaque monkey, illustrated on "flat map" reconstructions (Barbas, 1988) in which the dorsomedial portion of the cortex adjacent to the corpus callosum is at the top and the most ventral cortex at the base of the frontal lobe is shown at the bottom. Note labeling in ventral premotor cortex (area 6v) and frontal eye fields (area 8) ipsilaterally as well as extensive contralateral label. Abbreviations: ai = inferior arcuate sulcus; as = superior aracuate sulcus; ci = cingulate sulcus; lo = lateral orbital sulcus; mo = medial orbital sulcus; pr = principal sulcus; OFO and PrCO = architectonically defined transitional limbic areas. Adapted from Rodman and Nace (1997).

proposed that postnatal myelination is associated with chemical signals that contribute to the *termination* of critical period plasticity in visual cortex (Schoop, Gardziella, & Muller, 1997; also Daw, this volume), possibly by inhibiting the continued growth of neurites (Caroni & Schwab, 1988). Thus, although an adult pattern of cortical myelination may not be a unique or reliable index of mature function, its absence may be an important hint as to the prolongation or late emergence of some types of plasticity. Likewise, laminar patterns of postnatal myelin deposition may provide a useful guide as to the relative maturation of intracortical pathways and layers. Accordingly, we have set out to study the ontogeny of specific features of the intracortical myelination pattern in several extrastriate areas of the macaque (K. Carpenter & H. Rodman, unpublished data).

In adult monkeys, myelinated fibers in extrastriate areas are found within all cortical layers and are concentrated in several horizontal fiber plexi that are differentially distinct from area to area (e.g., Gattass, Sousa, & Gross, 1988; Lewis & Van Essen, 2000). In infants, however, myelinated fibers first appear at varying times after birth in the deepest layers and only gradually infiltrate the more superficial layers. Figure 3.3 compares the extension of myelinated fibers through the cortical layers for macaques of varying ages for the middle temporal area (MT) and anterior infant temporal cortex (ITa). Notably, there is virtually no detectable intracortical myelination in ITa at ages less than 6 weeks, when myelinated fibers have already begun to appear in the bottom cortical layers in MT. From 6 to 13 weeks, myelination in ITa lags behind that in MT. By 21 weeks (if not before), however, myelin extension in ITa has caught up to that in MT; extension in both areas then appears to plateau at 50 to 60% for several months until, sometime between 30 and 60 weeks, it reaches full (adult) extension in both areas, with sparse fibers reaching all the way to the pial surface. Thus, the myelin data for IT indicate a slow emergence of intracortical fibers relative to MT, a "catching-up" process between about 13 and 21 weeks (3 to 5 months), and an eventual rise to adult levels in the second half of the first year.

Studies of the Development of Neuronal Coding Properties in Extrastriate Cortex

Inferior Temporal Areas

Studies of the response properties of single neurons in the developing brain can provide not only a confirmation of whether the area in question is active and responsive to inputs from the environment but also an assessment of the degree to which the area has become "committed" to specific analyses, the strength of the signals produced, and details of coding

Neurobiology of Infant Vision

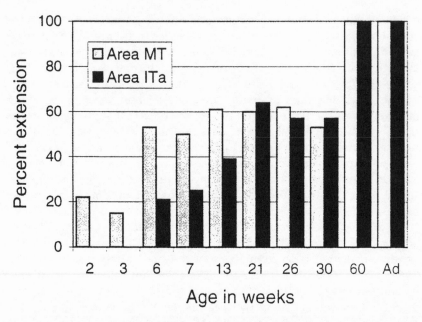

Age in weeks

Figure 3.3. Comparison of myelination in the anterior inferior temporal cortex (ITa) and the middle temporal area (MT) of developing macaque monkeys. Extension score represents the percent of the cortical traverse through which myelinated fibers were detectable at successive ages. Adult values (Ad) of 100% reflect the extension of myelinated profiles all the way to the pial surface (although they are sparse in the upper portion of the superficial layers). Measurements are derived from a total of 14 cases (two each for 6, 7, 13 weeks, and adult; one apiece at the other ages shown). K. Carpenter and H. Rodman (unpublished data).

properties that may or may not differ in important ways from the neural coding achieved by the same tissue in adulthood. However, there has been little empirical study of the physiological development of *any* primate cortex other than V1 at the single-neuron level, perhaps surprising in view of the strong current interest in infant perception and the controversial nature of "innateness" itself (Elman et al., 1996). Although critical immaturities (Brown, 1990) at earlier stations in the visual pathway determine the nature of the inputs received by anterior temporal visual areas, our strategy has been to study signals in anterior temporal areas including IT because, as described in the introduction, it is here that invariant object properties underlying the recognition process are extracted.

Basic single-unit properties. For practical reasons, our initial investigations of developing ventral temporal cortex (areas IT and STP [superior temporal polysensory area]) were made in anesthetized, immobilized infant macaque monkeys. Below about 4 months of age, it was virtually impossible to elicit responses, and spontaneously recorded action potentials were small and difficult to isolate. There was, however, a fairly abrupt emergence of responsiveness around 4 months; between 4 and 7 months, about half of neurons encountered were visually responsive, still significantly lower than that found in comparable adult subjects (Rodman, Skelly, & Gross, 1991). Surprised to find so little activity, we went on to test cells in awake infant monkeys trained to perform brief visual fixation. In these animals, the incidence of IT responsiveness (about 75% of cells) was no different than in adult monkeys—even for infants below 4 months! However, the strength of response (in spikes/second above baseline firing rate) was significantly lower in infant monkeys than in control adults viewing the same stimuli, and neural responses had longer, more variable latencies (Rodman, Ó Scalaidhe, & Gross, 1993). Response magnitude and mean latency of visual response were not correlated with age in days at time of recording for individual cells; this lack was possibly due to the small size of the overall sample and the fact that most of the data collected fell within the age window of 1.5 to 3.5 months.

An intentional focus on "high-level coding" notwithstanding, differences in responsiveness between adults and infants might be confounded by differences in sensitivity of the adult and infant visual systems to specific parameters such as size and contrast of the stimuli—that is, immaturities passed on from earlier levels of the visual pathway. Although we informally varied many of these parameters without obvious striking changes in response levels, we did not rule out the possibility that the infant neurons were more weakly sensitive to some components of the stimuli than others, relative to cells in adults. Taken as a whole, however, the results indicate that additional developmental changes in visual responsiveness take place in temporal cortex (IT and STP) even after 7 months of age in monkeys and leave open the question of the time course of changes prior to that point in the alert animal as well as the factors driving those changes on both stimulus and mechanistic levels.

Stimulus selectivity as measured by firing rate. Using mean firing rate as the response measure, our studies revealed the same general types of stimulus selectivity as seen in an adult control sample and previously documented in the literature (Figure 3.4). In alert monkeys, we found robust stimulus selectivity in IT even at the youngest ages tested (5 weeks). For example, cells in the infant sample were often tuned for the boundary curvature of closed shapes, as they are in adults (Schwartz et al., 1983). To compare the overall degree of selectivity in infant and adult monkeys, we performed a repeated-measures analysis of variance on response magnitudes for each cell across the different stimuli in the standard projected sets; the resulting distribution of F-ratios did not differ statistically between adult and infant samples. For both sets, the values were themselves highly significant.

As in adult temporal cortex, we found neurons selective for faces and

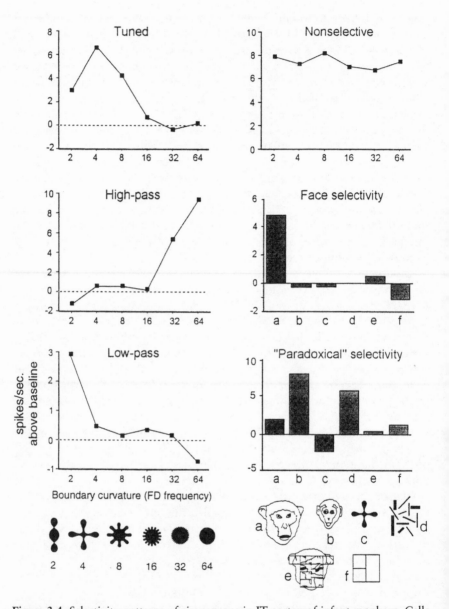

Figure 3.4. Selectivity patterns of six neurons in IT cortex of infant monkeys. Cells whose data are represented as line graphs were tested for sensitivity to boundary curvature (Fourier descriptor [FD] frequency, equivalent to number of lobes, stimuli shown at bottom left). As in adult macaques, we found examples of neurons that were tuned for FD frequency, behaved in high- or low-pass fashion, or did not show selectivity within the set of FDs tested. Other neurons (bar graphs) showing patterns of selectivity within the standard set of stimuli are shown at bottom right. See text for discussion of face selectivity and paradoxical selectivity.

aspects of face stimuli in infant monkeys under both awake and anesthetized conditions. We have documented these findings extensively elsewhere (Rodman, 1994; Rodman & Nace, 1997, Rodman, Ó Scalaidhe, & Gross, 1993), but a few points bear repeating here. The majority were found within IT proper, but a few were located within the upper bank of the floor of the STS, within STP, often together in pairs or small clumps, just as in adults. Although most responded to a variety of faces, and not to scrambles, a subset responded only to particular normal (unscrambled) faces within the sets tested. This behavior suggests that the response was not only based on some overall facial configuration but was at least influenced by other factors differentiating the "preferred" face from the others, such as the age or expression of the monkey depicted or specific structural features of the faces. For some, scrambled versions of a face elicited significant responses; a few did not respond to the scrambled version of the preferred face but could be activated by the eye region in isolation. These observations also indicate that components of the face (individual features) made a contribution to the response of at least some infant "face neurons." A few neurons showed sensitivity to one specific view of preferred stimulus faces, typically responding only to profiles. Moreover, although these cells appeared sensitive to viewing angle per se, they showed very similar responsiveness to the profile regardless of whether it faced left or right. Thus, these cells' response was probably not dependent upon the precise position of critical elements within the visual world.

Finally, as for neurons in adults, IT cells in infants sometimes exhibited *paradoxical selectivity* (Gross et al., 1993; see also Figure 3.4), in which strong responses are seen to a few stimuli that do not obviously share more common features than do the other stimuli tested. Overall, the large majority of visually responsive cells in infant temporal cortex have differential patterns of responding, which could contribute to ensemble coding of stimuli and which share some of the idiosyncrasies of adult coding patterns.

Temporal coding properties. Although visual neuroscience continues to use rate of firing as the most common measure of neural coding, it has become increasingly acknowledged that details of the temporal structure of responses also convey critical information and may in fact be the primary way that some cortical neurons encrypt their messages (reviewed in deCharms & Zador, 2000; Gawne, 1999). Thus, it is of interest that in adult IT many neurons show consistently different temporal response envelopes to different stimuli within a set (Richmond et al., 1987). Even though the responses we obtained in infants were rather weak overall, we found evidence for similar phenomena in infant IT (Figure 3.5). For example, latency to response often differed significantly for different stimuli; in some cases, excitation to one or more stimuli and inhibition to others, or mixed excitation/inhibition, were shown by single neurons. Whether these patterns are an integral part of the neural code used by IT neurons to enable rudi-

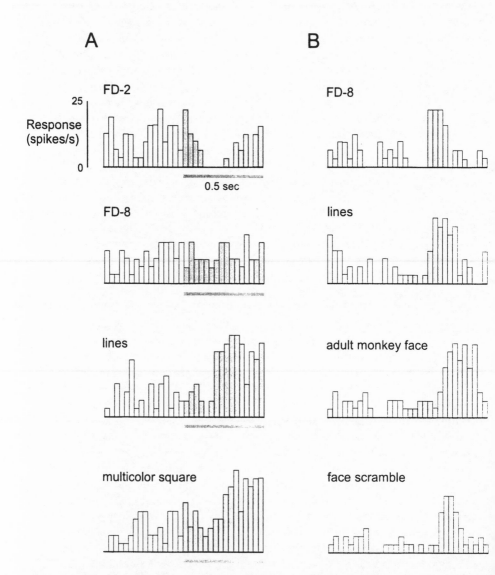

Figure 3.5. Post-stimulus-time histograms illustrating temporal patterns of responsiveness of two neurons in awake infant IT cortex to different stimuli. The line under the shaded portion of the histogram indicates the period during which the stimulus was presented, just after the animal attained fixation. Fourier descriptors (FDs) are illustrated in Figure 3.4. (**A**) Short-latency inhibitory response to FD-2, no net response to FD-8, and longer-latency excitatory responses to randomly oriented lines and a multicolored square. (**B**) Excitatory responses to different stimuli that differ in latency and/or duration.

mentary object recognition is not yet clear, but it is noteworthy that these differences in representation of different stimuli by IT neurons are available to potentially contribute to the encoding of stimulus identity within the first months of life.

Other Cortical Visual Areas

We also made a limited number of recordings in striate cortex and area MT in anesthetized animals (at 8 to 11 weeks of age) in the course of asking whether apparent suppression of responsiveness in IT under these conditions is area specific. Although we did not gather enough data to make quantitative statements about the tuning properties, response magnitudes, and other features of V1 and MT neurons in infants relative to adults, cardinal properties characteristic of adult neurons were present in our sample. Notably, cells in MT were predominantly direction-selective, as in adults, and tuning curves generated on the basis of computer-controlled stimulus presentation show selectivity roughly comparable to that of MT neurons in adults (Figure 3.6). Neurons in V1 were typically orientation tuned with small, discrete receptive fields.

Other Indices of Physiological Development of "Ventral Stream" Neocortex

ERP Studies Relevant to Object Recognition in Developing Humans

Although single-unit recording in infant monkeys presents a number of practical difficulties, it permits one to study the coding properties of individual neurons (or neuron clusters) within specific, localized cortical areas. In human infants, visual event-related potential (ERP) studies have contributed data complementary to those obtained in monkeys, with greater ease of acquisition (at least in some respects); however, ERP studies are characterized by poor (albeit improving) spatial resolution. For example (laying aside issues of localization), studies in 6-month-olds have shown differential electrophysiological signatures for the processing of faces and other objects as well as an effect of stimulus familiarity (de Haan & Nelson, 1999; also de Haan, this volume), observations that parallel the finding of distinct face-related unit responses in infant monkeys. ERP studies have also provided intriguing suggestions of differences between processing of the emotional content of faces in later development (5 to 7 years) and in adulthood (Kestenbaum & Nelson, 1992) and have significant implications for models of the development of face and object recognition and understanding the longtime course of emergence of some of the functions of temporal cortical visual streams.

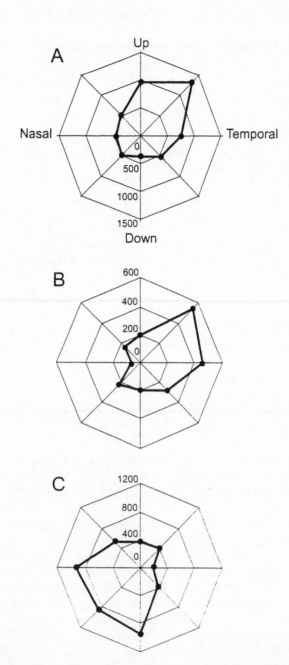

Figure 3.6. Polar tuning curves of three neurons in cortical visual area MT of infant monkeys, recorded under anesthesia. Numbers along the radius indicate response magnitude in percent of baseline spike rate. Maximal evoked firing rate: (**A**) 11.3 spikes/second; (**B**) 11.6 spikes/second; (**C**) 4.6 spikes/second. All three neurons had receptive fields within the central 10 degrees of the hemifield opposite the recording electrode.

Metabolic and Neurochemical Indices of Structural and Functional Maturation

In macaques, studies of energy utilization point to significant changes in the 2- to 6-month postnatal window (Jacobs et al., 1995), with ventral stream regions maturing slightly more slowly than dorsal visual areas associated with spatial functions (Distler et al., 1996). In a 2-deoxyglucose study, developing IT cortex showed activity levels that lagged behind those of posterior areas V2 and V4, which in turn lagged behind V1 (Bachevalier, Hagger, & Mishkin, 1991). For both humans and monkeys, the time course of postnatal metabolic changes has been suggested to correlate with changes in rates and stages of synaptogenesis and to reflect a critical confluence of developmental changes at about 4 months in monkeys and 1 year in humans. However, more recent positron emission tomography (PET) data in both humans (Chugani, 1998) and macaques (Moore et al., 1999) show that additional maturation of metabolic activity levels takes place in a variety of brain areas following a very protracted time course, with asymptotes in the late teenage years in humans.

Although there is a large literature on the development of expression of specific neurotransmitters, receptors, regulatory proteins, and other substances in primate cerebral cortex, relatively little of the relevant work has focused on visual areas outside V1 or the V1/V2 border. One general finding of significance is the concurrent overproduction of a variety of neurotransmitter receptors across the cortical mantle, in synchrony with overproduction of synaptic contacts, in the first 2 to 4 months postnatal (Lidow, Goldman-Rakic, & Rakic, 1991). Where studies have contrasted staining patterns, transmitter levels, or receptor binding in striate and cortex and other neocortical regions, a typical finding has been the relatively early emergence of an adultlike pattern in V1 and more diffuse labeling in association cortex, including extrastriate visual cortex, in the early postnatal period (reviewed in Rodman & Moore, 1997).

In at least one case, however, the picture differs (Berger et al., 1990). For the phosphoprotein DARPP-32, a substance associated with cells bearing D1 dopamine receptors, the widespread distribution seen in newborn or 6-week-old macaques is replaced by a much more restricted distribution in adults. Interestingly, while V1, V2, and parietal cortex retained few DARPP-reactive cells in adulthood, the anterior inferior temporal cortex, posterior orbitofrontal cortex, entorhinal cortex, and cingulate cortex— namely, the areas implicated in our own work or sources of feedback projections to them—retained the heavy staining seen in infancy.

In a more recent study, Oishi et al. (1998) measured the amount of messenger RNA (mRNA) for GAP-43, a growth-associated protein whose concentrations parallel the process of axonal elongation, in cortex of macaques at various pre- and postnatal stages. In all cortical areas examined (including V1, V2, posterior IT, and parietal cortex), GAP-43 mRNA concentrations were highest prenatally and asymptoted at adult levels by 2½ months postnatal. Both in infants and adults, levels were higher in so-called association areas, including IT, than in V1 or other primary or "low-order" regions. These data add to the evidence for a critical nexus of processes of structural development at 2 to 4 months postnatal in macaque temporal cortex. Overall, however, more work is needed to specify the time course of the expression of substances related to identified neuromodulatory systems and the formation of connections in relation to specific extrastriate areas at a larger set of critical points, or ranges, in early and later development.

WHAT BEHAVIOR TELLS US

Object recognition is a complex function, subsuming processing of stimulus features and extracting invariants, generating and storing representations of objects and features, and retrieving these representations in a myriad of contexts and often on the basis of partial information. As such, the problem of object recognition is both separately and jointly informed by considerations from the domains of elementary form processing, concept formation, and memory, each of which is well represented in the human developmental literature. In addition, the study of behavior and perception in young organisms is subject to the performance constraints imposed by motor immaturity. It is beyond the scope of the present account to specify all of the important insights deriving from these areas that have, in one form or another, influenced the present model. Instead, I aim to highlight those aspects for which at least rudimentary data exist for both human and nonhuman primates. Since much of our knowledge of detailed neural substrates derives from animal data, it is intended that this emphasis will maximally serve the goal of describing a framework informed by human cognition yet structured by known biology.

Featural Coding and Rudimentary Object Recognition

Zuckerman and Rock (1957) suggested that infants enter the world with some degree of innate visual knowledge as a product of adaptive evolution; Fantz (e.g., 1963) echoed these views and showed that human infants are born with some degree of pattern vision. Infant monkeys show simple form discrimination and a visual preference for novel patterns within the first month after birth (Bachevalier, 1990; Gunderson & Sackett, 1984; Zimmerman, 1961). However, they also show gradual changes in the types of stimuli preferred (Sackett, 1966).

The overall picture of the ontogeny of object recognition appears to depend on the strategies used to assess it in addition to the nature of the response required of the organism. In an admirable example of a comparative approach, Overman and Bachevalier and their associates showed that simple object learning capacity (concurrent discrimination task) appears early in ontogeny in both human (12 to 32 months) and rhesus monkey (3 months) (Bachevalier & Mishkin, 1984; Overman et al., 1992). Further, this capacity shows an early sex difference in both species (Overman et al., 1996). However, a more cognitively taxing delayed-nonmatch-to-sample (DNMS) object recognition task was not possible until much later in ontogeny in both. On the other hand, when a more primitive response measure (preferential looking) is used to assess recognition of visual objects, evidence of visual recognition can be obtained in the first weeks of life in both humans (Pascalis & de Schonen, 1994) and monkeys (Bachevalier, 1990; Gunderson & Sackett, 1984). Thus, visual recognition abilities appear present in rudimentary form early in life in primates and then take a very long time to mature completely (Carey, 1992; M. Johnson, 1994), with the outcome of testing highly dependent on the precise nature of the behavioral instrument used to elicit and measure capacity.

Complex Object Perception and Recognition

One aspect of complex object processing that has received a great deal of attention is the perception and recognition of faces (Rodman, 1999; also de Haan, this volume). Adult primates—both humans and monkeys—are highly skilled at recognizing and differentiating novel and familiar faces (Farah et al., 1998; Perrett & Mistlin, 1990) and show stereotyped patterns of eye movements when viewing faces (Nahm et al., 1997; Yarbus, 1967). Early studies indicated a lag between birth in humans and the appearance of face discrimination capacity; for example, Maurer and Barrera (1981) showed that while 1-month-olds looked equally at normal and scrambled schematic faces, 2-month-olds looked significantly longer at the normal schematic face configuration (see also M. Johnson, 1994). Other early studies (e.g., Haaf, Smith, & Smitty, 1983) did not find evidence for such a preference until about 4 months. On the other hand, when dynamic stimuli were used, evidence for selective attention to facial configurations was reported even in newborns, who track such stimuli with eye and head movements (Goren, Sarty, & Wu, 1975; Maurer & Young, 1983). Changes in face processing appear to persist well beyond infancy. Such changes include increased sensitivity to configurational information (as evidenced by the gradual emergence of the "inversion effect," the tendency for face processing to be disproportionately impaired by stimulus inversion), the emergence of hemispheric specialization for face processing, and an apparent dip in sensitivity in early adolescence (reviewed in Carey, 1992; Chung & Thomson, 1995).

Less is known about the ontogeny of face processing in nonhuman primates, but there is evidence for early sensitivity, as well as developmental changes. Much as very young human infants appear to be preferentially sensitive to face shapes, infant monkeys respond socially to pictures of monkeys (e.g., Mendelson, 1982) and show a preference for the normal configuration of facial features (Lutz et al.,1998) in the first weeks. By 3 to 7 weeks, they show sensitivity to the angle of gaze displayed in stimulus faces, which provides important social information (Mendelson, Haith, & Goldman-Rakic, 1982).

TOWARD A BIOLOGICALLY PLAUSIBLE FRAMEWORK FOR THE DEVELOPMENT OF OBJECT RECOGNITION

Theoretical Advances

Overall, there has been a relative paucity of theory within the domain of infant object recognition that has included neurobiological grounding as a primary goal or constraint. However, there are some notable exceptions. Atkinson (1984, 1992), building on and advancing the ideas of Bronson (1974), suggested that the differential functioning of subsystems within the visual pathways more generally could be used to explain some features of visual development in humans. In so doing, Atkinson called attention specifically to two processes (development of selectively tuned populations of neurons for different visual features and development of eye movement control mechanisms) and two pathways (the so-called parvocellular and magnocellular systems that originate in retinogeniculocortical projections). In the 1990s, M. Johnson and colleagues (1990, 1994; Johnson & Vecera, 1993; Morton & Johnson, 1991) advanced a similarly "maturational" framework, further incorporating the idea of the sequential maturation of brain pathways beyond the first cortical stage (V1) to explain specific developmental changes in visual orienting, visual attention, and complex object perception (face recognition) over the first half-year to year of life. More recently, influenced by ideas on the epigenetic nature of development (e.g., Gottlieb, 1992) and data on infant frontal lobe function, M. Johnson (2000) modified the framework to focus on the gradual postnatal specialization of multiple pathways in parallel and the implications for immature behavioral action. These approaches provide both a starting point and an inspiration for the model described below.

A Proposed Framework for the Development of Object Recognition

Based on the data reviewed above, I have sought to construct a theoretical framework for understanding and generating predictions about the development of brain mechanisms of object recognition in primates. The framework is specifically concerned with the development of those aspects of visual object recognition for which the adult primate brain has specialized circuits in which neurons have selectivity for high-level features and are physically localized into clumps, columns, or regions, or what we have termed *relatively dedicated circuitry*. Face recognition is one example of a domain that is subserved by this type of circuitry (Desimone, 1991; Rodman, 1999); the recognition of alphanumeric characters (Allison et al., 1994); highly trained novel objects (Logothetis, Pauls, & Poggio, 1995); and familiar classes with which expertise is achieved at the subordinate level (Gauthier & Tarr, 1997) are others. The term *relatively dedicated* refers to the notion that within these processing units the majority of neurons, while engaging in ensemble coding of individual objects, do not participate in coding as wide a variety of types of patterns as do other cells in surrounding tissue but are involved primarily in analyzing one class of objects.

As for the accounts mentioned above, this framework is a maturational one, in the sense that it posits that maturation of circuits within identified cortical areas, sets of areas, or pathways enables the appearance of functional change. In other words, it seeks to specify intrinsic processes and phenomena during normal development that occur in an experience-independent or experience-expectant fashion to lay a species-typical foundation for eventual mature functioning. In particular, it concurs with the notion of *partial functioning* of substrate espoused by M. Johnson (2000) and further seeks to begin hypothesizing and identifying mechanisms that change the nature and degree of functioning as the individual develops.

The Nature of Relatively Dedicated Circuitry

The nature of relatively dedicated circuitry is best defined by the processes by which we propose that it arises. In this view, relatively dedicated representation of a class of stimuli is dependent on extensive examination of the stimuli in a spatially directed format (e.g., by eye movements and/ or manual examination) that provides feedback to stabilize functional interactions between ensembles of neurons in "high-order" sensory regions and their inputs and outputs. Moreover, this spatially formatted interaction is proposed to be extensive enough to produce relatively dedicated representation of object classes *only* for those classes made up of exemplars that are highly similar and behaviorally significant to the individual. Moreover, we believe that while the domains for which animals develop relatively dedicated circuitry are highly experience dependent and differ from individual to individual, strong commonalities are shown both within and across species (e.g., faces in primates and some other groups) to the extent that common niches and experiences are involved.

Genesis of Relatively Dedicated Circuitry during Development

A major challenge is to specify how relatively dedicated circuitry arises in development. I propose the following two critical components. First, the model specifies an early "bootstrapping"[3] operation, corresponding to mechanisms that are very important to the early postnatal development and stabilization of circuitry early but that become progressively less important (or are perhaps even overwritten) in time. Second, I suggest that there is only a very gradual emergence of true adultlike plasticity at both behavioral and neural levels as the organism learns about new behaviorally significant *categories* of objects and regularities in its own environment and applies that knowledge to new instances. In other words, I propose that the infant primate brain, on the one hand, makes use of strategies that are less available or important later in life and, on the other, shows less overall efficiency of learning. Specific mechanisms are proposed below.

An "Innate" Advantage for Some Classes of Objects?

Data discussed in "Complex Object Perception and Recognition" have been interpreted to mean that primates have special sensitivity to face stimuli or facelike configurations at or close to birth. Numerous authors (e.g., Morton & Johnson, 1991) have postulated an inborn predisposition to attend to face stimuli that functions to provide stimulation to cortical mechanisms, which in turn would gradually allow the subject to learn specific faces. Whether such a predisposition is based on a prototype directing the infant to look at facelike configurations or a matching between the spatial distribution of stimulus energy present in faces and the infant's visual psychophysics (Kleiner, 1993; see also de Haan, this volume) remains unresolved. In either case, an assumption of the framework is that in toto the visual system of the newborn primate does include a functional bias toward visual examination of facelike stimuli.

Mechanisms

Components of the Bootstrapping Operation

First, it is suggested that the *temporal lobe including neocortex* does itself contribute to the directing of attention by providing rudimentary information about object properties from birth on. More specifically, cortical neurons even in "higher" areas should be operational and show stimulus selectivity even in neonatal monkeys. Thus, an important component of the current framework is that part of the bootstrapping operation consists of an inherent, if weak, responsivity on the part of neurons in the cortical tissue that eventually performs the full analysis of complex objects (such as rudimentary selectivity for face stimuli) for a subset of neurons.

Second, I propose that *motor feedback* (especially from scanning eye movements) as an animal interacts with a stimulus should be especially effective in development as a signal for "stamping in" activation patterns within areas involved in representing the stimulus and in enabling association of the separate parts of an object seen on sequential fixations. As a subject views salient features of an object, the fovea falls in rapid succession on components that will later be treated as a perceptual whole. Even considering that metrics of saccadic eye movements are immature early in infancy (Lucchetti & Cevolani, 1992), and that significant improvements in scanning efficency take place in the early postnatal period (Johnson & Johnson, 2001), infant monkeys and humans alike show reproducible patterns of visual exploration of stimuli with eye movements. Motor feedback signaling a series of sequential fixations within the central visual field could thus be a powerful, if primitive, cue that features comprising a coherent whole are present there. In fact, the notion of a close linkage of pattern and face recognition with the use of specific scanpaths is not a new one (e.g., Noton & Stark, 1971; Rizzo, Hurtig, & Damasio, 1987; Yarbus, 1967).

Third, it is proposed that *relative motion of an object and its background* should be an especially reliable cue for delimiting objects early in life and that the developing object recognition system should be more sensitive to this cue than later in life. Knowing where one object begins and another ends is critical in the process of building representations of object identity. The relative motion of an object and its background provides a powerful cue for the segmentation of an image into objects. Humans are sensitive to this cue early in life (Spitz, Stiles, & Siegel 1993; Wattam-Bell, 1996); in fact, common motion plays a privileged role in perception of object unity by infants, relative to other synchronous changes (Jusczyk et al., 1999). By 2 to 3 months, human infants can use kinetic visual information to perceive contours and object boundaries (Arterberry & Yonas, 2000; Bertenthal, Proffitt, & Kramer, 1987; Johnson & Mason, 2002) and later "identify" them by differential viewing in a habituation paradigm when static (Kaufmann, 1995). In other studies, human infants show sensitivity to more complex types of relative motion, including biological motion and the perception of surfaces in depth, when tested at 3 to 4 months (e.g., Fox & McDaniel, 1982; Johnson & Aslin, 1998). In adult primates, relative motion is explicitly encoded by cells of the dorsal visual stream areas (Allman, Miezin, & McGuinness, 1985). I propose that this information is also explicitly coded by these areas in infants and furthermore made available to temporal cortical areas as a source of confirming information about object boundaries.

Finally, the framework suggests that pure *temporal contiguity of stimuli* is likewise a cue that the object recognition system makes special use of early in life for formation of associations between components of a stimulus that make up an object. Stimulus features that are foveated in rapid succession, in combination with saccadic eye movements of small to medium size (and perhaps lack of head and neck movements), have an enhanced likelihood of being parts of the same object. Thus, a mechanism for association and subsequent development of conjoint selectivity dependent on temporal contiguity alone (Stryker, 1991) is proposed to be an important component of the process by which inferior temporal circuits that parse the visual world arise in the absence of extensive contextual or "top-down" influences instructing the animal what the viewed object is.

Developmentally Delayed Plasticity

However, while stimulus features viewed in close physical and temporal proximity are likely to be parts of the same object (especially if they move in concert), this is not a guarantee. Aside from the proposals for the nature of relatively dedicated circuitry and the components of the bootstrapping operation, a major novel feature of this model is that some types of learning-related alterations in the temporal neocortex should be minimal or absent, or more dependent on repeated visual experience, early in life. Interestingly, lesion-behavior studies in monkeys indicate that IT cortex does not actually "commit" to its obligatory contribution to object recognition until sometime after infancy. Some sparing of form and object discrimination and recognition capacity is obtained when damage to this tissue takes place as late as a year of age (Bachevalier, 1990; Raisler & Harlow, 1965). This sparing recalls that seen after early lesions to dorsolateral frontal cortex (Goldman, 1971), except that substantial ability is still seen even when the monkeys are tested years after early inferior temporal cortex damage (Malkova, Mishkin, & Bachevalier, 1995). Sparing or reassignment of function after an early lesion implies that other brain regions are capable of taking over for the excised circuits and suggests that the mechanisms permitting function may not yet have been fully established in the region removed, although the sparing may also reflect a critical period for compensation by other tissue. While recovery after early lesions is not a focus of this framework, it does propose that delayed commitment of IT to object recognition is at least an important basis of the sparing seen after early damage.

In adult monkeys, temporal cortex neurons show a variety of types of plasticity that have been proposed as neural correlates of object learning (reviewed in Erickson, Jagadeesh, & Desimone, 2000; Rodman & Nace, 1997) and include rapid and relatively passive changes in responsiveness and selectivity as well as more complex types of learning. Such stimulus-specific adaptation may function to improve processing of novel images by reducing interference from activity elicited from familiar ones, as Ringo (1996) and others have suggested, and these simpler forms of plasticity may be amenable to study even in very young subjects. Without the benefit of category knowledge, rapid shifts of responsiveness or formation of associations between stimuli that underlie plasticity may actually be counterproductive. I propose that rapid reconfiguration of response properties is developmentally delayed, producing less efficient plasticity in some cases, and constitutes a neural correlate of the delayed contribution of this region to object recognition. Furthermore, I suggest that the developmental delay in plasticity is achieved by a slow maturation of expression of receptor mechanisms and neurochemical substrates controlling rapid shifts in neuronal excitability.

IMPLICATIONS OF SPECIFIC ANATOMICAL AND PHYSIOLOGICAL MECHANISMS FOR THE MODEL

The Question of Early Cortical Contributions

Several authors have argued that in humans, circuits directing visual attention to significant objects are primarily or exclusively subcortical in the first several months and only come to include a significant cortical component by 2 to 4 months of age (e.g., Atkinson, 1984; Dubowitz et al., 1986; M. Johnson, 1990). This contention is supported by a variety of data indicating significant changes in a variety of indices at this stage (see also "Relation to Milestones in Development"). Other authors (e.g., Slater, Morison, & Somers, 1988) have argued for a significant measure of visual cortical function at birth, albeit supplemented by subcortical orienting mechanisms.

"Low-Order" Cortical Areas

The question of early cortical contributions to visual function in humans has drawn heavily on behavioral and electrophysiological evidence for orientation discrimination. To the extent that segmentation of an object on the basis of oriented contours is a feature of the object recognition process, early cortical processing of orientation in "low-order" visual areas such as V1 and V2 would support the proposal of rudimentary object analysis by cortical circuits early in life. Evidence for orientation processing has been documented in human newborns using a habituation paradigm (Slater, Morison, & Somers, 1988) and by 6 weeks in visual-evoked potential studies (Braddick, Wattam-Bell, & Atkinson, 1986) At the single-unit level, selectivity for orientation is found close to or at birth in macaques (Wiesel & Hubel, 1974). Similarly, studies on the development of binocularity (stereopsis), long considered a critical sign of cortical function, have shown binocular disparity tuning to be present in an adultlike proportion of V1 cells at birth (Chino et al., 1997), even though stereovision appears abruptly only at about 4 weeks of age (O'Dell & Boothe, 1997). However, the overall responsiveness of these neurons was low, paralleling our own infant data in IT, although responses could be evoked under anesthesia close to birth in V1, whereas they could not be in IT even at the age of several months.

Association Cortex

Studies reviewed earlier of both anatomy and physiology of developing inferior temporal cortex lead to two clear conclusions. First, basic properties are present within the first several months of life in the monkey (although we do not yet know what happens earlier). Second, this tissue undergoes a very long period of postnatal maturation in which feedback connections are refined, myelin is deposited on intrinsic axons, metabolic rates increase, and visually triggered firing rates reach adult levels. In contrast, the "lower-order" areas thus far studied (MT and V1) appear more mature at comparable ages in terms of visually driven activity, myelination, and neurochemistry. Frontal areas, on the other hand (and as might be expected), lag behind temporal "association" cortex in terms of these measures.

The studies reviewed above are consistent with both an early rudimentary functioning of both low-order *and* temporal cortex and a long period of development of adultlike capacity and learning-dependent plasticity. The physiological studies indicate that adultlike patterns of response are present by a month or two of age but leave open the question of the neonatal state, the question of whether selectivity early in life depends upon similar stimulus features as in adulthood, and whether rapid shifts in selectivity (plasticity) are developmentally delayed, as hypothesized. The time course of development of adultlike capacity now needs to be specified, along with determining the mechanisms by which the system achieves adult plasticity.

Role of Influences from Outside the Ventral Temporal Cortex in Jump-Starting the Object Recognition Process

Feedback Systems

In numerous species and systems, both refinement and loss or elimination of transient or "exuberant" connections have been shown to take place in development, and both have been invoked as important mechanisms by which remodeling of circuits allows experience to influence function (reviewed in Innocenti, 1982, 1995). One of the postulates of the framework is that motor feedback (as an animal visually "samples" a stimulus) is used heavily in development as a signal for configuring temporal cortex circuitry for object recognition. This hypothesis predicts that feedback pathways, especially from motor systems, should be different early in life and is supported by our earlier finding of greater connectivity with motor, contralateral, and frontal areas in infants. Feedback projections have also been seen as critical for the process of *reentry* (Edelman, 1987), a proposed mechanism by which processing in one area can influence processing in others to bind or correlate features of an object with one another and with context (Tononi, Sporns, & Edelman, 1992). Thus, a more fine-grained analysis of the ontogeny of feedback circuits may provide additional clues for which types of information are used to help configure object recogniton circuitry as the system organizes itself in part from within.

Motion Processing and the Relative Pace of Development of Processing Streams

Another of the proposals of the framework described above is that information about relative motions of contours is a crucially important signal in segmenting the object landscape early in life. Accordingly, an associated prediction is that some of the signals from extrastriate areas analyzing visual motion should become operational prior to those in the ventral stream that become crucial for object recognition. In monkeys, our own neurophysiological findings (discussed above) and the metabolic data (Distler et al., 1996) support a slightly earlier maturation of dorsal versus ventral areas. The relative pace of development of the so-called magnocellular and parvocellular geniculocortical streams, which map only loosely at best onto dorsal and ventral cortical processing, has been a central issue in theoretical reviews of primate visual development. On the basis of rate of development of anatomical inputs and staining properties of subdivisions of V1 and of physiological properties in the lateral geniculate nucleus, we have suggested (Rodman & Moore, 1997) that dorsal stream areas primarily driven by magno inputs attain functional maturity somewhat ahead of ventral stream areas. Similarly, M. Johnson (1990) proposed that a "broadband-MT" pathway for visual orienting becomes functional prior to other cortico-cortical pathways. Furthermore, Dobkins, Anderson, and Lia (1999) have shown differences in human infant luminance and chromatic contrast sensitivity functions that suggest earlier development of magno-dominated pathways. On the other hand, Atkinson (1992) reviewed data indicating that infants show sensitivity to changes of orientation and to color differences before they show differential responses to the direction of movement and disparity changes and concluded that parvocellular-based systems for color and form analysis are functional earlier postnatally than magnocellular-based systems for encoding location, motion, and depth.

Such inconsistency may be resolved by an evolving view in which neural subsystems themselves consist of multiple processing pathways that have different developmental trajectories (Banton & Bertenthal, 1997; M. Johnson, 2000; Teller, 2000). In other words, it may be less appropriate (or useful) to ask about the relative pace of development of dorsal and ventral streams than about the relative pace of development of task-specific capacities and neural circuits thought to underlie them and interact with other such circuits. In the case of motion processing, studies in human infants show sensitivity to translational or rotational motion close to birth (Banton & Bertenthal, 1997); moreover, episodes of visual pursuit reflect target speed at 1 month, interpreted as reflecting a cortical contribution to motion processing (Phillips et al., 1997). Other types of motion sensitivity, including that for various types of relative motion, appear slightly later (see also "Mechanisms"). Although little is known about the development of relative motion processing at either the behavioral or neurophysiological level in infant monkeys, its relatively early appearance in humans is consistent with its incorporation into the framework given here.

PREDICTIONS FOR EXPERIMENTATION

Response Properties

As described above, an important component of the model is that part of the "bootstrapping" operation consists of a weak inherent (i.e., present in the neonatal state) selectivity for complex objects or features in the cortical areas that encode complex object properties in the adult animals. Accordingly, we would expect to find that neurons in areas such as IT and STP are weakly responsive and stimulus selective from birth on and that a subset will be selective for face stimuli, as in older animals. An interesting (but not obligatory) possibility that might derive from the notion of an inherent, evolved "template" for face recognition is that a *larger* proportion will be selective for aspects of face stimuli in the neonatal state than later on.

Another prediction centers on the proposed role of eye movement feedback in bootstrapping the specialized circuitry that will come to subserve responses to faces and other complex, socially relevant objects and scenes. If this feedback is especially crucial early in ontogeny, we might expect to see differences in eye movement modulation of ongoing spike activity in temporal neocortex relative to that seen in adults. Such modulation would presumably be maximal during or following scanning sequences involving moderate-size eye movements within the central visual field (consistent with examining a unitary object). Alternatively, there might be a systematic relationship between onset of individual saccades and response modulation, such that the performance of an eye movement (or fixation) per se gates or plays a permissive role in the firing of the neuron. Such modulation could be especially effective in infancy since infant temporal cortex neurons apparently have a higher threshold for activation (low spontaneous and evoked rates of activity).

Physiological Plasticity

Many of the types of plasticity observed in temporal cortex cells of adult monkeys involve changes in population response patterns over weeks or months, or upon performance of a relatively difficult learned task such as DNMS, and as such are not amenable to study in infant monkeys. However, rapid and relatively passive changes in responsiveness and selectivity have also been reported, such as passive habituation to a repeated stimulus, or shifts in selectivity for stimuli within a repeated set, which may actually represent primitive memory mechanisms (Miller, Li, & Desimone, 1991; Rolls et al., 1989). According to the framework given here, shifts of selectivity should be slower to develop (i.e., take more presentations) and/or be less pronounced in younger subjects. On the other hand, if temporal contiguity is an important cue utilized by the bootstrapping operation, then some associative mechanisms (i.e., emergence of conjoint selectivity for stimuli presented close together in time—such as the average time between fixations of gaze on the different portions of an object) may be equally or even more efficient in the early postnatal period as later on.

Structural and Neurochemical Correlates

The present framework specifically postulates a developmental delay of plasticity in ventral temporal cortex as a result of slow maturation of mechanisms permitting rapid shifts of neuronal excitability. In a variety of systems, activation of the NMDA subtype of glutamate receptor has been proposed or implicated in Hebbian modification resulting from coherent patterns of synaptic activity (e.g., Singer & Artola, 1991; and see Grossberg, this volume). In primary visual cortex, NMDA receptor binding density shows a course that correlates with the time course of the critical period for columnar plasticity (Trepel et al., 1998). One might expect, thus, that a region with delayed developmental plasticity would show a delay in NMDA receptor expression. On the other hand, calcium binding proteins such as calbindin D-28K are proposed to buffer Ca^{++} influx and thus neuronal excitability (Baimbridge, Celio, & Rogers, 1992). Calbindin D-28K in particular is distributed in brain in a fashion complementary to that of cytochrome-rich and highly active patches (Allman & Zucker, 1990). Accordingly, one might expect a relatively mature or even intensified pattern of calbindin immunoreactivity early in life in an area designed to delay plasticity. Interestingly, calbindin immunoreactivity is associated with reduction of some types of plasticity in the hippocampal system, and Ca^{++} buffering more generally is strongly implicated in metaplasticity, the phenomenon whereby recent prior stimulation alters the subsequent susceptibility of connections to modifications such as LTP and LTD (Abraham & Bear, 1996). In addition, because (according to our model) face processing draws on the relatively dedicated circuitry organized by motor feedback, we predict that face "clumps" should be especially rich in feedback inputs from motor and frontal areas in infants.

FURTHER CONSTRAINTS AND CONSIDERATIONS

Relations to Processes at Other Levels of Analysis

As various authors have clearly argued and illustrated, each level of analysis in developmental studies is constrained by the maturity of the inputs to the process or region in question. For reasons detailed in previous sections, the physiology and anatomy of the temporal lobe (in particular the neocortex) have been selected as the level of focus, rather than the level of behavior or earlier visual processing. With regard specifically to temporal lobe contributions, the focus of the framework is to specify developmental changes in response properties, plasticity, and anatomical substrates within temporal lobe areas associated with object recognition. However, in the larger picture, specifying constraints contributing to immature response patterns is an important part of the goal of understanding cortical and cognitive development. For example, in monkeys, both positional discrimination (vernier acuity) and visual resolution (grating acuity) develop over the first year of life, albeit with differences in pace; similar functions obtain for humans in approximately the first 5 years (e.g., Teller et al., 1978, reviewed in Kiorpes & Movshon, 1989; Teller, 2000). Ultimately, the spatial resolving power of the visual system in toto will define whether individual visual features (such as the elements of a pattern) can be separately encoded (and bound together) by the organism at a given stage of postnatal life and must be taken into account in considering how precisely a test stimulus can be represented.

Relation to Milestones in Development

One of the more salient and interesting patterns to emerge from the human data is a confluence of changes that take place or commence within a window between about 2 and 4 months of age. This pattern includes changes in object and pattern perception (S. Johnson, 1996; Morton & Johnson, 1991), scanning of compound forms (Haith, 1986), changes in oculomotor behavior (Gilmore & Johnson, 1997; Johnson & Johnson, 2001; Phillips et al., 1997; also see Gilmore, this volume), and the emergence of active exploration of self-contingent behavior (Rochat, 1998). The specific cues utilized to achieve the perception of the unitary nature of an object also change in this 2- to 4-month window in human infants, corresponding to a marked improvement in ability to extract meaningful information from this stimulus array (reviewed in S. Johnson, 2001).

Although a 1:4 ratio of monkey:human perceptual development has been established for functions such as stereopsis and acuity (Teller, 2000), sufficient data do not yet exist to argue strongly for an overall focus of change at what would be the equivalent monkey age of about 2 to 4 weeks.

Future studies of the development of object recognition in nonhuman primate models will need to be alert to the possibility of particular changes in behavior and perception at about this time, as well as in neural underpinnings. For example, an important early developmental milestone in human form perception is the so-called *externality effect*, the tendency of human infants less than 2 months of age to look at the boundaries or external features of stimuli rather than at internal details, followed by a switch to looking more at internal features starting at about 2 months (Haith, 1986). While shifts in featural scanning do occur in infant monkeys between 1 and 3 weeks of age, they follow a different topography, producing more, rather than fewer, fixations of the external contour with increasing age within this window (Mendelson, Haith, & Goldman-Rakic, 1983).

The Role of Emotion

In adult primates, the emotional context in which stimuli are embedded is a powerful determinant of the efficiency with which objects and events are encoded. Whether the impact of emotional state plays a comparable or (probably) even stronger role in "gating" such storage in infancy, and precisely how, remains to be specified in our model. However, changing interactions between temporal cortical areas and both the amygdala and more anterior cortical regions presumably play a role. In both infant and adult primates, the amygdala has been implicated in assigning emotional valence to stimuli and experience, even showing some single unit activity selective for faces (Tovee, 1995). Studies by other labs have already illustrated that circuits involving interactions between inferior temporal areas and the amygdala undergo considerable postnatal reorganization, under normal conditions as well as subsequent to early injury (Webster, Ungerleider, & Bachevalier, 1991b).

One of the more striking findings from our anatomical studies was the presence of "exuberant" connectivity with frontal areas and the nonvisual regions such as the insula and cingulate cortex. On a speculative note, one specific role for feedback from nonvisual areas (including premotor, polysensory, and limbic) may be as a marker for the internal construction of a bodily state consistent with the emotion of a viewed individual (Adelmann & Zajonc, 1989; Adolphs et al., 2000; Damasio, 1994) and may thus provide a mechanism for efficient representation and retrieval (i.e., recognition) of facial expressions and similar intentional information conveyed by body posture. Immature patterns of feedback connections from precisely these areas early in life may indicate either a functional immaturity or an early boosting of IT processing by such outside influences. As Barbas has shown (e.g., 1988; Rempel-Clower & Barbas, 2000), the patterns of corticocortical projections linking frontal and temporal association cortices are characterized by exquisitely specific areal variations in terms of both origin and termination. In addition, frontal cortex itself undergoes an extremely protracted time course of ontogenetic change (Goldman-Rakic, 1987; Goldman-Rakic, Bourgeois, & Rakic, also see 1997; Thatcher, 1997; Finlay, Clancy, & Kingsbury, this volume), and a closer analysis of the refinement of its connectivity with IT will likely provide further clues as to the relative importance of signals related to emotion, motor activity, memory, and attention in the genesis of object recognition.

SUMMARY

Nonhuman primates provide a model system for studying the development of object recognition in which behavioral data from humans and monkeys alike can be viewed in the light of specific structural and physiological phenomena and used to generate predictions for further research at both behavioral and neural levels. Ideally, this interaction can then serve as the basis for the construction and refinement of biologically plausible theoretical accounts that propose specific neural mechanisms and make further predictions for empirical testing. Existing data on the development of temporal cortex circuits that underlie object recognition in mature primates show rudimentary capacity to code object properties in the period of infancy encompassing approximately 1 to 4 months after birth coupled with a weakness of overall signal strength and an ongoing structural refinement evident at a variety of levels of analysis. These data, in concert with data on behavioral development, have led to the development of a theoretical framework in which an intrinsic developmental delay and/or damping of overall plasticity is proposed to complement the use of several specific mechanisms for forming correct associations and generating a class of circuitry dedicated to representing ecologically important objects. Reconsideration of the behavioral literature in the light of the framework also underscores the need for additional studies in the infant monkey model close to birth as well as later in ontogeny to further establish the correspondence between milestones in human and monkey development and in maturation of neural circuits. Finally, the behavioral and neuroscience literature bearing on the framework suggests the need to account for the influence of emotion and other cognitive factors in the model and in the generation of mature object representations.

NOTES

1. As has been discussed by Elman et al. (1996), among others, the notion of "innateness" is intrinsically problematic because it suggests a precisely specified and developmentally obligatory outcome, whereas more modern views stress the highly dynamic and emergent nature of phenotypes and the intrinsic and extrinsic con-

straints on gene expression (e.g., Gottlieb, 1992). Thus, for the remainder of this chapter, the term *innate* will be avoided, although I will use the descriptor *inherent* to refer to aspects of structure or function that can reasonably, albeit not unfailingly, be expected to appear at birth in an organism with a species-typical prenatal environment.

2. Although the completion of neurogenesis early in life has been a core assumption in neuroscience for a century or more, it now appears that at least a small number of new cells are born and incorporated into existing structures even in adult mammals, into a variety of areas including neocortex (Gross, 2000).

3. By "bootstrapping" I refer to a function whereby the visual recognition system "gets itself going" to form object representations without yet having had experience of the significance of objects to help direct attention to them.

REFERENCES

Abraham, W.C., & Bear, M.F. (1996). Metaplasticity: The plasticity of synaptic plasticity. *Trends in Neurosciences, 19*, 126–130.

Adelmann, P.K., & Zajonc, R.B. (1989). Facial efference and the experience of emotion. *Annual Review of Psychology, 40*, 249–280.

Adolphs, R., Damasio, H., Tranel, D., Cooper, G., & Damasio, A.R. (2000). A role for somatosensory cortices in the visual recognition of emotion as revealed from three-dimensional lesion mapping. *Journal of Neuroscience, 20*, 2683–2690.

Allison, T., McCarthy, G., Nobre, A., Puce, A., & Belger, A. (1994). Human extrastriate visual cortex and the perception of faces, words, numbers and colors. *Cerebral Cortex, 4*, 544–554.

Allman, J., Miezin, F., & McGuinness, E. (1985). Stimulus-specific responses from beyond the classical receptive field: Neurophysiological mechanisms for local-global comparisons on visual neurons. *Annual Review of Neuroscience, 8*, 407–430.

Allman, J., & Zucker, S. (1990). Cytochrome oxidase and functional coding in primate striate cortex: A hypothesis. *Cold Spring Harbor Symposia on Quantitative Biology, 55*, 979–982.

Arterberry, M.E., & Yonas, A. (2000). Perception of three-dimensional shape specified by optic flow by 8-week-old infants. *Perception and Psychophysics, 62*, 550–556.

Atkinson, J. (1984). Human visual development over the first 6 months of life: A review and a hypothesis. *Human Neurobiology, 3*, 61–74.

Atkinson, J. (1992). Early visual development: Differential functioning of parvocellular and magnocellular pathways. *Eye, 6*, 129–135.

Bachevalier, J. (1990). Ontogenetic development of habit and memory formation in primates. In A. Diamond (Ed.), *Development and neural bases of higher cognitive functions* (pp. 457–484). New York: Academic Press.

Bachevalier, J., Hagger, C., & Mishkin, M. (1991). Functional maturation of the occipitotemporal pathway in infant rhesus monkeys. In N.A. Lassen, M.E. Raichle, & L. Friberg (Eds.), *Brain work and mental activity* (pp. 231–242). Copenhagen: Munksgaard.

Bachevalier, J., & Mishkin, M. (1984). An early and a late developing system for learning and retention in infant monkeys. *Behavioral Neuroscience, 98,* 770–778.

Bachevalier, J., & Mishkin, M. (1994). Effects of selective neonatal temporal lobe lesions on visual recognition memory in rhesus monkeys. *Journal of Neuroscience, 14,* 2128–2139.

Baimbridge, K.G., Celio, M.R., & Rogers, J.H. (1992). Calcium-binding proteins in the nervous system. *Trends in Neurosciences, 15,* 303–308.

Banton, T., & Bertenthal, B.I. (1997). Multiple developmental pathway for motion processing. *Optometry and Vision Science, 74,* 751–760.

Barbas, H. (1988). Anatomic organization of basoventral and mediodorsal visual recipient prefrontal regions in the rhesus monkey. *Journal of Comparative Neurology, 276,* 313–342.

Berger, B., Febvret, A., Greengard, P., & Goldman-Rakic, P.S. (1990). DARPP-32, a phosphoprotein enriched in dopaminoceptive neurons bearing dopamine D1 receptors: Distribution in the cerebral cortex of the newborn and adult rhesus monkey. *Journal of Comparative Neurology, 299,* 327–348.

Bertenthal, B.I., Proffitt, D.R., & Kramer, S.J. (1987). Perception of biomechanical motions by infants: Implementation of various processing constraints. *Journal of Experimental Psychology, 13,* 577–585.

Braddick, O.J., Wattam-Bell, J., & Atkinson, J. (1986). Orientation-specific cortical responses develop in early infancy. *Nature, 320,* 617–619.

Bronson, G. (1974). The postnatal growth of visual capacity. *Child Development, 45,* 873–890.

Brown, A. (1990). Development of visual sensitivity to light and color vision in human infants: A critical review. *Vision Research, 30,* 1159–1188.

Callaway, E. (1998). Prenatal development of layer-specific local circuits in primary visual cortex of the macaque monkey. *Journal of Neuroscience, 18,* 1505–1527.

Carey, S. (1992). Becoming a face expert. *Philosophical Transactions of the Royal Society of London, 335,* 95–103.

Caroni, P., & Schwab, M.E. (1988). Two membrane protein fractions from rat central myelin with inhibitory properties for neurite growth and fibroblast spreading. *Journal of Cell Biology, 106,* 1281–1288.

Chino, Y.M., Smith, E.L., Hatta, S., & Cheng, H. (1997). Postnatal development of binocular disparity sensitivity in neurons of the primate visual cortex. *Journal of Neuroscience, 17,* 296–307.

Chugani, H.T. (1998). A critical period of brain development: Studies of cerebral glucose utilization with PET. *Preventive Medicine, 27,* 184–188.

Chung, M-S., & Thomson, D.M. (1995). Development of face recognition. *British Journal of Psychology, 86,* 55–87.

Damasio, A.R. (1994). *Descartes' error: Emotion, reason, and the human brain.* New York: Avon Books.

deCharms, R.C., & Zador, A. (2000). Neural representation and the cortical code. *Annual Review of Neuroscience, 23,* 613–647.

de Haan, M., & Nelson, C.A. (1999). Brain activity differentiates face and object processing in 6-month-old infants. *Developmental Psychology, 35,* 1113–1121.

Desimone, R. (1991). Face-selective cells in the temporal cortex of monkeys. *Journal of Cognitive Neuroscience, 3*, 1–8.

Distler, C., Bachevalier, J., Kennedy, C., Mishkin, M., & Ungerleider, L.G. (1996). Functional development of the corticocortical pathway for motion analysis in the macaque monkey: A 14C-2-deoxyglucose study. *Cerebral Cortex, 6*, 184–195.

Dobkins, K.R., Anderson, C.M., & Lia, B. (1999). Infant temporal contrast sensitivity functions (tCSFs) mature earlier for luminance than for chromatic stimuli: Evidence for precocious magnocellular development? *Vision Research, 39*, 3223–3239.

Dubowitz, L.M.S., deVries, L., Mushin, J., & Arden, G.B. (1986). Visual function in the newborn infant: Is it cortically mediated? *Lancet, 1*, 1139–1141.

Edelman, G.M. (1987). *Neural Darwinism.* New York: Basic Books.

Elman, J., Bates, E.A., Johnson, M.H., Karmiloff-Smith, A., Parisi, D., and Plunkett, K. (1996). *Rethinking innateness: A connectionist perspective on development.* Cambridge, MA: MIT Press.

Erickson, C.A., Jagadeesh, B., & Desimone, R. (2000). Learning and memory in the inferior temporal cortex of the macaque. In M. Gazzaniga (Ed.-in-Chief), *The new cognitive neurosciences* (pp. 743–752) Cambridge, MA: MIT Press.

Fantz, R.L. (1963). Pattern vision in newborn infants. *Science, 140*, 296–297.

Farah, M.J. (1990). *Visual agnosia: Disorders of object recognition and what they tell us about normal vision.* Cambridge, MA: MIT Press.

Farah, M.J., Wilson, K.D., Drain, M., & Tanaka, J.N. (1998). What is "special" about face perception?. *Psychological Review, 105*, 482–498.

Flechsig, P. (1901). Developmental (myelogenetic) localisation of the cerebral cortex in the human subject. *Lancet, 2*, 1027–1029.

Fox, R., & McDaniel, C. (1982). The perception of biological motion by human infants. *Science, 218*, 486–487.

Gattass, R., Sousa, A.P.B., and Gross, C.G. (1988). Visuotopic organization and extent of V3 and V4 of the macaque. *Journal of Neuroscience, 8*, 1831–1845.

Gauthier, I., & Tarr, M.J. (1997). Becoming a "Greeble" expert: Exploring mechanisms for face recognition. *Vision Research, 12*, 1673–1682.

Gauthier, I., Tarr, M.J., Anderson, A.W., Skudlarski, P., & Gore, J.C. (1999). Activation of the middle fusiform "face area" increases with expertise in recognizing novel objects. *Nature Neuroscience, 2*, 568–573.

Gawne, T.J. (1999). Temporal coding as a means of information transfer in the primate visual system. *Critical Reviews in Neurobiology, 13*, 83–101.

Gilmore, R.O., & Johnson, M.H. (1997). Body-centered representations for visually guided action emerge during early infancy. *Cognition, 65*, B1–B9.

Goldman, P.S. (1971). Functional development of the prefrontal cortex in early life and the problem of neuronal plasticity. *Experimental Neurology, 32*, 366–387.

Goldman-Rakic, P.S. (1987). Development of cortical circuitry and cognitive functions. *Child Development, 58*, 642–691.

Goldman-Rakic, P.S., Bourgeois, J.P., & Rakic, P. (1997). Synaptic substrate of cognitive development: Life-span analysis of synaptogenesis in the prefrontal cortex. In N.A. Krasnegor, G.R. Lyon, & P.S. Goldman-Rakic (Eds.), *De-*

velopment of the prefrontal cortex: Evolution, neurobiology and behavior (pp. 27–47). Baltimore: Brookes Publishing.

Goodale, M.A., & Milner, A.D. (1992). Separate visual pathways for perception and action. *Trends in Neuroscience, 15,* 20–25.

Goren, C.C., Sarty, M., & Wu, P.Y.K. (1975). Visual following and discrimination of face-like stimuli by newborn infants. *Pediatrics, 56,* 544–549.

Gottlieb, G. (1992). *Individual development and evolution.* New York: Oxford University Press.

Gross, C.G. (1973). Inferotemporal cortex and vision. In E. Stellar & J.M. Sprague (Eds.), *Progress in physiological psychology* (Vol. 5, pp. 77–124). New York: Academic Press.

Gross, C.G. (2000). Neurogenesis in the adult brain: Death of a dogma. *Nature Reviews Neuroscience, 1,* 67–73.

Gross, C.G., Rodman, H.R., Gochin, P.M., & Colombo, M.W. (1993). Inferior temporal cortex as a pattern recognition device. In E. Baum (Ed.), *Computational learning and cognition* (pp. 44–73). Philadelphia: SIAM Press.

Gunderson, V.M., & Sackett, G.P. (1984). Development of pattern recognition in infant pigtailed macaques (*Macaca nemestrina*). *Developmental Psychology, 20,* 418–426.

Haaf, R., Smith, P., & Smitty, S. (1983). Infant responses to face-like patterns under fixed-trial and infant-control procedures. *Child Development, 54,* 172–177.

Haith, M.M. (1986). Sensory and perceptual processes in early infancy. *Journal of Pediatrics, 109,* 158–171.

Huttenlocher, P.R., & Dabholkar, A. (1997). Regional differences in synaptogenesis in human cerebral cortex. *Journal of Comparative Neurology, 387,* 167–178.

Innocenti, G.M. (1982). Development of interhemispheric cortical connections. *Neurosciences Research Progress Bulletin, 20,* 532–540.

Innocenti, G.M. (1995). Exuberant development of connections, and its possible permissive role in cortical evolution. *Trends in Neuroscience, 18,* 397–402.

Jacobs, B., Chugani, H.T., Allada, V., Chen, S., Phelps, M.E., Pollack, D.B., & Raleigh, M.J. (1995). Developmental changes in brain metabolism in sedated rhesus macaques and vervet monkeys revealed by positron emission tomography. *Cerebral Cortex, 5,* 222–233.

Johnson, M.H. (1990). Cortical maturation and the development of visual attention in early infancy. *Journal of Cognitive Neuroscience, 2,* 81–95.

Johnson, M.H. (1994). Brain and cognitive development in infancy. *Current Opinion in Neurobiology, 4,* 218–225.

Johnson, M.H. (2000). Functional brain development in infants: Elements of an interactive specialization framework. *Child Development, 71,* 75–81.

Johnson, M.H., & Vecera, S.P. (1993). Cortical parcellation and the development of face processing. In B. de Boysson-Bardies, S. de Schonen, P. Jusczyk, P. MacNeilage, & J. Morton (Eds.), *Developmental neurocognition: Face and speech processing in the first year of life* (pp. 135–148). Dordrecht: Kluwer Academic Publishers.

Johnson, S.P. (1996). Habituation patterns and object perception in young infants. *Journal of Reproductive and Infant Physiology, 14,* 207–218.

Johnson, S.P. (2001). Visual development in human infants: Binding features, surfaces and objects. *Visual Cognition, 8,* 565–578.

Johnson, S.P., & Aslin, R.N. (1998). Young infants' perception of illusory contours in dynamic displays. *Perception, 27,* 341–353.

Johnson, S.P., & Johnson, K.L. (2001). Early perception-action coupling: Eye movements and the development of object perception. *Infant Behavior and Development, 23,* 461–483.

Johnson, S.P., & Mason, U. (2002). Perception of kinetic illusory contours by 2-month-old infants. *Child Development, 73,* 22–34.

Jusczyk, P.W., Johnson, S.P., Spelke, E.S., & Kennedy, L.J. (1999). Synchronous change and perception of object unity: Evidence from adults and infants. *Cognition, 71,* 257–288.

Kaufmann, F. (1995). Development of motion perception in early infancy. *European Journal of Pediatrics, 154,* S48–S53.

Kestenbaum, R., & Nelson, C.A. (1992). Neural and behavioral correlates of emotion recognition in children and adults. *Journal of Experimental Child Psychology, 54,* 1–18.

Kiorpes, L., & Movshon, J.A. (1989). Differential development of two visual functions in primates. *Proceedings of the National Academy of Sciences (USA), 86,* 8998–9001.

Kleiner, K.A. (1993). Specific vs. non-specific face recognition device. In B. de Boysson-Bardies, S. de Schonen, P. Jusczyk, P. MacNeilage, & J. Morton (Eds.), *Developmental neurocognition: Face and speech processing in the first year of life* (pp. 103–108). Dordrecht: Kluwer Academic Publishers.

Kobatake, E., Wang, G., & Tanaka, K. (1998). Effects of shape-discrimination training on the selectivity of inferotemporal cells in adult monkeys. *Journal of Neurophysiology, 80,* 324–330.

Konner, M. (1991). Universals of brain development in relation to brain myelination. In K.R. Gibson & A.C. Petersen, (Eds.), *Brain maturation and cognitive development: Comparative and cross-cultural perspectives* (pp. 181–223). New York: deGruyter.

Kuroiwa, J., Inawashiro, S., Miyake, S., & Aso, H. (2000). Self-organization of orientation maps in a formal neuron model using a cluster learning rule. *Neural Networks, 13,* 31–40.

Lewis, J.W., & Van Essen, D.C. (2000). Mapping of architectonic subdivisions in the macaque monkey, with emphasis on parieto-occipital cortex. *Journal of Comparative Neurology, 428,* 79–111.

Lidow, M.S., Goldman-Rakic, P.S., & Rakic, P. (1991). Synchronized overproduction of neurotransmitter receptors in diverse regions of the primate cerebral cortex. *Proceedings of the National Academy of Sciences (USA), 88,* 10218–10221.

Logothetis, N., Pauls, J., Poggio, T. (1995). Shape representation in the inferior temporal cortex of monkeys. *Current Biology, 5,* 552–563.

Lucchetti, C., & Cevolani, D. (1992). The effects of maturation on spontaneous eye movements in the macaque monkey. *Electroencephalography and Clinical Neurophysiology, 85,* 220–224.

Lutz, C.K., Lockard, J.S., Gunderson, V.M., & Grant, K.S. (1998). Infant monkeys' visual responses to drawings of normal and distorted faces. *American Journal of Primatology, 44,* 169–174.

Malkova, L., Mishkin, M., & Bachevalier, J. (1995). Long-term effects of selective neonatal temporal lobe lesions on learning and memory in monkeys. *Behavioral Neuroscience, 109,* 212–226.

Mareschal, D., & Johnson, S.P. (2002). Learning to perceive object unity: A connectionist acccount. *Developmental Science, 5,* 151–172.

Maurer, D., & Barrera, M. (1981). Infants' perception of natural and distorted arrangements of a schematic face. *Child Development, 47,* 523–527.

Maurer, D., & Young, R.E. (1983). Newborn's following of natural and distorted arrangements of facial features. *Infant Behavior and Development, 6,* 127–131.

Mendelson, M.J. (1982). Clinical examination of visual and social responses in infant rhesus monkeys. *Developmental Psychology, 18,* 658–664.

Mendelson, M.J., Haith, M.H., and Goldman-Rakic, P.S. (1982). Face scanning and responsiveness to social cues in infant rhesus monkeys. *Developmental Psychobiology, 18,* 222–228.

Mendelson, M.J., Haith, M.H., & Goldman-Rakic, P.S. (1983). Scanning of compound geometric forms in infant rhesus monkeys. *Developmental, Psychology, 19,* 387–397.

Mesulam, M.-M., & Mufson, E.J. (1982). Insula of the Old World monkey: III: Efferent cortical output and comments on function. *Journal of Comparative Neurology, 21,* 38–52.

Miller, E.K., Li, L., & Desimone, R. (1991). A neural mechanism for working and recognition memory in inferior temporal cortex. *Science, 254,* 1377–1379.

Miyashita, Y. (2000). Visual associative long-term memory: Encoding and retrieval in the inferotemporal cortex of the primate. In M. Gazzaniga (Ed.-in-Chief), *The new cognitive neurosciences* (pp. 379–392). Cambridge, MA: MIT Press.

Moore, A.H., Cherry, S.R., Pollack, D.B., Hovda, D.A., & Phelps, M.E. (1999). Application of positron emission tomography to determine cerebral glucose utilization in conscious infant monkeys. *Journal of Neuroscience Methods, 88,* 123–133.

Morton, J., & Johnson, M.H. (1991). CONSPEC and CONLERN: A two-process theory of infant face recognition. *Psychological Review, 98,* 164–181.

Nahm, F.K.D., Perret, A., Amaral, D.G., & Albright, T.D. (1997). How do monkeys look at faces? *Journal of Cognitive Neuroscience, 9,* 611–623.

Noton, D., & Stark, L. (1971). Scanpaths in saccadic eye movements while viewing and recognizing patterns. *Vision Research, 11,* 929–942.

O'Dell, C., & Boothe, R.G. (1997). The development of stereoacuity in infant rhesus monkeys. *Vision Research, 37,* 2675–2684.

Oishi, T., Higo, N., Umino. Y., Matsuda, K., & Hayashi, M. (1998). Development of GAP-43 mRNA in the macaque cerebral cortex. *Developments in Brain Research, 109,* 87–97.

Overman, W., Bachevalier, J., Schumann, E., & Ryan, P. (1996). Cognitive gender differences in very young children parallel biologically based cognitive gender differences in monkeys. *Behavioral Neuroscience, 110,* 673–684.

Overman, W., Bachevalier, J., Turner, M., & Peuster, A. (1992). Object recognition versus object discrimination: Comparison between human infants and infant monkeys. *Behavioral Neuroscience, 106,* 15–29.

Pascalis, O., & de Schonen, S. (1994). Recognition memory in 3- to 4-day-old human neonates. *Neuroreport, 5*, 1721–1724.

Paus, T., Zijendebos, A., Worsley, K., Collins, D.L., Blumenthal, J., Giedd, J.N., Rapoport, J.L., & Evans, A.C. (1999). Structural maturation of neural pathways in children and adolescents: In vivo study. *Science, 283*, 1908–1911.

Perrett, D.I., & Mistlin, A.J. (1990). Perception of facial characteristics by monkeys. In W.C. Stebbins & M.A. Berkeley (Eds.), *Comparative perception, Vol. II: Complex signals* (pp. 187–215). New York: Wiley.

Phillips, J.O., Finnochio, D.V., Ong, L., & Fuchs, A. (1997). Smooth pursuit in 1-to-4-month-old human infants. *Vision Research, 37*, 3009–3020.

Plunkett, K., & Marchman, V. (1993). From rote learning to system building: Acquiring verb morphology in children and connectionist nets. *Cognition, 48*, 21–69.

Preuss, T.M., & Goldman-Rakic, P.S. (1991). Myelo- and cyto-architecture of the granular frontal cortex and surrounding regions in the strepsirhine primate *Galago* and the anthropoid primate *Macaca. Journal of Comparative Neurology, 310*, 429–474.

Raisler, R.L., & Harlow, H.F. (1965). Learned behavior following lesions of posterior association cortex in infant, immature, and preadolescent monkeys. *Journal of Comparative and Physiological Psychology, 60*, 167–174.

Rakic, P., Bourgeois, J.P., Eckenhoff, M.E.F., Zecevic, N., & Goldman-Rakic, P.S. (1986). Concurrent overproduction of synapses in diverse regions of the primate cerebral cortex. *Science, 232*, 232–235.

Rempel-Clower, N.L., & Barbas, H. (2000). The laminar pattern of connections between prefrontal and anterior temporal cortices in the Rhesus monkey is related to cortical structure and function. *Cerebral Cortex, 10*, 851–865.

Richmond, B.J., Optican, L.M., Podell, M., & Spitzer, H. (1987). Temporal encoding of two-dimensional patterns by single units in primate inferior temporal cortex. I. Response characteristics. *Journal of Neurophysiology, 57*, 132–146.

Ringo, J.L. (1996). Stimulus-specific adaptation in inferior temporal and medial temporal cortex of the monkey. *Behavioral Brain Research, 76*, 191–197.

Rizzo, M., Hurtig, R., & Damasio, A.R. (1987). The role of scanpaths in facial recognition and learning. *Annals of Neurology, 22*, 41–45.

Rochat, P. (1998). Self-perception and action in infancy. *Experimental Brain Research, 123*, 102–109.

Rodman, H.R. (1994). Development of inferior temporal cortex in the monkey. *Cerebral Cortex, 5*, 484–498.

Rodman, H.R. (1999). Face recognition. In R.A. Wilson & F.C. Keil (Eds.), *The MIT encyclopedia of cognitive science* (pp. 309–311). Cambridge, MA: MIT Press.

Rodman, H.R., & Consuelos, M.J. (1994). Cortical projections to anterior inferior temporal cortex in infant macaque monkeys. *Visual Neuroscience, 11*, 119–133.

Rodman, H.R., & Moore, T. (1997). Development and plasticity of extrastriate visual cortex in monkeys. In J.H. Kaas, K. Rockland, & A. Peters (Eds.), *Cerebral cortex, Vol. 12: Extrastriate cortex.* New York: Plenum.

Rodman, H.R., & Nace, K.L. (1997). Development of neuronal activity in cortical regions underlying visual recognition in monkeys. In N.A. Krasnegor, G.R. Lyon, & P.S. Goldman-Rakic (Eds.), *Development of the prefrontal cortex: Evolution, neurobiology and behavior* (pp. 167–190). Baltimore: Brookes Publishing.

Rodman, H.R., Ó Scalaidhe, S.P., & Gross, C.G. (1993). Response properties of neurons in temporal cortical visual areas of infant monkeys. *Journal of Neurophysiology, 70,* 1115–1136.

Rodman, H.R., Skelly, J.P., & Gross, C.G. (1991). Stimulus selectivity and state dependence of activity in inferior temporal cortex in infant monkeys. *Proceedings of the National Academy of Sciences, 88,* 7572–7575.

Rolls, E.T., Baylis, G.C., Hasselmo, M.E., and Nalwa, V. (1989). The effect of learning on the face selective responses of neurons in the cortex in the superior temporal sulcus of the monkey. *Experimental Brain Research, 76,* 153–164.

Sackett, G.P. (1966). Development of preference for differentially complex patterns of infant monkeys. *Psychonomic Science, 6,* 441–442.

Schoop, V.M., Gardziella, S., & Muller, C.M. (1997). Critical period-dependent reduction of the permissiveness of cat visual cortex tissue for neuronal adhesion and neurite growth. *European Journal of Neuroscience, 9,* 1911–1922.

Schwartz, E.L., Desimone, R., Albright, T.D., & Gross, C.G. (1983). Shape recognition and inferior temporal neurons. *Proceedings of the National Academy of Sciences (USA), 80,* 5776–5778.

Singer, W., & Artola, A. (1991). The role of NMDA receptors in use-dependent plasticity of the visual cortex. In H.V. Wheal & A.M. Thomson (Eds.), *Excitatory amino acid synaptic function* (pp. 333–353). London: Academic Press.

Slater, A., Morison, V., & Somers, M. (1988). Orientation discrimination and cortical function in the human newborn. *Perception, 17,* 597–602.

Sorenson, K.M., & Rodman, H.R. (1996). The lateral geniculate nucleus does not project to area TE in infant or adult macaques. *Neuroscience Letters, 217,* 5–8.

Spitz, R.V., Stiles, J., & Siegel, R.M. (1993). Infants' use of relative motion as information for form: Evidence for spatiotemporal integration of complex motion displays. *Perception & Psychophysics, 53,* 190–199.

Stryker, M.P. (1991). Temporal associations. *Nature, 354,* 108–109.

Swindale, N.V. (1992). A model for the coordinated development of columnar systems in primate striate cortex. *Biological Cybernetics, 66,* 217–230.

Teller, D.Y. (2000). Visual development: Psychophysics, neural substrates, and causal stories. In M. Gazzaniga (Ed.-in-Chief), *The new cognitive neurosciences* (pp. 73–81). Cambridge, MA: MIT Press.

Teller, D.Y., Regal, D.M, Videen, T.O., & Pulos, E. (1978). Development of visual acuity in infant monkeys (*Macaca nemestrina*) during the early postnatal weeks. *Vision Research, 18,* 561–566.

Thatcher, R.W. (1997). Human frontal lobe development: A theory of cyclical cortical reorganization. In N.A. Krasnegor, G.R. Lyon, & P.S. Goldman-Rakic (Eds.), *Development of the prefrontal cortex: Evolution, neurobiology and behavior* (pp. 85–113). Baltimore: Brookes Publishing.

Tillmann, B., Bharucha, J.J., & Bigand, E. (2000). Implicit learning of tonality: A self-organizing approach. *Psychological Review, 107,* 885–913.

Tononi, G., Sporns, O., & Edelman, G.M. (1992). Reentry and the problem of integrating multiple cortical areas: Simulation of dynamic integration in the visual system. *Cerebral Cortex, 2,* 310–335.

Tovee, M.J. (1995). Face recognition. What are faces for? *Current Biology, 5,* 480–482.

Trepel, C., Duffy, K.R, Pegado, V.D., & Murphy, K.M. (1998). Patchy distribution of NMDAR1 subunit immunoreactivity in developing visual cortex. *Journal of Neuroscience, 18,* 3404–3415.

Ungerleider, L.G., & Mishkin, M. (1982). Two cortical visual systems. In D.J. Ingle, M.A. Goodale, & R.J.W. Mansfeld (Eds.), *Analysis of visual behavior* (pp. 549–586). Cambridge, MA: MIT Press.

Van der Knaap, M.S., Valk, J., Bakker, C.J., Schooneveld, M., Faber, J.A.J., Willemse, J., & Gooskens, R.H. (1991). Myelination as an expression of the functional maturity of the brain. *Developmental Medicine and Child Neurology, 33,* 849–857.

Wattam-Bell, J. (1996). Visual motion processing in one-month-old infants: Habituation experiments. *Vision Research, 36,* 1679–1685.

Webster, M.J., Ungerleider, L.J., & Bachevalier, J. (1991a). Connections of inferior temporal areas TE and TEO with medial temporal-lobe structures in infant and adult monkeys. *Journal of Neuroscience, 11,* 1095–1116.

Webster, M.J., Ungerleider, L.J., & Bachevalier, J. (1991b). Lesions of inferior temporal area TE in infant monkeys alter cortico-amygdalar projections. *Journal of Neuroscience, 11,* 1095–1116.

Webster, M.J., Ungerleider, L.J., & Bachevalier, J. (1995). Transient subcortical connections of inferior temporal areas TE and TEO in infant macaque monkeys. *Journal of Comparative Neurology, 352,* 213–226.

Weiskrantz, L., & Saunders, R.C. (1984). Impairments of visual object transforms in monkeys. *Brain, 107,* 1033–1072.

Wiesel, T.N., & Hubel, D.H. (1974). Ordered arrangement of orientation columns in monkeys lacking visual experience. *Journal of Comparative Neurology, 158,* 307–318.

Yakovlev, P.I., & LeCours, A.R. (1967). The myelogenetic cycles of regional maturation of the brain. In A. Minkowski (Ed.), *Regional maturation of the brain in early life* (pp. 3–70). Philadelphia: Davis.

Yarbus, A.L. (1967). *Eye movements and vision.* New York: Plenum.

Zimmerman, R.R. (1961). Analysis of discrimination learning capacities in the infant rhesus monkey. *Journal of Comparative and Physiological Psychology, 54,* 1.

Zuckerman, C.B., & Rock, I. (1957). A re-appraisal of the roles of past experience and innate organizing processes in visual perception. *Psychological Bulletin, 54,* 269–296.

Chapter 4

Development and Neural Bases of Infant Visual Recognition Memory

Michelle de Haan

ABSTRACT

Infants arrive in the world with the ability to learn from their visual experience. A striking example is the rapidity with which newborns learn to recognize the mother's face: From only hours after birth, they look longer at her face than at the face of a stranger (Bushnell, Sai, & Mullin, 1989; Pascalis et al., 1995). Results from behavioral studies of the development of recognition memory demonstrate many similarities in the characteristics of infant and adult recognition memory, suggesting that there is a remarkable continuity in this ability. However, hypotheses of the neural bases of the development of recognition memory suggest that in spite of the surface similarities there may be important changes in the neural systems mediating recognition from infancy to adulthood. This chapter reviews investigation of both the behavioral expression and neural bases of recognition memory during infancy and considers how these apparent discrepancies might be resolved.

The ability to respond differently to a stimulus or event because it has been experienced before is a basic aspect of memory that is present very early in life. For example, 2- to 4-day-old infants who have repeatedly heard a particular song during pregnancy show signs of orientation when they hear this song but not when they hear other ones (Hepper, 1988, 1991). While methodological constraints make similar prenatal experiments in the visual domain challenging, infants do show evidence of recognizing familiar visual stimuli, such as the mother's face, from the earliest moments tested after birth (e.g., Bushnell, Sai, & Mullin, 1989). The fact that recognition memory is present from birth and that infants' recognition abilities are related to measures of their intellectual function later in life (Rose & Feldman, 1997) suggest that it may present a basic aspect of cognition that is continuous from infancy and adulthood. Yet studies of the neural bases of memory have led investigators to suggest that recognition memory undergoes qualitative change during infancy (Nelson, 1995; Schacter & Moscovitch, 1984). The aim of this chapter is to provide a selective review of development of visual recognition memory, focusing on findings addressing key questions, emphasizing gaps in our knowledge, and pointing to important areas for future investigation. The chapter is divided into two main parts, the first discussing how long infants can remember and the factors that influence remembering and the second on the possible neural bases of infant recognition memory and its relation to adult recognition memory.[1]

HOW LONG CAN INFANTS REMEMBER?

The question of how long infants can remember what they experience is of fundamental importance to the study of cognitive development. In order to be able to learn about the world and form stable representations of their experiences, infants must be able to retain information for more than just a few seconds or minutes. Several techniques have been devised to investigate infants' long-term recognition abilities.

Looking Time Measures

The most common techniques used to study infants' visual recognition memory are habituation, familiarization, and visual-paired comparisons (reviewed in Bornstein, 1985). These techniques are based on infants' tendency to look longer at a novel stimulus than at one with which they have become familiar (for a more detailed description of these techniques, see Table 4.1). Memory for the familiar stimulus is inferred from the differential looking to the novel compared to the familiar stimulus. Occasionally, infants show a preference for the *familiar* rather than the novel stimulus. Both novelty and familiarity preferences are generally taken as evidence of recognition. A number of explanations have been put forth to account for why infants sometimes show preference for novelty and sometimes for familiarity. The age of the infant (Hunt, 1963), the length of the learning period (Richards, 1997; Sophian, 1980), the infant's affect during learning (Nachman, Stern, & Best, 1986), and the delay between learning and memory testing (Bahrick & Pickens, 1995) can all affect the direction of the looking preference (reviewed in Pascalis & de Haan, in press). For example, 5- to 9-month-olds who show neutral affect during familiarization tend to learn more quickly and show novelty preferences during memory testing, while infants who show positive affect during familiarization tend to learn

Table 4.1
Techniques for Studying Infant Memory Based on Infant Visual Attention

Technique	Description
Habituation-to-Criterion	The infant is exposed to a stimulus either repeatedly or continuously until the time he or she spends looking at it falls below a criterion defined by the experimenter (e.g., until the length of two consecutive looks is less than 50% of the length of the first two looks).
Dishabituation	Following habituation, the infant is presented with a novel stimulus. Dishabituation is said to occur if the infant looks longer at the novel stimulus than at either (1) the familiar stimulus during the last trial(s) of habituation or (2) the familiar stimulus when it is presented again following habituation. Memory for the familiar stimulus is inferred if the infant shows dishabituation to the novel stimulus.
Familiarization	The infant is exposed to a stimulus for a fixed amount of time that is defined by the experimenter. This can be either a fixed amount of time actually looking at the stimulus or a fixed amount of real time regardless of looking.
Visual Paired Comparison	Following habituation or familiarization, the infant is exposed to a novel stimulus paired with the familiar stimulus. Usually the test pair is presented twice with the position of the stimuli reversed left to right across trials to control for any bias the infant may have to look to a particular side of the screen. Memory for the familiar stimulus is inferred if the infant looks longer at the novel than the familiar stimulus.

more slowly and show familiarity preferences during memory testing (Rose, Futterweit, & Jankowski, 1999).

Infants only a few days old look longer at a novel than a familiar face following habituation-to-criterion, both when memory is tested immediately after habituation (Slater, Morison & Rose, 1983) and when a 2-minute delay is imposed between habituation and test (Pascalis & de Schonen, 1994). Some studies have found that 3- to 6-month-olds also show impressive memories and are able to remember visual stimuli for days to weeks. In two studies investigating delayed recognition of faces, 3- and 6-month-olds looked longer at a novel than a familiar face following either a 2-minute (Cornell, 1974; Pascalis et al., 1998) or a 24-hour delay (Pascalis et al., 1998), and in a third study 6-month-olds looked longer at novel than familiar faces following a 2-week delay (Fagan, 1974). In three studies investigating delayed recognition of moving patterns, 3-month-olds looked longer at familiar than novel patterns after a 1-month (Courage & Howe,

1998) or 3-month (Bahrick, Hernandez-Reif, & Pickens, 1997; Bahrick & Pickens, 1995) delay. In contrast, the results of other studies suggest that infants' memories are not so robust and may persist only minutes or seconds. Cornell (1974) found that 5-month-old infants showed no novelty preference after a 2-minute delay, Pancratz and Cohen (1970) found that 4-month-olds showed a novelty preference immediately after familiarization but not after a 5-minute delay, and Diamond (1995) found that 4-month-olds allocated a significantly greater proportion of their looking to a novel stimulus following a 10-second, but not a 15-second, delay. These discrepant findings are likely due to methodological factors that are discussed below.

Delayed Nonmatch-to-Sample

In the delayed nonmatch-to-sample procedure, participants are first presented with an object and then, after a delay, are tested with the familiar object together with a novel one. During testing they are rewarded for choosing the novel object by reaching for it. A unique pair of objects is used for each trial. Once the rule is mastered, recognition abilities can be tested by increasing the delay between presentation and test or by increasing the number of items to be remembered. Success on this task emerges slowly over the first years of life. Children younger than 12 to 15 months of age have great difficulty learning the task even with relatively short delays (Overman et al., 1992). By 18 to 32 months of age, infants are able to learn the task, although slowly, and are able to tolerate delays of 5 seconds (Diamond, 1990), 10 seconds (Overman et al., 1992), or 30 seconds (Diamond, 1990). Once infants are able to perform the task at the shorter delay of 5 seconds, they are also able to tolerate the longer delay of 30 seconds.

Conjugate Reinforcement

The conjugate reinforcement procedure is an operant conditioning procedure in which the infant learns to move his or her leg to make a mobile move (see Rovee-Collier [1990, 1997] for review and details). The infant is placed in a crib that has a mobile suspended from a stand clamped to the rail. A ribbon is tied on one end to the mobile and on the other to the infant's ankle. During a baseline phase the ribbon is not connected to the mobile, and the infant's unlearned kick rate is measured. Then follows the acquisition phase during which the ribbon is connected to the mobile so that the infant's kicking moves the mobile. After some delay, the infant's retention of the conditioned response is assessed by reexposing the infant to the mobile and measuring the kicking response when the ribbon is not connected to the mobile. Differences in kicking between the baseline or the end of the learning phase and the retention phase are taken as evidence of memory.

Recognition memory can be tested by comparing the infant's kicking response when he or she is exposed to the familiar mobile or testing context and a novel mobile or testing context. For example, 3-month-olds show memory for 6 to 8 days after training when tested with the familiar mobile but show no evidence of memory even 1 day after training when tested with a novel mobile (Rovee-Collier & Sullivan, 1980); Sullivan, Rovee-Collier, & Tynes, 1979). This result suggests that infants recognized the familiar mobile and discriminated it from the novel one. Convergent evidence using looking time measures indicates that infants also show differential looking to the two mobiles: They look longer at the familiar than the novel mobile (Wilk, Klein, & Rovee-Collier, 2000, cited in Rovee-Collier, 2001). Indeed, infants seem to encode a very specific representation of the training mobile as well as the context in which training occurred. For example, if more than just a single object is altered in a five-object training mobile, 2- to 3-month-olds' otherwise near-perfect retention at 1 day's delay is abolished (Hayne et al., 1986), and if the crib liner is altered, 6-month-olds' otherwise near-perfect retention is abolished (even with the familiar mobile; Borovsky & Rovee-Collier, 1990).

However, as delay increases, infants' responding begins to change such that after several days their response to a novel mobile is as strong as to the familiar one (Rovee-Collier & Sullivan, 1980). This result is interpreted as reflecting infants' gradual forgetting of the specific details of the training experience, so that with increasing delay the contents of the infants' memories change and they are responding to the general rather than to the specific stimulus (Rovee-Collier & Sullivan, 1980). In other words, after several days, infants no longer recognize the specific mobile that they saw during training but remember more generally that they saw a mobile.

Event-Related Potentials

Event-related potentials (ERPs) are changes in brain activity that are time-locked to the presentation of a particular stimulus. ERPs consist of a series of positive and negative deflections called components that are thought to reflect particular aspects of stimulus processing (for recent reviews of use of ERPs to study cognitive development, see Johnson et al., 2001; Nelson & Monk, 2001; Taylor & Baldeweg, in press). They provide precise data on the timing of stimulus-evoked brain events and some information about its neural source. ERPs are thought to reflect primarily the activity of pyramidal cells in the cortex and hippocampus that fire together in response to the event (Allison, 1984). Because the changes in brain activity elicited by an event are small in size relative to ongoing brain activity, the event-related potential is typically averaged over a number of stimulus presentations. Through the averaging process, brain activity that is time-locked to the presentation of the stimulus is retained and background activity that occurs randomly with respect to the onset of the stimulus averages to small values.

ERPs are recorded from electrodes that are simply placed on the scalp and held in place by one of various methods (see Johnson et al., 2001; or Thomas & Casey, in press). They are ideal for studying the neural correlates of cognition in young infants because they are noninvasive and because they do not require participants to make any overt response. While behavioral measures such as looking time or leg kicking tend to best reflect the outcome of the cognitive process (e.g., the stimulus was recognized or not), ERPs document neural activity on a millisecond-by-millisecond basis from the moment the infant first sees the stimulus.

The earliest component in the infant ERP that differs consistently for novel compared to familiar stimuli is the negative component (Nc). This component is typically most prominent over frontocentral electrodes and peaks about 600 milliseconds after visual stimulus onset in 6-month-olds (e.g., de Haan & Nelson, 1997; 1999; see Figure 4.1). According to one view, the Nc reflects processes involved in orienting attention to novelty (Courchesne, Ganz, & Norcia, 1981; Nelson, 1994). This view is supported by studies showing that in infants as young as 1 month of age (Karrer & Monti, 1995) the amplitude of the Nc is larger for stimuli that occur infrequently in a series than for those that occur frequently (Ackles & Cook, 1998; Courchesne, Ganz, & Norcia, 1981; Karrer & Ackles, 1987). However, others have argued that the Nc may reflect processes involved more generally in engagement of sustained attention rather than in selective attention to novelty (Richards, 2001). This view is supported by recent results showing that the amplitude of the Nc is greater to both novel and familiar stimuli during periods of sustained attention than during periods of inattention (Richards, 2000).

A few studies suggest that the Nc may also reflect some aspects of memory. In 6-month-olds, the Nc is larger for primed than unprimed upright faces (Webb & Nelson, 2001). Priming is a type of implicit memory, which in adults is often measured as speeded responding to previously presented material that occurs even when the material is not actually recognized as having been seen before. The Nc is also larger in 6-month-olds for the mother's face and the infant's own toy than for novel faces or toys (de Haan & Nelson, 1997, 1999). Whether this response reflects the attention-getting properties of salient stimuli such as the mother's face or implicit memory for these stimuli is not clear.

The Nc does not seem to index processes related to delayed recognition memory (Carver, Bauer, & Nelson, 2000; Nelson et al., 1998; Pascalis et al., 1998). Instead, slow wave activity following the Nc differentiates novel and familiar stimuli when a delay is involved (see Figure 4.1). In three

The Infant Event-Related Potential During a Visual Recognition Task

Nc (negative component)
-middle latency response
occurring 400 to 800 msec
after stimulus onset
-attentional response

PSW (positive slow wave) ——
- later latency response
occurring 800 to 1,700 msec
after stimulus onset
-memory updating

NSW (negative slow wave) - - -
- later latency response
occurring 800 to 1,700 msec
after stimulus onset
-detection of novelty

Return to baseline ——
- later latency response
occurring 800 to 1,700 msec
after stimulus onset
-present for stimuli not
requiring memory updating
and not detected as novel

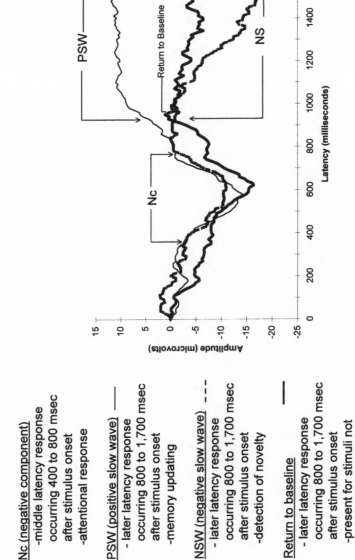

Figure 4.1. Components typically observed in the infant ERP during visual recognition memory tasks. From de Haan and Nelson (1997).

studies examining delayed recognition, infants were either familiarized (Carver, Bauer, & Nelson, 2000) or habituated (Nelson et al., 1998; Pascalis et al., 1998) to visual stimuli and following a delay were presented with an ERP test in which novel and familiar items were presented intermixed. Three-month-olds show a positive slow wave for a novel stimulus when tested 2 minutes after habituation (Pascalis et al., 1998), 8-month-olds show a positive slow wave to a familiar stimulus when tested 1 or 5 minutes after habituation (Nelson et al., 1998), and 9-month-olds show a positive slow wave to a familiar stimulus when tested 1 week after familiarization (Carver, Bauer, & Nelson, 2000). Nelson (1994) has suggested that the positive slow wave represents the updating of memory for a stimulus that is only partially encoded. Thus, in these studies, the 8- and 9-month-olds may have been updating a decaying memory for the familiar stimulus, while the 3-month-olds may have been attempting to encode the novel stimulus and updating their as yet incomplete representation of it.

WHAT FACTORS INFLUENCE HOW LONG BABIES REMEMBER?

The studies reviewed above show that in the first year of life infants are able to recognize familiar stimuli even when a delay is imposed between the learning episode and memory test. However, estimates of the duration of infants' long-term recognition memory vary greatly from none to a few seconds or minutes to days and weeks. In particular, the discrepancy between the slow development of performance on the delayed nonmatch to sample task and the earlier development of performance on other tasks led to the conclusion that the delayed nonmatch to sample task was dependent on a different, later-developing recognition memory system (e.g., Bachevalier & Mishkin, 1984). However, subsequent investigations have suggested that it is not infants' recognition abilities that limit their performance on this task but rather their difficulties with other aspects of the task such as relating the stimulus to the reward (Diamond, 1995). This section will provide an overview of factors that affect whether infants show delayed recognition by providing illustrative examples rather than an exhaustive review. The focus will be on *delayed* recognition, and thus studies of immediate recognition will only be mentioned to illustrate specific points.

Type of Learning Experience

Quantity of Experience

The length of the learning experience is known to influence whether babies show immediate recognition memory (Rose et al., 1982), but does it also influence how long they remember? Rose (1981) found that both 6-

and 9-month-olds show novelty preferences immediately following a brief familiarization, but only 9-month-olds continue to do so after a few minutes' delay. Six-month-olds do show novelty preferences following habituation to criterion even after delays of many hours (e.g., Pascalis et al., 1998). Together, these results suggest that younger babies may need longer exposure during learning than do older babies to remember over delays.

A widely held model of infant recognition is that each time a visual stimulus is encountered a mental representation is formed that becomes progressively more detailed. If the infant "notices" new details (i.e., the mental representation is not complete), then the infant will continue looking, but if the representation is complete, then the stimulus is no longer attended. This model accounts for why infants look longer at novel stimuli: because there is little or no new information to encode from familiar stimuli but much new information to encode from novel stimuli. Thus, with more time to encode a stimulus a more detailed representation can be formed that may be more resistant to forgetting. This effect interacts with age, so that as processing speed becomes faster with age, a more detailed representation can also be formed more quickly.

Quality of Experience

Mass versus distributed exposure. Not only may the quantity of experience influence infants' memory, but so may the way it is presented. For example, as for adults (e.g., Schwartz, 1975), distributed rather than massed exposure during learning facilitates infants' delayed recognition. This was demonstrated in a study in which 6-month-olds were famliarized to a face for four 5-second trials that were separated by either a 3-second (massed exposure) or 1-minute (distributed exposure) intertrial interval, and then their memories were tested at 5 seconds, 1 minute, 5 minutes, or 1 hour delay (Cornell, 1980). Infants from both groups showed evidence of recognition at the 5-second delay, but only infants who were given distributed exposure did so at longer delays.

Single versus multiple exemplars. Another important aspect of the learning experience is the range of different stimuli present. Studies show that following exposure to different, but related, examples during learning, infants as young as 3 months of age form perceptual categories (e.g., a perceptual representation of "dog" and not just representations of each individual dog; reviewed in Quinn, 1998). Formation of perceptual categories may facilitate subsequent encoding of other members of the same category. For example, several studies show that adults form a prototypic representation of facial features and their relative positions based on the faces they experience, and one way they can encode new faces is in terms of how they deviate from this prototype (Benson & Perrett, 1991; Rhodes, 1993). It is thought that this type of encoding allows processing of key features that are most useful for discriminating among faces and in this way is important for adults' ability to remember hundreds of different facial identities. That the prototype is likely based on the individual's experience with faces in the visual environment is supported by studies showing other-race and other-species effects: Adults are worse at recognizing novel members of other races or other species than at recognizing novel members of their own race and species, presumably because the latter can be more easily related to the prototype formed from faces seen most frequently in their daily experience (Rhodes et al., 1989).

To test whether young infants form similar perceptual categories based on the faces they see, in one study (de Haan et al., 2001) 1- and 3-month-old infants were familiarized to four individual faces and then tested with two types of visual-paired comparison trials: (1) one to determine whether the baby recognized a computer-generated "average" prototype of the four faces and (2) one to verify that the baby could remember an individual face. Only 3-month-olds showed evidence of recognizing the average of the four faces seen during familiarization (see Figure 4.2). They showed this by looking longer at the familiar individual face than at the average of the four faces during the first test, presumably because, like adults, they found the average prototype looked more familiar even than the individual face they had seen before. Infants at both ages demonstrated that they recognized individual faces by looking longer at the novel face than one of the familiar faces during the second test (see Figure 4.2). These results suggest that while infants can memorize individual faces from birth (Pascalis & de Schonen, 1994), only by some time between 1 and 3 months of age are they beginning to be able to relate information from separate encounters with different faces to form a mental prototype. In other words, only at this time will their previous experience with faces affect how they encode a new face.

Perceptual categories may allow more efficient encoding of individual members of a category by "alerting" the infant to key features that normally individuate members of the category. This would allow encoding of a smaller number of features that are most relevant for discriminating individuals rather than a large number of features that may or may not be useful—and as a result enhance recognition. However, further investigation is needed to determine whether infants retain perceptual categories over time. Most studies of infants' formation of perceptual categories have focused on the types of information that infants can categorize rather than on memory and therefore have tested infants immediately after familiarization without imposing delays. If infants are able to retain this category information over time, it would support the view that perceptual categories play a role in facilitating infants' encoding of new category exemplars.

Interference. Several studies have investigated whether material presented between learning and the recognition test affects infants' delayed recognition. Generally, these studies show that infant recognition memory is re-

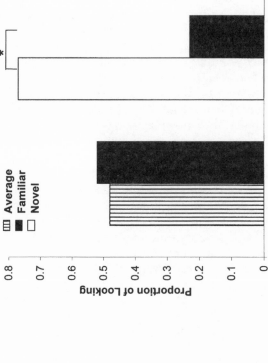

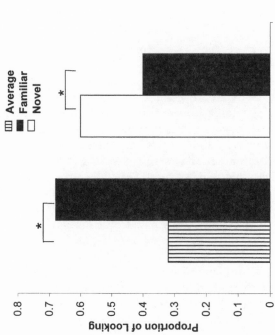

Figure 4.2. Proportion of looking during the two test trials for 1-month-olds and 3-month-olds. Three-month-olds show evidence of recognizing both the average prototype of the faces seen during familiarization and the individual faces, while 1-month-olds appear to recognize only the individual faces and not the prototype. Reprinted with kind permission from de Haan, M., Johnson, M.H., Maurer, D., & Perrett, D.I. (2001). Recognition of individual faces and average face prototypes by 1- and 3-month-old infants. *Cognitive Development, 16,* 659–678. Copyright 2001, Elsevier Science, Ltd., The Boulevard, Langford Lane, Kidlington OX5 1GB, UK.

markably immune to the potentially detrimental effects of interference. For example, Rose (1981) found that 9-month-olds were able to show recognition after a few minutes delay even when interfering material was presented during the delay. A series of experiments by Fagan (1973, 1977) indicates that forgetting is induced by interference only when stimuli very similar to the trained stimulus are presented shortly after study.

Reactivation. When infants fail to show evidence of memory, is their memory completely inaccessible, or can it be reactivated by a brief reminder? The results of one study (Bahrick, Hernandez-Reif, & Pickens, 1997) suggest the latter. In that study, infants were given a "reminder" (a brief exposure of a static picture of the moving stimulus seen during familiarization) of a familiar stimulus that they appeared to have forgotten. This reminder proved effective in reinstating a novelty preference, showing that the memory was not completely forgotten. Similar results are found using the conjugate reinforcement procedure, where brief exposure to the distinctive crib liner in which training occurred or to the mobile (without the infant controlling its movement) results in reactivation of otherwise forgotten memories in 3-month-olds at 2, 3, or 4 weeks after the training phase (Hayne, Rovee-Collier, & Perris, 1987; Sullivan, 1982).

Reactivation may play an important role in infant memory. Repeated reactivations of the memory may help to sustain and consolidate it so that even if infants' memories are not long lasting, they are able to sustain representations over long periods of time.

Age

Does the ability to recognize an item following a delay improve with age? Rose (1981) found that following brief familiarization both 6- and 9-month-olds showed a novelty preference when no delay was imposed, but only 9-month-olds did so following a few minutes' delay. Diamond (1995) found that following familiarization 4-month-olds spent a great proportion of time looking at novel rather than familiar stimuli after a delay of 10 seconds but not longer, 6-month-olds after delays of 10 seconds and 1 minute, and 9-month-olds after delays of 10 seconds, 15 seconds, 1 minute, 3 minutes, and 10 minutes. Thus, with age there appears to be a slowing of the rate of forgetting such that infants become able to tolerate increasing delays between learning and recognition testing and still show evidence of recognition (for similar conclusions based on studies of elicited imitation see Bauer [1995] and of conjugate reinforcement see Rovee-Collier & Shyi [1992]).

The results of ERP studies (Nelson & Collins, 1991, 1992) also indicate that there may be changes in the rate of memory decay between 6 to 8 months. In these studies, 6- and 8-month-olds were first familiarized to two faces and then presented with a series of stimuli in which one of the familiar faces occurred frequently (60%) and one occurred infrequently (20%), with the remaining trials showing trial-unique novel stimuli (20%). Six-month-olds showed a positive slow wave for the infrequently occurring familiar stimulus, a return-to-baseline for the frequently occurring familiar stimulus, and a negative slow wave for the novel stimuli (see Figure 4.1). The positive slow wave was interpreted as representing the updating of an incomplete stimulus representation, the return to baseline represents a recognition of a fully encoded stimulus, and the negative slow wave a detection of novelty (without further encoding). Thus, 6-month-olds retained an intact representation of the familiar stimulus that occurred frequently during test but not of the one that occurred infrequently. This suggests that their memory for the infrequently occurring familiar stimulus had already begun to decay. In contrast, 8-month-olds showed a return-to-baseline response for both familiar stimuli and a negative slow wave for the novel stimuli. This suggests that 8-month-olds had been able to retain an intact representation of both familiar stimuli, even the one that occurred infrequently during test. Together, these results suggest that there may be a decrease in the rate of memory decay between 6 and 8 months of age. While this ERP study focused on immediate recognition, a more rapid rate of memory decay will presumably also influence whether a stimulus is recognized following a delay.

One concern with the studies reviewed above showing less forgetting in older than younger infants is that these differences might reflect differences in learning rather than differences in forgetting per se (for discussion, see Howe & Courage, 1997). For example, if older and younger children are given the same learning experience, younger children may forget more because they learned more slowly and had a less complete representation of the to-be-remembered materials. Developmental studies of forgetting can address this potential confound by using learning to criterion designs (rather than a number of trials or fixed familiarzation) that are more likely to ensure equal learning at different ages and by testing knowledge after learning. For example, in the study by Rose (1981), both 6- and 9-month-old infants had learned enough to show a novelty preference at immediate test but only the 9-month-olds after a delay. This and other studies that have systematically addressed the question (e.g., Howe & Courage, 1997) support the view that there are developmental decreases in the rate of forgetting independent even when the confounding influence of age differences in learning is controlled.

Is Memory for Faces "Special"?

Studies with animals suggest that unlearned biases may play a role in infant learning and memory (e.g., in birdsong see Marler [1997] and in imprinting see McCabe & Nicol [1999]). Human newborns arrive in the world with an apparently unlearned tendency to orient to faces (reviewed in Johnson & Morton, 1991). There are different views as to the basis of this response. According to one view, newborns' apparent preference for faces is actually due to more general constraints in their visual information processing (e.g., Banks & Salapatek, 1981; Simion et al., 2001). In this hypothesis, there is no aspect of the system that is responding specifically to faces; instead, the preferential orienting of the newborn to faces is just a consequence of more general mechanisms guiding visual attention. According to a different view, infants from birth have a preference for facelike stimuli that is based not only on the visibility of the stimuli but on a more specific knowledge of the configuration of the face (Johnson & Morton, 1991). For example, in the CONSPEC hypothesis, a specific subcortical mechanism, CONSPEC, causes newborns to orient to patterns with elements in a facelike arrangement (Morton & Johnson, 1991).

Whichever explanation for infants' enhanced attention to faces is correct, one consequence could be that infants are better at learning and remembering faces than other stimuli. This is predicted from the studies reviewed above relating increased exposure at learning to better recognition. Babies' special attention to faces may make it easier for them to form lasting representations of faces than other stimuli that are less attention-getting.

Few studies have directly compared infants' memory for faces and objects, but existing results suggest that memory for faces differs from memory for objects. The results of one behavioral study to directly investigate this question support this view: Six-month-old infants are able to recognize faces after a delay of 2 weeks but are able to recognize patterns only after a delay of 2 days (Fagan, 1972). Results of two other studies indirectly suggest that infants may also be able to remember more individual faces than objects. The study of infants' ability to form a mental prototype described above indicates that, following exposure to four individual faces, both 1- and 3-month-olds were able to recognize the individual faces (de Haan et al., 2001). In other words, the infants appeared to have a memory "span" of at least four faces. The results of another recent study of infants' memory span for patterns indicate that only 25% of 5- to 7-month-olds were able to keep three to four items in memory (Rose, Feldman, & Jankowski, 2001). The comparison must be made cautiously because of procedural differences, but the pattern of results suggests that infants may have a greater memory span for faces than other visual patterns.

The results of the only ERP study to compare infants' responses to faces and objects suggest that the neural correlates of recognition also differ for the two. In this study, 6-month-olds' ERPs were recorded while they viewed computer images of either their mother's face and a stranger's face or their own toy and a novel toy (de Haan & Nelson, 1999). For both faces and toys, the familiar item elicited a larger Nc (see "Event-Related Potential" section above for explanation of this ERP component) than the novel item. However, for faces this occurred over the right, but not the left, hemisphere, while for objects this occurred over both right and left sides. These results suggest that a different configuration of neural generators was active during face compared to object recognition.

ARE THERE MULTIPLE PHASES IN INFANT RECOGNITION MEMORY?

In adults, there is evidence to suggest that there are multiple phases of memory. In this view, short-term memory (seconds to minutes) is mediated by different systems than long-term memory (years; see, e.g., McCarthy & Warrington, 1992), which may in turn be mediated by different systems than very long term memory (decades; see, e.g., Haist, Bowden Gore, & Mao, 2001). A multiphase model has also been proposed for infant memory that describes different states of accessibility of infant memory over time and how this relates to their preferences in looking time procedures. According to this model: (1) infants' memories become increasingly inaccessible with greater delays between familiarization and test, and (2) differences in the accessibility of the memory are reflected in different patterns of infant looking to the novel and familiar stimuli at test (Bahrick, Hernandez-Reif, & Pickens, 1997; Bahrick & Pickens, 1995). Four phases of infant looking/memory are proposed: *recent memory*, when memory is maximally accessible and a novelty preference are shown; *transient memory*, when no preference is shown; *remote memory*, when memory is less accessible and a familiarity preference is shown; *inaccessible memory*, when the memory is inaccessible and no preferences are shown. Investigations based on the looking time four-phase model of infant memory have found results consistent with the predicted pattern of infant looking preferences (Bahrick, Hernandez-Reif, & Pickens, 1997; Bahrick & Pickens, 1995; Courage & Howe, 1998). For example, following familiarization to a moving stimulus, 3-month-old infants show novelty preferences after a 1-minute delay, no preference at 1 day or 2 weeks, and familiarity preferences at longer delays of 1 and 3 months (Bahrick, Hernandez-Reif, & Pickens, 1997; Bahrick & Pickens, 1995). To date, these investigations have focused almost exclusively on 3-month-olds' recognition of moving stimuli, and the possibility of age-related changes in forgetting has not been pursued.

Summary

From the first days of life infants are able to recognize a visual stimulus they have recently seen, and by the first half-year of life they are able to remember over delays of days or even weeks. Numerous factors such as the quantity and quality of the encoding experience, the nature of the stimuli, and the presence of reminders influence infants' recognition. The results of studies investigating the factors that affect infant memory point to many similarities in the functioning of infant and adult memory (Rovee-Collier, 1997). Perhaps one of the more notable differences is the apparently greater sensitivity of infant memory to changes in context between learning and test (e.g., Hayne, Boniface, & Barr, 2000).

More studies have focused on documenting how such factors affect whether infants can remember at all than on age-related changes in how long they can remember. Studies that have looked for age-related changes in recognition do suggest that with increasing age infants are able to re-member over longer delays. The contribution of encoding, storage, and retrieval factors to this change is not clear. Collectively, the studies suggest that infants may be most likely to show evidence of recognition if they are given relatively prolonged, distributed exposure to a face and are tested for recognition by pairing the familiar face with one that looks distinct from it.

WHAT IS THE NEURAL BASIS OF INFANT RECOGNITION MEMORY?

The results of many studies of infant recognition memory, and infant memory more generally, have highlighted the similarities in the character-istics of infant and adult memory, leading investigators to argue that "there seems to be considerable invariance in memory development, at least at the level of basic processes and mechanisms. That is, whatever these 'basics' necessary for storage and retrieval of information are, they are clearly pres-ent and operating in the first year of life" (Howe & Courage, 1997, p. 157). In contrast, investigations into the neural bases of memory development have tended to focus on differences between infants and older children and adults and on seeming discontinuities in memory such as infantile amnesia (e.g., Nelson, 1995). This section will discuss four hypotheses regarding the possible neural bases of infant memory. This discussion will be focused at the systems level (where in the brain storage occurs) rather than at the molecular level (the mechanisms whereby memories are stored and main-tained). Prior to such a change in focus, it is necessary to consider briefly current thinking about the neural underpinnings of the distinction between explicit and implicit memory in adults.

Adult Memory

In adults, memory is not a unitary function but can be divided into dif-ferent components. One such distinction is between explicit or declarative memory and implicit or nondeclarative memory. Explicit memory depends on the hippocampus and anatomically related structures in the medial tem-

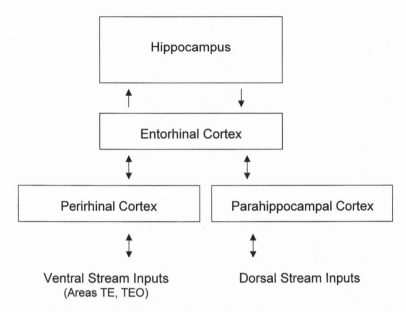

Figure 4.3. Schematic diagram of the connections of the medial temporal hippocampal system (filled boxes). Adapted from Mishkin et al. (1997).

poral lobe (see Figure 4.3) and diencephalon and is characterized by relatively rapid learning and (at least in adult humans) conscious recollection of previous experiences. Recall and recognition memory in adults are both considered tests of explicit memory. Implicit memory involves a number of abilities that are independent of the medial temporal lobe and are expressed as skills or habits, some of which are characterized by relatively slow learning over repeated experiences without specific memory of the learning experience. Implicit memory is typically measured by changes in performance (e.g., decreased reaction time). Investigations of the neural bases of memory development have been largely aimed at determining whether the different components of memory observed in adults develop at different times and/ or at different rates.

The distinction between explicit and implicit memory arose from studies of patients with damage to the medial temporal region of the brain (Squire, 1992). The first of these patients whose memory was studied quantitatively was HM, who showed a profound anterograde amnesia (difficulty in remembering things that occurred after the onset of the illness) following bilateral removal of the medial temporal regions for treatment of intractable epilepsy (Milner, Corkin, & Teuber, 1968; Scoville & Milner, 1957). HM and other patients with similar or more circumscribed medial temporal damage show deficits in declarative memory. For example, HM could neither remember his new address nor be trusted to find his way home alone even 1 year after moving house (Milner, 1966). However, such patients retain some other learning abilities, collectively called implicit memory, such as priming, simple conditioning, and motor learning (Squire & Knowlton, 1995). For example, HM was able to learn to trace a drawing when looking in a mirror rather than looking at his hand and retained his learning over days (Milner, 1965). Another aspect of memory that is relatively unaffected is immediate memory. For example, HM has a normal auditory and visual immediate memory span (Drachman & Arbit, 1966; see also Baddeley & Warrington, 1970). Thus, short-term memory (memory for roughly 20 to 30 seconds) appears to be mediated by neural structures independent of the medial temporal lobes.

Hypotheses of the Neural Bases of Memory Development

Investigations of the neural bases of human memory development have been largely aimed at determining whether the different components of memory observed in adults develop at different times and/or at different rates. In adults the different components of memory are not isolated but interact with each other (Thompson & Kim, 1996). For example, even in a relatively simple learning situation such as Pavlovian trace conditioning (when a short period of no stimuli intervenes between presentation of the conditioned stimulus and unconditioned stimulus), both cerebellar ("implicit") and hippocampal-based ("explicit") memory systems are involved. If different components of memory emerge at different times, studying development could provide an opportunity to study these components in isolation in a way not possible in healthy adults.

Implicit Memory Hypothesis

Schacter and Moscovitch (1984) were among the first to suggest that while implicit memory is present from early in infancy, explicit memory does not begin to emerge until approximately 8 to 12 months of age. In other words, true recognition memory is not present before this time. This view was based in part on investigations showing that adult monkeys with hippocampal lesions are impaired on the delayed nonmatch to sample task (Mahut, Zola-Morgan, & Moss, 1982; Zola-Morgan & Squire, 1986; Zola-Morgan, Squire, & Amaral, 1989). Based on these findings, infants' poor performance was attributed to the immaturity of the hippocampus (Bachevalier & Mishkin, 1984; Nadel & Zola-Morgan, 1984; Schacter & Moscovitch, 1984). If this is true, it follows that procedures in which infants *do* show evidence of memory, such as visual-paired comparisons and conjugate reinforcement, must be implicit.

However, subsequent investigations suggest that this view is not an accurate description of infant memory. First, there is increasing evidence that in humans and other primates the hippocampus is mature relative to other cortical areas involved in memory (though it continues to develop until at least 5 years of age in humans; reviewed in Seress, 2001). Second, further investigation with the delayed nonmatch to sample task led to the conclusion that recognition memory per se does not limit infants' performance of the task. Instead, other demands of the task, such as relating a stimulus to reward (Diamond, 1995), are likely the reason(s) for the protracted course of development.

This leaves open the possibility that explicit memory may be functioning early in life. This possibility was supported by a study showing that adults with hippocampal damage show impaired delayed recognition in the visual-paired comparison task (McKee & Squire, 1993). A later study showed that in healthy adults novelty preferences in the visual-paired comparison task are correlated with reaction times and confidence judgments in recognition memory tasks but not with priming (Manns, Stark, & Squire, 2000). These results provide further support for the view that the visual-paired comparison task taps the explicit, medial temporal lobe–based memory rather than implicit memory (Manns, Stark, & Squire, 2000). The fact that young infants *do* show evidence of delayed recognition on this task suggests that the hippocampus must be sufficiently mature early in life to mediate at least some aspects of explicit memory. Direct support for the view that success on the visual-paired comparison task depends on the integrity of the hippocampus in infants comes from a study showing that infant monkeys with damage to the medial temporal lobe show impaired delayed recognition both when tested as infants and when tested as adults (Bachevalier, Brickson, & Hagger, 1993; Pascalis & Bachevalier, 1999). However, in these studies the lesions included not only the hippocampal formation but also amygdala and surrounding tissues, and it is not certain whether lesions during infancy restricted to the hippocampus would also impair performance as they do in adults (Zola et al., 2000).

It is not entirely clear whether the hippocampus's contribution to performance in the visual-paired comparison task is in recognition memory or in orienting to novelty. One way to test these alternatives is to examine performance with little or no delay between learning and visual-paired comparison memory testing. If the hippocampus is involved in orienting to novelty per se, then individuals with hippocampal damage should perform poorly even if no delay is involved; conversely, if the hippocampus is involved in recognition memory, then these individuals should perform normally with no delay but poorly with delay. The results of studies of monkeys with hippocampal damage support the second option: These monkeys perform normally on the visual-paired comparison task at zero or very short delays (e.g., 1-second delay in Zola et al., 2000) but are impaired at longer delays. These results suggest that hippocampal damage does not impair the ability to respond to novelty but does impair memory. However, the results of neuroimaging studies with human adults suggest that the hippocampus plays an important role in encoding and responding to stimulus novelty per se (Dolan & Fletcher, 1997; Elliott & Dolan, 1998; Strange et al., 1999), even in tasks where (like visual-paired comparisons) there is not intention or objective requirement to retrieve (Rugg et al., 1997; Schacter et al., 1996). One possible explanation is that the hippocampus is normally involved in novelty detection (and so is activated in neuroimaging studies) but is not necessary (and so novelty detection is not impaired when it is damaged). A second possible explanation is that different parts of the hippocampus are involved in recognition and novelty detection. This possibility is support by a recent neuroimaging study in adults suggesting that the anterior hippocampus responds to novelty, while the posterior hippocampus responds to familiarity (Strange et al., 1999).

Whatever the exact role of the hippocampus, collectively the results of studies with human and monkeys indicate that a form of medial temporal lobe–based recognition memory is present early in life. Thus, more recent theories of the development of infant memory have postulated that an "infant form" of explicit memory is present already early in life. This system is thought to coexist with developing implicit memory systems, although the degree of interaction between these systems is not clear. These theories are thus converging closer to the view derived from the behavioral literature that emphasizes continuity in memory processes over development.

Preexplicit Memory Hypothesis

According to this view, in addition to implicit memory, there is a form of "preexplicit" memory that develops within the first few months of life (Nelson, 1995; Nelson & Webb, in press). This type of memory is largely based on the infant's response to novelty and is observed in procedures like the visual-paired comparison. As infants approach 1 year or so of age, development of regions within the temporal cortex, in particular, area TE (the area in the inferior temporal cortex that is one of the final stations of the ventral visual "what" pathway at which a complete representation of a visual object is synthesized; Nelson, 1995), may allow emergence of more adultlike memory. This is seen in abilities such as improved performance on the delayed nonmatch to sample task and delayed cross-modal recognition of objects. As these cortical regions and their connections mature, dramatic improvements in explicit memory are observed (Nelson, 1995).

The Subcortical-Cortical Model

This model is similar to the preexplicit memory model in that it proposes an early appearing hippocampal memory system that is later supplemented by temporal cortical regions. It differs from those described above in that it attempts to specifically account for the development of adults' expertise in face recognition by focusing on unlearned biases in brain systems that can affect the type of material infants learn and remember. This model was initially based on investigations of development of recognition of conspecifics in the domestic chick. Imprinting is the process by which young, precocial birds, such as domestic chicks, recognize and develop a social attachment for the first conspicuous object that they see after hatching. In the laboratory, newly hatched domestic chicks will imprint onto a variety of objects such as moving colored balls and cylinders. Even after only a few hours of exposure to such a stimulus, chicks will come to prefer it to any other object.

A variety of evidence suggests that there are two independent neural systems that underlie filial preference in the chick (Horn 1985; Johnson, Bolhuis, & Horn, 1985). The first is a specific predisposition for the young chick to orient toward objects resembling conspecifics. This system appears to be specifically tuned to the correct spatial arrangement of elements of the head and neck region (Johnson & Horn, 1988) but not to the color or size (see Johnson & Bolhuis, 1991). While the stimulus configuration triggering the predisposition is not species or genus specific, it is sufficient to pick out the mother hen from other objects the chick is likely to see in the first few days after hatching. The second system is the one that actually learns about the objects to which the young chick attends and is subserved by a particular area of the chick forebrain called the intermediate and medial hyperstriatum ventrale (IMHV). Studies using autoradiographic, biochemical, lesion, and electrophysiological techniques have established the IMHV is crucially involved in visual imprinting (for recent reviews, see Horn, 1998). For example, bilateral lesions to IMHV placed before or after training severely impair preference for the trained object in subsequent choice tests but do not affect several other types of visual or learning tasks Johnson & Horn, 1986, 1987; (McCabe et al., 1982). In the natural environment, the first system ensures that the second system mediated by the IMVH acquires information about the particular individual mother hen close by.

The results of these investigations led to the development of a two-process theory of development of face recognition in human infants. According to this theory (Johnson & Morton, 1991), distinct brain systems are proposed to underlie development of face processing in infancy: (1) CONSPEC, a system operating from birth that functions to bias the newborn to orient toward faces and (2) CONLERN, a later-emerging system sensitive to the effects of experience through passive exposure. In this model, CONSPEC is mediated by primitive, possibly largely subcortical, circuits, whereas CONLERN is mediated by developing cortical circuits in the ventral visual pathway. The purpose of CONSPEC is to fine-tune the still-plastic cortical circuits underlying CONLERN and thereby contribute to the development of cortical areas specialized for face processing.

In the initial formulation of the theory (Johnson & Morton, 1991), CONLERN begins to influence behavior at 6 to 8 weeks of age and allows emergence of the ability to recognize the identity of individual faces. However, subsequent studies demonstrated that even newborn infants show evidence of recognizing the facial identity (Bushnell, Sai, & Mullin, 1989; Pascalis et al., 1995). In order to take these findings into account, Johnson and de Haan (2001) revised the original theory and proposed that prior to the specialization of cortical circuits for faces these stimuli can be processed and recognized in the same general-purpose way as other visual patterns. This provides some basis for the ability to recognize a number of individual faces from early in life. This more limited ability is then supplemented with the emergence of CONLERN at 6 to 8 weeks of age, when more adultlike processing of faces begins to emerge

Familiarity-Based Memory Hypothesis

A slightly different formulation of the preexplicit memory theory is that infant recognition memory is based on the familiarity subcomponent of recognition memory. In adults, recognition memory consists of both familiarity- and recollection-based components. Familiarity-based recognition is experienced as a "feeling of knowing" that a stimulus has been experienced before, without necessarily remembering the details of the experience. This type of recognition is thought to be mediated by subhippocampal cortex (Vargha-Khadem, Gadian, & Mishkin, 2001). In contrast, recollection-based recognition is experience as recognition that is accompanied by specific memory of having experienced the stimulus before and is often accompanied by memory of details of the encoding context. This type of recognition is thought to be mediated by the hippocampus (Vargha-Khadem, Gadian, & Mishkin, 2001). In the familiarity-based memory hypothesis, infants have implicit memory and a familiarity-based recognition memory (presumably mediated by subhippocampal regions), and only later in development do hippocampally mediated recollection-based recognition (and recall) emerge.

This familiarity-based recognition hypothesis is similar to the preexplicit memory hypothesis in that both suggest that a partial form of explicit memory is operating early in life. It differs from the preexplicit memory hypothesis in that it points to the parahippocampal regions, in particular, the perirhinal cortex, as important for recognition. Recent research with animal models of memory supports the view that the parahippocampal region of the medial temporal lobe is particularly critical for recognition memory. Selective damage to this area (including the entorhinal, perirhinal, and parahippocampal cortex) in rats or monkeys results in deficits in visual recognition memory, while damage to the hippocampus results in only mild or no impairment on the same tasks (reviewed in Mishkin, Vargha-Khadem, & Gadian, 1998; Mishkin et al., 1997). Damage to the perirhinal cortex even in infant monkeys results in deficits in recognition later in life (Malkova et al., 1998). Indeed, performance on the visual-paired comparison test has also been found sensitive to lesion of the perirhinal cortex lesion (Clark et al., 1996, 1997).

The cognitive profile of patients with amnesia due to bilateral hippocampal damage sustained early in life also suggests that the parahippocampal regions mediate recognition memory (Baddeley, Vargha-Khadem, & Mishkin, 2001; Gadian et al., 2000; Vargha-Khadem, Gadian, & Mishkin, 2001; Vargha-Khadem et al., 1997). If the hippocampus is critical for recognition memory, these children would be expected to perform very poorly on recognition tasks. However, these children show deficits mainly in delayed recall, with relatively intact recognition memory.[2] For example, whereas they perform close to the lowest possible level on delayed recall tests, their immediate recall and immediate or delayed recognition of the same materials are at or close to the normal level (with the exception of cross-modal memory; Baddeley, Vargha-Khadem, & Mishkin, 2001; Vargha-Khadem et al., 1997). Thus, these patients appear to have relatively intact recognition memory in spite of hippocampal damage. The intact recognition demonstrated by the developmental amnesics is thought to be mediated by the parahippocampal regions (Vargha-Khadem, Gadian, & Mishkin, 2001). In this view, developmental amnesics have intact familiarity-based recognition (mediated by parahippocampal regions) that is sufficient for good performance on tests of recognition but have impaired recollection-based recognition and recall memory (mediated by hippocampus). In other words, developmental amnesics might have a more "infant-like" organization of memory systems. If so, study of both these patients and developing infants provides the unique opportunity of assessing the characteristics of familiarity-based memory in isolation from recollection-based memory in a way not possible in adults.

Which Model?

The relative contributions of the hippocampus and perirhinal cortex to recognition memory in adults remains unresolved (Murray & Bussey, 1999); thus it is not surprising that their involvement in infant recognition memory is also not clearly established. The evidence from studies of the visual-paired comparison task provides compelling evidence that the medial temporal lobe is functioning from early in life and plays a role in mediation of infant memory. If the hippocampus functions early in life primarily to orient the infant toward novelty (Nelson, 1995), then the familiarity-based memory function of the perirhinal cortex may develop at the same time or be responsible for improvements in infant memory in the second half of the first year (Bachevalier, 2001). Unlearned biases, such as the bias to orient to faces, may result in faster development of recognition abilities for these stimuli. Among the proposed roles of the perirhinal cortex in adults is in encoding of visual features and complex conjunctions between them

(Murray & Bussey, 1999) and the ability to recognize an object regardless of viewpoint, size, and so on. Thus, development in the perirhinal cortex may also contribute to infants' visual recognition abilities by allowing them to form perceptual categories and to form more effective memory representations of complex objects and categories through processing of conjunction of features. These functions are similar to those proposed for the CONLERN system in the two-process theory of face recognition (Johnson & de Haan, 2001).

CONCLUSIONS

From the first days of life, infants are able to recognize a visual stimulus they have recently seen, and by the first half-year of life they are able to recognize it even days or weeks later. However, whether or not recognition is observed depends heavily on the characteristics of the learning and recognition testing procedures. Collectively the studies suggest that infants may be most likely to show evidence of recognition if they are given relatively prolonged, distributed exposure to a face and are tested for recognition with a pair of faces that are distinct from one another—and if they still appear to forget, a reminder can help. However, further systematic study of how these various factors influence *delayed* recognition at different ages will be informative, as the majority of studies have focused mainly on immediate memory and single age groups.

Four possible models of infants' memory were presented. Evidence from studies of the neural bases of memory make the implicit memory hypothesis unlikely. While implicit memory is likely operating early in infancy, it is not likely the only type of memory. The weight of evidence pointing to the importance of the hippocampus for memory assessed in visual-paired comparisons appears more in favor of the preexplicit memory view than the familiarity-based memory view. However, in the studies of infant monkeys, lesions were not confined strictly to the hippocampus and included surrounding tissue. Moreover, these hypotheses are not mutually exclusive and may complement one another. The current emphasis on the existence of at least precursor forms of explicit memory in infants converges with the view formulated from behavioral studies of some continuities in memory processes from infancy to adulthood.

Formulating theories based on the pattern of performance of adults with brain damage or older children who experienced brain damage as children can be informative. Moreover, the idea that development consists of different adultlike abilities "switching on" at different times is appealing because it would provide the opportunity to study certain abilities in isolation in a way that is not possible in adults. However, this perspective can lead to false conclusions about the nature of infant memory. The same task may normally be mediated by different neural structures in infants and adults;

thus neuropsychological models of infant memory based on studies of adults with brain lesions may not apply to infants. Evidence from studies of infant monkeys shows that the connectivity of key structures in the medial temporal lobe memory system, including the perirhinal cortex, differs from that in adults in that there are some connections present in infants but not adults and some connections present at both ages but more widespread in infants (Webster, Ungerleider, & Bachevalier, 1991; cf. Rodman and also Finlay, Clancy, & Kingsbury, this volume). The brain is also capable of remarkable plasticity, so models of infant memory based on the effects of early lesions on functioning later in life may also not be representative of the neural organization at the earlier time point. These considerations emphasize the importance of developing models of infant memory based on studies of infants, as those based on adult models of memory will likely fail to capture unique characteristics of the developing system. Continued research applying neuroimaging techniques (reviewed in Thomas & Casey, in press) and neural network models of memory (reviewed in Hasselmo & McClelland, 1999) to questions of development are promising approaches.

NOTES

1. As the topic of this chapter is visual recognition memory, it will focus on studies that allow conclusions about infants' recognition (usually by comparing responses to novel and familiar stimuli) rather than on memory more generally. Thus, it will not cover studies of infants' delayed imitation or other paradigms that do not assess recognition memory per se.

2. This syndrome differs from amnesia observed in adults in several aspects, but relevant to this topic is that, unlike adult amnesics, who have deficits in both recall and recognition memory, the amnesic children display clear deficits only in delayed recall, showing comparatively preserved recognition memory.

REFERENCES

Ackles, P.K., & Cook, K.G. (1998). Stimulus probability and event-related potentials of the brain in 6-month-old human infants: A parametric study. *International Journal of Psychophysiology, 29*, 115–143.

Allison, T. (1984). Recording and interpreting event-related potentials. In E. Donchin (Ed.), *Cognitive psychophysiology: Event-related potentials and the study of cognition* (pp. 1–36). Hillsdale, NJ: Lawrence Erlbaum.

Bachevalier, J. (2001). Neural bases of memory development: Insights from neuropsychological studies in primates. In C.A. Nelson & M. Luciana (Eds.), *Handbook of developmental cognitive neuroscience* (pp. 365–379). Cambridge, MA: MIT Press.

Bachevalier, J., Brickson, M., & Hagger, C. (1993). Limbic-dependent recognition memory in monkeys develops early in infancy. *NeuroReport, 4*, 77–80.

Bachevalier, J., & Mishkin, M. (1984). An early and a late developing system for learning and retention in infant monkeys. *Behavioral Neuroscience, 98,* 770–778.

Baddeley, A., Vargha-Khadem, F., & Mishkin, M. (2001). Preserved recognition in a case of developmental amnesia: Implications for semantic memory? *Journal of Cognitive Neuroscience, 13,* 357–369.

Baddeley, A.D., & Warrington, E.K. (1970). Amnesia and the distinction between long- and short-term memory. *Journal of Verbal Learning and Verbal Behavior, 9,* 176–189.

Bahrick, L.E., Hernandez-Reif, M., & Pickens, J.N. (1997). The effect of retrieval cues on visual preferences and memory in infancy: Evidence for a four-phase attention function. *Journal of Experimental Child Psychology, 67,* 1–20.

Bahrick, L.E., & Pickens, J.N. (1995). Infant memory for object motion across a period of three months: Implications for a four-phase attention function. *Journal of Experimental Child Psychology, 59,* 343–371.

Banks, M., & Ginsburg, A.P. (1985). Infant visual preferences: A review and new theoretical treatment. *Advances in Child Development and Behavior, 19,* 207–246.

Banks, M., & Salapatek, P. (1981). Infant pattern vision: A new approach based on the contrast sensitivity function. *Journal of Experimental Child Psychology, 31,* 1–45.

Bauer, P.J. (1995). Recalling past events: From infancy to early childhood. *Annals of Child Development, 11,* 25–71.

Benson, P.J., & Perrett, D.I. (1991). Perception and recognition of photographic quality facial caricatures: Implications for recognition of natural images. *European Journal of Cognitive Psychology, 3,* 105–135.

Bornstein, M.H. (1985). Habituation as a measure of visual information processing in human infants: Summary, systematization and synthesis. In G.H Gottlieb & N.A. Krasnegor (Eds.), *The measurement of audition and vision in the first year of postnatal life: A methodological overview* (pp. 253–300). Norwood, NJ: Ablex Press.

Borovsky, D., & Rovee-Collier, C. (1990). Contextual constraints on memory retrieval at six months. *Child Development, 61,* 1569–1583.

Bushnell, I.W.R., Sai, R., & Mullin, J.T. (1989). Neonatal recognition of the mother's face. *British Journal of Developmental Psychology, 7,* 3–15.

Carver, L.J., Bauer, P.J., & Nelson, C.A. (2000). Associations between infant brain activity and recall memory. *Developmental Science, 3,* 234–246.

Clark, R.E., Teng, E., Squire, L.R., & Zola, S. (1996). The visual-paired-comparison task and the medial temporal lobe memory system. *Society for Neuroscience Abstract, 22,* 281.

Clark, R.E., Teng, E., Squire, L.R., & Zola, S. (1997). Perirhinal damage impairs memory in visual-paired comparison task. *Society for Neuroscience Abstract, 23,* 12–18.

Cornell, E.H. (1974). Infants' discrimination of photographs of faces following redundant presentations. *Journal of Experimental Child Psychology, 18,* 98–106.

Cornell, E.H. (1980). Distributed study facilitates infants' delayed recognition memory. *Memory & Cognition, 8,* 539–542.

Courage, M.L., & Howe, M.L. (1998). The ebb and flow of infant attentional preferences: Evidence for long-term recognition memory in 3-month-olds. *Journal of Experimental Child Psychology, 70,* 26–53.

Courchesne, E., Ganz, L., & Norcia, A.M. (1981). Event-related potentials to human faces in infants. *Child Development, 52,* 804–811.

de Haan, M., Johnson, M.H., Maurer, D., & Perrett, D.I. (2001). Recognition of individual faces and average face prototypes by 1- and 3-month-old infants. *Cognitive Development, 16,* 659–678.

de Haan, M., & Nelson, C.A. (1997). Recognition of the mother's face by six-month-old infants: A neurobehavioral study. *Child Development, 68,* 187–210.

de Haan, M., & Nelson, C.A. (1999). Brain activity differentiates face and object processing by 6-month-old infants. *Developmental Psychology, 34,* 1114–1121.

Diamond, A. (1990). Rate of maturation of the hippocampus and the developmental progression of children's performance on the delayed non-matching to sample and visual-paired comparison tasks. In A. Diamond (Ed.), *The development and neural bases of higher cognitive functions. Annals of the New York Academy of Sciences Vol. 608* (pp. 394–433). New York: New York Academy of Sciences.

Diamond, A. (1995). Evidence of robust recognition memory early in life even when assessed by reaching behavior. *Journal of Experimental Child Psychology, 59,* 419–456.

Dolan, R.J., & Fletcher, P.C. (1997). Dissociating prefrontal and hippocampal function in episodic memory encoding. *Nature, 388,* 582–585.

Drachman, D., & Arbit, K. (1966). Memory and the hippocampal complex. *Archives of Neurology, 15,* 52–61.

Elliott, R., & Dolan, R.J. (1998). Neural response during preference and memory judgements for subliminally presented stimuli: A functional neuroimaging study. *Journal of Neuroscience, 18,* 4697–4704.

Fagan, J.F. (1972). Infants' recognition memory for faces. *Journal of Experimental Child Psychology, 14,* 453–476.

Fagan, J.F. (1973). Infants' delayed recognition memory and forgetting. *Journal of Experimental Child Psychology, 16,* 424–450.

Fagan, J.F. (1974). Infant recognition memory: The effects of length of familiarisation and type of discrimination task. *Child Development, 45,* 351–356.

Fagan, J.F. (1977). Infant recognition memory: Studies in forgetting. *Child Development, 48,* 68–78.

Fagan, J.F. (1978). Facilitation of infants' recognition memory. *Child Development, 49,* 1066–1075.

Gadian, D.G., Aicardi, J., Watkins, K.E., Porter, D.A., Mishkin, M., & Vargha-Khadem, F. (2000). Developmental amnesia associated with early hypoxic-ischaemic injury. *Brain, 123,* 499–507.

Haist, F., Bowden Gore, J., & Mao, H. (2001). Consolidation of human memory over decades revealed by functional magnetic resonance imaging. *Nature Neuroscience, 4,* 1139–1145.

Hasselmo, M.E., & McClelland, J.L. (1999). Neural models of memory. *Current Opinions in Neurobiology, 9,* 184–188.

Hayne, H., Boniface, J., & Barr, R. (2000). The development of declarative memory in human infants: Age-related changes in deferred imitation. *Behavioral Neuroscience, 114,* 77–83.

Hayne, H., Greco, L., Earley, P., Griesler, P., & Rovee-Collier, C. (1986). The ontogeny of early event memory: II. Encoding and retrieval by 2- and 3-month-olds. *Infant Behavior and Development, 9,* 441–460.

Hayne, H., Rovee-Collier, C., & Perris, E.E. (1987). Categorization and memory retrieval by three-month-olds. *Child Development, 58,* 750–760.

Hepper, P.G. (1988). Foetal "soap" addiction. *Lancet, 1,* 1347–1348.

Hepper, P.G. (1991). An examination of fetal learning before and after birth. *Irish Journal of Psychology, 12,* 95–107.

Horn, G. (1985). *Memory, imprinting, and the brain: An inquiry into mechanisms.* Oxford: Clarendon Press.

Horn, G. (1998). Visual imprinting and the neural mechanisms of recognition memory. *Trends in Neurosciences, 21,* 300–305.

Howe, M.L., & Courage, M.L. (1997). Independent paths in the development of infant learning and forgetting. *Journal of Experimental Child Psychology, 67,* 131–163.

Hunt, J.M. (1963). Piaget's observations as a source of hypotheses concerning motivation. *Merrill-Palmer Quarterly, 9,* 263–275.

Johnson, M.H., & Bolhuis, J.J. (1991). Imprinting, predispositions and filial preference in the chick. In R.H. Andrew (Ed.), *Neural and behavioral plasticity* (pp. 133–156). Oxford: Oxford University Press.

Johnson, M.H., Bolhuis, J.J., & Horn, G. (1985). Interaction between acquired preferences and developing predispositions during imprinting. *Animal Behavior, 33,* 1000–1006.

Johnson, M.H., & de Haan, M. (2001). Developing cortical specialisation for visual-cognitive function: The case of face recognition. In J.L. McClelland & R.S. Seigler (Eds.), *Mechanisms of cognitive development: Behavioral and neural perspectives* (pp. 253–270). Mahwah, NJ: Lawrence Erlbaum Associates.

Johnson, M.H., de Haan, M., Oliver, A., Smith, W., Hatzakis, H., Tucker, L.A., & Csibra, G. (In press). Recording and analyzing high density ERPs with infants using the geodesic sensor net. *Developmental Neuropsychology, 19,* 295–323.

Johnson, M.H., & Horn, G. (1986). Dissociation of recognition memory and associative learning by a restricted lesion of the chick forebrain. *Neuropsychologia, 24,* 329–340.

Johnson, M.H., & Horn, G. (1987). The role of a restricted region of the chick forebrain in the recognition of individual CONSPECifics. *Behavioral Brain Research, 23,* 269–275.

Johnson, M.H., & Horn, G. (1988). The development of filial preferences in the dark-reared chick. *Animal Behavior, 36,* 675–683.

Johnson, M.H., & Morton, J. (1991). *Biology and cognitive development: The case of face recognition.* Oxford: Blackwell.

Karrer, R., & Ackles, P.K. (1987). Visual event-related potentials of infants during a modified oddball procedure. *Electroencephalography and Clinical Neurophysiology, 49* (Suppl)., 603–608.

Karrer, R., & Monti, L.A. (1995). Event-related potentials of 4–7-week-old infants in a visual recognition memory task. *Electroencephalography and Clinical Neurophysiology, 94,* 414–424.

Kleiner, K.A., & Banks, M.S. (1987). Stimulus energy does not account for 2-month-olds' face preferences. *Journal of Experimental Psychology: Human Perception and Performance, 13,* 594–600.

Mahut, H., Zola-Morgan, S., & Moss, M. (1982). Hippocampal resections impair associative learning and recognition memory in the monkey. *Journal of Neuroscience, 2,* 1214–1229.

Malkova, L., Pixely, G.L., Webster, M.J., Mishkin, M., & Bachevalier, J. (1998). The effects of early rhinal cortex lesions on visual recognition memory in rhesus monkeys. *Society for Neuroscience Abstracts, 24,* 1906.

Manns, J.R., Stark, E.L., & Squire, L.R. (2000). The visual-paired-comparison task as a measure of declarative memory. *Proceedings of the National Academy of Science (USA), 97,* 12375–12379.

Marler, P. (1997). Three models of song learning: Evidence from behavior. *Journal of Neurobiology, 33,* 501–516.

McCabe, B.J., Cipolla-Neto, J., Horn, G., & Bateson, P.P.G. (1982). Amnesiac effects of bilateral lesions placed in the hyperstriatum ventrale of the chick after imprinting. *Experimental Brain Research, 48,* 13–21.

McCabe, B.J., & Nicol, A.U. (1999). The recognition memory of imprinting: Biochemistry and electrophysiology. *Behavioral Brain Research, 98,* 253–260.

McKee, R.D., & Squire, L.R. (1993). On the development of declarative memory. *Journal of Experimental Psychology: Learning, Memory and Cognition, 19,* 397–404.

Milner, B. (1965). Visually-guided maze learning in man: Effects of bilateral hippocampal, bilateral frontal and unilateral cerebral lesions. *Neuropsychologia, 3,* 317–338.

Milner, B. (1966). Amnesia following operations on the temporal lobes. In C.W.M. Whitty & O.L. Zangwill (Eds.), *Amnesia* (pp. 109–133). London: Butterworth.

Milner, B., Corkin, S., & Teuber, H.-L. (1968). Further analysis of the hippocampal amnesic syndrome: 14-year follow-up of H.M. *Neuropsychologia, 6,* 215–234.

Mishkin, M., Suzuki, W., Gadian, D.G., & Vargha-Khadem, F. (1997). Hierarchical organization of cognitive memory. *Philosophical Transactions of the Royal Society London B, 352,* 1461–1467.

Mishkin, M., Vargha-Khadem, F., & Gadian, D.G. (1998). Amnesia and the organisation of the hippocampal system. *Hippocampus, 8,* 212–216.

Morton, J., & Johnson, M.H. (1991). CONSPEC and CONLERN: A two-process theory of infant face recognition. *Psychological Review, 2,* 164–181.

Murray, E.A., & Bussey, T.J. (1999). Perceptual-mnemonic functions of the perirhinal cortex. *Trends in Cognitive Sciences, 3,* 142–151.

Nachman, P.A., Stern, D.N., & Best, C. (1986). Affective reactions to stimuli and infants' preference for novelty and familiarity. *Journal of the American Academy of Child Psychiatry, 25,* 801–804.

Nadel, L., & Zola-Morgan, S. (1984). Infantile amnesia: A neurobiological perspective. In M. Moscovitch (Ed.), *Infant memory* (pp. 145–172). New York: Plenum.

Nelson, C.A. (1994). Neural correlates of recognition memory in the first postnatal year of life. In G. Dawson & K. Fischer (Eds.), *Human behavior and the developing brain* (pp. 269–313). New York: Guilford Press.

Nelson, C.A. (1995). The ontogeny of human memory: A cognitive neuroscience perspective. *Developmental Psychology, 31,* 723–738.

Nelson, C.A., & Collins, P.F. (1991). Event-related potential and looking-time analysis of infants' responses to familiar and novel events: Implications for recognition memory. *Developmental Psychology, 27,* 50–58.

Nelson, C.A., & Collins, P.F. (1992). Neural and behavioral correlates of recognition memory in 4- and 8-month-old infants. *Brain & Cognition, 19,* 105–121.

Nelson, C.A., & Monk, C. (2001). The use of event-related potentials in the study of cognitive development. In C.A. Nelson & M. Luciana (Eds.), *Handbook of developmental cognitive neuroscience* (pp. 125–136). Cambridge, MA: MIT Press.

Nelson, C.A., Thomas, K.M., de Haan, M., & Wewerka, S.S. (1998). Delayed recognition memory in infants and adults as revealed by event-related potentials. *International Journal of Psychophysiology, 29,* 145–165.

Nelson, C.A., & Webb, S.J. (In press). A cognitive neuroscience perspective on early memory development. In M. de Haan & M.H. Johnson (Eds.), *The cognitive neuroscience of development.*

Overman, W.H. (1990). Performance on traditional matching to sample, non-matching to sample, and object discrimination tasks by 12- to 32-month-old children. In A. Diamond (Ed.), *The development and neural bases of higher cognitive functions. Annals of the New York Academy of Sciences, Vol. 608* (pp. 394–433). New York: New York Academy of Sciences. 365–393.

Overman, W.H., Bachevalier, J., Turner, M., & Peuster, A. (1992). Object recognition versus object disrimination: Comparison between human infants and infant monkeys. *Behavioral Neuroscience, 106,* 15–29.

Pancratz, C.N., & Cohen, L.H. (1970). Recovery of habituation in infants. *Journal of Experimental Child Psychology, 9,* 208–216.

Pascalis, O., & Bachevalier, J. (1999). Neonatal aspiration lesions of the hippocampal formation impair visual recognition memory when assessed by paired-comparison task but not by delayed nonmatching-to-sample task. *Hippocampus, 9,* 609–616.

Pascalis, O., & de Haan, M. (In press). Recognition memory and novelty preference: What model? In H. Hayne & J. Fagen (Eds.), *Progress in infancy research* (Vol. 3).

Pascalis, O. de Haan, M., Nelson, C.A., de Schonen, S. (1998). Long-term recognition assessed by visual-paired comparison in 3- and 6-month-old infants. *Journal of Experimental Psychology: Learning, Memory and Cognition, 24,* 249–260.

Pascalis, O., & de Schonen, S. (1994), Recognition memory in 3- to 4-day-old human neonates. *NeuroReport, 5,* 1721–1724.

Pascalis, O., de Schonen, S., Morton, J., Deruelle, C., & Fabre-Grent, M. (1995).

Mother's face recognition by neonates: A replication and an extension. *Infant Behavior and Development, 18,* 79–95.

Quinn, P.C. (1998). Object and spatial categorisation in young infants: "What" and "where" in early visual perception. In A. Slater (Ed.), *Perceptual development: Visual, auditory and speech perception in infancy* (pp. 131–165). Hove, UK: Psychology Press.

Rhodes, G. (1993). Configural coding, expertise, and the right hemisphere advantage for face recognition. *Brain & Cognition, 22,* 19–41.

Rhodes, G., Tan, S., Brake, S., & Taylor, K. (1989). Race sensitivity in face recognition: An effect of different encoding processes. In A.F. Bennett & K.M. McConkey (Eds.), *Cognition in individual and social contexts* (pp. 83–90). Amsterdam: Elsevier.

Richards, J.E. (1997). Effects of attention on infants' preference for briefly exposed visual stimuli in the paired-comparison recognition-memory paradigm. *Developmental Psychology, 33,* 22–31.

Richards, J.E. (2000). *The effect of attention on the recognition of brief visual stimuli: An ERP study.* Paper presented at the International Conference on Infancy Studies, Brighton, UK, July.

Richards, J.E. (2001). Attention in young infants: A developmental psychophysiological perspective. In C.A. Nelson & M. Luciana (Eds.), *Handbook of developmental cognitive neuroscience* (pp. 321–338). Cambridge, MA: MIT Press.

Rose, S.A. (1981). Developmental changes in infants' retention of visual stimuli. *Child Development, 52,* 227–233.

Rose, S.A., & Feldman, J.F. (1997). Memory and speed: Their role in the relation of infant information processing to later IQ. *Child Development, 68,* 630–641.

Rose, S.A., Feldman, J.F., & Jankowski, J.J. (2001). Visual short-term memory in the first year of life: Capacity and recency effects. *Developmental Psychology, 37,* 539–549.

Rose, S.A., Futterweit, L.R., & Jankowski, J. (1999). The relation of affect to attention and learning in infancy. *Child Development, 70,* 549–559.

Rose, S.A., Gottfried, A.W., Melloy-Carminar, P., & Bridger, W.H. (1982). Familiarity and novelty preference in infant recognition memory: Implications for information processing. *Developmental Psychology, 18,* 704–713.

Rovee-Collier, C. (1990). The "memory system" of prelinguistic infants. In A. Diamond (Ed.), *The development and neural bases of higher cognitive functions. Annals of the New York Academy of Sciences, Vol. 608* (pp. 517–542). New York: New York Academy of Sciences.

Rovee-Collier, C. (1997). Dissociations in infant memory: Rethinking the development of implicit and explicit memory. *Psychological Review, 104,* 467–498.

Rovee-Collier, C. (2001). Information pick-up by infants: What is it, and how can we tell? *Journal of Experimental Child Psychology, 78,* 35–49.

Rovee-Collier, C., & Shyi, G. (1992). A functional and cognitive analysis of infant long-term retention. In M.L. Howe, C.H. Brainerd, & V.F. Reyna (Eds.), *Development of long-term retention* (pp. 3–55). New York: Spinger.

Rovee-Collier, C.K., & Sullivan, M.W. (1980). Organization of infant memory.

Journal of Experimental Psychology: Human Learning and Memory, 6, 798–807.

Rugg., M.D., Fletcher, P.C., Frith, C.D., Frackowiak, R.S.J., & Dolan, R.J. (1997). Brain regions supporting intentional and incidental memory: A PET study. *NeuroReport, 8,* 1283–1287.

Schacter, D.L., Alpert, N.M., Savage, C.R., Rauch, S.L., & Albert, M.S. (1996). Conscious recollection and the human hippocampal formation: Evidence from positron emission tomography. *Proceedings of the National Academy of Sciences (USA), 93,* 321–325.

Schacter, D.L., & Moscovitch, M. (1984). Infants, amnesics and dissociable memory systems. In M. Moscovitch (Ed.), *Infant memory* (pp. 173–216). New York: Plenum.

Schwartz, M. (1975). The effect of constant vs. varied encoding and massed vs. distributed presentations on recall of paired associates. *Memory & Cognition, 3,* 390–394.

Scoville, W.B., & Milner, B. (1957). Loss of recent memory after bilateral hippocampal lesions. *Journal of Neurology, Neurosurgery & Psychiatry, 20,* 11–21.

Seress, L. (2001). Morphological changes of the human hippocampal formation from midgestation to early childhood. In C.A. Nelson & M. Luciana (Eds.), *Handbook of developmental cognitive neuroscience* (pp. 45–58). Cambridge, MA: MIT Press.

Simion, F., Macchi Cassia, V., Turati, C., & Valenza, E. (2001). The origins of face perception: Specific vs. non-specific mechanisms. *Infant and Child Development, 10,* 59–65.

Slater, A., Morison, V., & Rose, D. (1982). Visual memory at birth. *British Journal of Psychology, 73,* 519–525.

Sophian, C. (1980). Habituation is not enough: Novelty preferences, search and memory in infancy. *Merrill-Palmer Quarterly, 26,* 239–257.

Squire, L.R. (1992). Declarative and nondeclarative memory: Multiple brain systems supporting learning and memory. *Journal of Cognitive Neurscience, 4,* 232–243.

Squire, L.R., & Knowlton, B.J. (1995). Memory, hippocampus, and brain systems. In M. Gazzaniga (Ed.), *The cognitive neurosciences* (pp. 825–837). Cambridge, MA: MIT Press.

Stanton, M.E. (2000). Multiple memory systems, development, and conditioning. *Behavioral Brain Research, 110,* 25–37.

Strange, B.A., Fletcher, P.C., Henson, R.N.A., Friston, K.J., & Dolan, R.J. (1999). Segregating the functions of the human hippocampus. *Proceedings of the National Academy of Sciences (USA), 96,* 4034–4039.

Sullivan, M.W. (1982). Reactivation: Priming forgotten memories in human infants. *Child Development, 53,* 516–523.

Sullivan, M.W., Rovee-Collier, C.K., & Tynes, D.M. (1979). A conditioning analysis of infant long term memory. *Child Development, 50,* 152–162.

Taylor, M., & Baldeweg, T. (In press). Basic principles and applications of EEG, ERPs, and intracranial methods. *Developmental Science.*

Thomas, K.M., & Casey, B.J. (In press). Methods for imaging the developing brain.

In M. de Haan & M.H. Johnson (Eds.), *The cognitive neuroscience of development*.

Thompson, R.F., & Kim, J.J. (1996). Memory systems in the brain and localization of a memory. *Proceedings of the National Academy of Sciences (USA), 93*, 13438–13488.

Valenza, E., Simion, F., Cassia, V.M., & Umilta, C. (1996). Face preference at birth. *Journal of Experimental Psychology: Human Perception and Performance, 22*, 892–903.

Vargha-Khadem, F., Gadian, D.G., & Mishkin, M. (2001). Dissociations in cognitive memory: The syndrome of developmental amnesia. *Philosophical Transactions of the Royal Society, London, 356*, 1–6.

Vargha-Khadem, F., Gadian, D.G., Watkins, K.E., Connelly, A., Van Paesschen, W., & Mishkin, M. (1997). Differential effects of early hippocampal pathology on episodic and semantic memory. *Science, 277*, 376–380.

Webb, S., & Nelson, C.A. (2001). Perceptual priming for upright and inverted faces in infants and adults. *Journal of Experimental Child Psychology, 79*, 1–22.

Webster, M.J., Ungerleider, L.G., & Bachevalier, J. (1991). Connections of inferior temporal areas TE and TEO with medial temporal-lobe structures in infant and adult monkeys. *Journal of Neuroscience, 11*, 1095–1116.

Zola, S.M., Squire, L.R., Teng, E., Stefanacci, L., Buffalo, E.A., & Clark, R.E. (2000). Impaired recognition memory in monkeys after damage limited to the hippocampal region. *Journal of Neuroscience, 20*, 451–463.

Zola-Morgan, S., & Squire, L.R. (1986). Memory impairment in monkeys following lesions limited to the hippocampus. *Behavioral Neuroscience, 100*, 155–160.

Zola-Morgan, S., Squire, L.R., & Amaral, D.G. (1989). Lesions of the hippocampal formation but not lesions of the fornix or mamillary nuclei produce long-lasting memory impairment in monkeys. *Journal of Neuroscience, 9*, 897–912.

Chapter 5

Where Are They Going?
The Perception of Information about
Visual Direction in Young Infants

Rick O. Gilmore

ABSTRACT

Recent evidence suggests that young infants' abilities to perceive information about different aspects of visual direction may have a prolonged developmental time course. Specifically, 3- to 5-month-old infants may represent the static direction of simple visual targets in a primitive eye-centered coordinate system and may not discriminate direction of observer motion information from optic flow especially well. Subsequent changes in these abilities are probably due to the joint influence of perceptual, experiential, and neurological factors, in particular, development in regions of the visual cortex that process multimodal spatial information. Taken together, these studies of static and dynamic visual direction suggest that spatial processing may function quite differently in very young infants compared with older children or adults, and they illustrate how an integrated multilevel approach to the development of spatial vision in early infancy might proceed.

INTRODUCTION

Many forms of human perceptual, cognitive, and motor behavior depend upon information about spatial relationships, such as the direction and distance of objects or surfaces in the environment. Current accounts of spatial processing in adults highlight the importance of circuits in the cerebral cortex associated with the dorsal visual processing stream (Andersen, 1997; Milner & Goodale, 1995; Ungerleider & Mishkin, 1982). While there is considerable complexity in the circuitry, the dorsal visual processing stream originates in areas V1 and V2 of visual cortex and projects to regions in the posterior superior temporal and parietal lobes. These areas appear to represent spatial relationships in multiple, interacting coordinate systems in which visual and nonvisual sources of information are systematically integrated (Andersen, 1997; Stein, 1992). Multiple dorsal stream systems contribute to processing associated with movement of the arms, head, and eyes (Andersen, 1997; Milner & Goodale, 1995), as well. Several dorsal stream regions, especially those involved in motion processing, are heavily interconnected with a companion ventral stream that projects toward regions in the inferior occipital and temporal lobes. The ventral stream appears functionally specialized for processing shape, color, and form. While many details about how processing within and between the two streams operates remain poorly understood, dorsal stream systems clearly play a central role in visual processing related to spatial relationships and action planning.

However, neuroanatomical (Conel, 1939–1967; Huttenlocher, 1990; Huttenlocher & Dabholkar, 1997), neurophysiological (Chugani & Phelps, 1986; Chugani, Müller, & Chugani, 1996), and behavioral (Atkinson, 1984; Bronson, 1982; Johnson, 1990) evidence suggests that many cortical areas, including primary visual cortex and the dorsal stream systems to which it projects, may not be functionally mature at birth but instead develop rapidly over the first several months of life. Accordingly, spatial processing may function quite differently in very young infants compared with older children or adults (Newcombe & Huttenlocher, 2000; Yonas & Granrud, 1985), due at least in part to changes in the functional maturity of neural circuitry associated with visual perception and action planning (Gilmore & Johnson, 1997a, 1997b). If this is so, then a complete account of the development of spatial perception and action planning in infancy should, among other objectives, aim to associate specific changes in infants' behavior with developments in visual processing systems that have relatively well-defined functional characteristics. This goal is an ambitious one, and it has not yet been achieved. However, this chapter will describe recent research that attempts to illustrate some of the strengths of an integrated approach to the question of how certain aspects of spatial vision develop in early infancy.

One way to cast the goal of spatial perception is to specify that its aim is to determine the locations and paths of objects relative to the viewer, or conversely, of the viewer relative to the environment, in a spherical coordinate system centered on the viewer. In this characterization, there are essentially two dimensions of direction, azimuth and elevation, and one of distance. Over the past 20 years or so, a number of authors have advanced our understanding of infants' sensitivity to various forms of information about depth, such as binocular disparity (Birch, Gwiazda, & Held, 1982; Held, Birch, & Gwiazda, 1980), motion-related cues (Craton & Yonas,

1990; Nañez, 1987; Schmuckler & Li, 1998; von Hofsten, Kellman, & Putaansuu, 1992), and pictorial information (Yonas, Arterberry, & Granrud, 1987; Yonas & Granrud, 1985). While there is some evidence that infants can discriminate the rudimentary features of certain pictorial depth relations (Bhatt & Waters, 1998) within the first 3 months, the bulk of the evidence suggests that there is a specific sequence in the emergence of sensitivity to depth information. Sensitivity to motion-defined changes in depth emerges first, within the first 2 to 3 months of life. Binocular processing of retinal disparity information emerges somewhat later, between 3 and 5 months of age, and not until infants are 5 to 7 months old does reliable evidence emerge that pictorial cues to depth are actively perceived and used to guide behavior.

Furthermore, while the biological underpinnings of many other aspects of depth perception are beyond our current understanding, several authors have sought to associate certain changes in infants' sensitivity to depth information to specific biological milestones. The sudden onset and rapid development of stereoacuity is one example. It has been argued that the formation of eye-specific processing regions or ocular dominance columns in primary visual cortex is the principal neural event associated with the onset of stereopsis (Held, 1985). We now know that in both the cat (Pettigrew, 1974) and monkey (LeVay, Wiesel, & Hubel, 1980) the process of ocular dominance column segregation continues for several weeks postnatally, and the completion of segregation occurs at about the time of the onset of stereopsis (O'Dell, Quick, & Boothe, 1991; Timney, 1981). As a result, it appears that the onset of binocular stereo vision may be quite closely associated with the completion of ocular dominance formation, although questions about why binocular function appears so abruptly in the face of gradual ocular dominance formation, among others, remain. More detailed discussions of these and related findings regarding changes in infants' spatial vision can be found elsewhere (Atkinson, 2000; Kellman & Banks, 1998).

In this chapter, I will discuss recent behavioral evidence concerning the development of young infants' abilities to perceive spatial aspects of the visual environment that have received relatively less attention both in terms of behavioral measures and neural correlates. In particular, I will focus on two lines of research related to the development of *direction perception* in the earliest months of postnatal life. The results will suggest that, like the case of sensitivity to depth information, notable changes occur in the first 6 months of life in infants' abilities to perceive and act upon information about visual direction. Moreover, while multiple factors almost certainly play a role in shaping processes of change, both aspects of direction perception activate specific, higher-order visual processing systems in adults. Accordingly, these aspects of spatial perception may, like the case of stereo vision, serve as instructive test cases for testing hypotheses about the link between behavioral change and development in specific biological substrates.

THE DEVELOPMENT OF DIRECTION PERCEPTION

How do infants perceive the direction of objects in the environment? The perception of direction may appear to be a simpler problem than the perception of depth since the normal optical projection onto the retina preserves direction information both locally and globally. Nevertheless, the perception of static direction and the perception of dynamic direction—the paths of self and object motion—are not as simple as they first appear. The human eyes, head, and body move, and each of these relatively independent types of movements changes visual information about direction in different ways. Some simple examples will help illustrate the point. An object that is on the left side of my visual field will move to the right side of my visual field if I move my eyes far to the left. When defining the visual direction of the object, do I specify it as on the left or on the right? Similarly, a large rotation of my head in one direction will induce a nearly uniform movement of the entire visual field in the opposite direction at approximately the same angular speed as my head movement. The pattern of visual movement is almost identical to that which would be induced if the visual world rotated around my head. How does the perceiver discriminate these situations from one another? The answers to both questions, of course, are (1) that information about visual direction is defined relative to specific coordinate systems or *frames of reference*; (2) that the perception of visual direction involves visual and *nonvisual* sources of information, namely, from proprioception; and (3) that the perception of visual direction may depend, in part, on what sort of action depends on the information. The same visual target can be to the right or left of my visual field, depending on where I fixate, but remain in the same position relative to my head or body. Perceiving visual direction relative to my visual field may be useful in planning head and eye movements, whereas perceiving direction relative to my body, which requires combining visual information with eye and head movement information, may be useful for planning other actions such as arm or body movements. In short, the perception of direction information is complicated by the problem of defining the frame or frames of reference, by the requirement that visual and nonvisual information be integrated, at least in some cases, and by task demands.

Perceiving Static Direction

Most previous developmental research on the topic has indicated that infants younger than 6 months old initially perceive spatial locations using body-centered coordinates, sometimes called egocentric coordinates (Rieser,

1979). Gradually, sensitivity to direction information that is based on stable features of the environment, such as the location of specific cues or features, emerges (Acredolo, 1990; Piaget & Inhelder, 1948). This evidence largely comes from a series of studies in which infants are trained to make a specific looking response to one location, then are displaced to another location, and the pattern of their subsequent behavior is measured. The striking finding from tests using this paradigm (reviewed in Acredolo, 1990; Bremner, 1978) was that 9- to 11-month-old infants who were displaced by 180° from their original orientation toward a target window continued to look in the "incorrect" direction relative to their bodies, not the "correct" direction. Related research has shown, however, that infants' performance is improved when they are tested in familiar environments as opposed to the laboratory (Acredolo, 1979) and that infants as young as 6.5 months can discriminate changes in visual direction that are caused by self-movement from those that are caused by object movement (Kaufman & Needham, 1999). Related data from a task in which infants watch objects being buried and then retrieved from consistent or inconsistent locations in a sandbox apparatus show that the ability to discriminate direction information in environment-relative terms might emerge as young as 5 months (Newcombe & Huttenlocher, 2000). These data seem to suggest that body-centered and limited environment-centered coding of direction information emerge relatively early in the first year of life, at least under some conditions. However, it is not known whether these representations for action are prespecified and present from birth or whether they emerge gradually over the first year from an even more primitive coordinate system.

One way to address this question is to examine the development of a behavior that allows the influence of body-centered and non-body-centered sources of information about spatial location to be distinguished. The double-step saccade paradigm permits precisely this type of investigation (Aslin & Shea, 1987; Becker & Jürgens, 1979; Groll & Ross, 1982; Hallett & Lightstone, 1976a, 1976b). In this paradigm, participants are instructed to look at sequences of visual targets that flash briefly in a dark visual field; the second stimulus appears and disappears before or during the response to the first stimulus. The position of a target relative to the fovea, that is, its *eye-centered* position, is sufficient for planning a response to the first but not the second target. This is because the first eye movement shifts the center of gaze and, with it, the second target's position on the retina. Accordingly, to make an accurate *sequence* of saccades, participants in the double-step paradigm must incorporate additional nonvisual information, such as eye or head position, in planning their eye movements. Adults and school-age children make accurate saccades to both targets in most circumstances (Aslin & Shea, 1987; Becker & Jürgens, 1979; Groll & Ross, 1982; Hallett & Lightstone, 1976a, 1976b). This suggests that adults and older children do not represent visual target locations in eye-centered coordinates. Instead, these participants use either head-centered representations, which combine visual position with signals specifying eye position (Mays & Sparks, 1980), or eye-centered representations, which incorporate the effects of planned eye movements (Duhamel, Colby, & Goldberg, 1993).

In order to determine what spatial representations guide the perception of visual direction from the earliest months of life, Mark Johnson and I (Gilmore & Johnson, 1997a, 1997b) adapted the double-step paradigm for infants. We hypothesized that young infants would be more likely than older infants to code the location of visual targets in strictly visual or eye-centered coordinates. This prediction was based on the presumption that coding locations in head- or body-centered coordinates would require the accurate integration of visual information about target position and non-visual information about eye or head movements. The integration of these two sources of information presumably depends upon circuitry in the cortex that is initially immature. Specifically, we predicted that body-centered representations for visual targets would gradually strengthen in influence over the first several months of life but that initially visually based representations of location would dominate saccade planning.

In a series of experiments, we observed an increase with age in the prevalence of body-centered saccade sequences. Infants 3 to 5 months of age were more likely to make saccade sequences based on visual or eye-centered information alone, but 6- to 7-month-olds were more likely to base their responses on body-centered position information. The combined results supported the hypothesis that there is a shift in the representation that infants use in coding the direction of visual targets during the first several months after birth. The systematic integration of visual and eye position or movement information is associated with processing in the dorsal visual processing stream (Andersen, 1997; Andersen et al., 1993), specifically in eye movement–related areas LIP and 7a of the macaque monkey and analogous areas in humans. In particular, some human adults with lesions to parietal lobe structures make eye movement sequence errors that suggest the processing of body-centered direction is severely impaired (Duhamel et al., 1992). Accordingly, these results suggested to us that an eye-centered representation of visual direction dominates spatial perception and saccade planning in very young infants, due, at least in part, to immaturity in dorsal stream processing systems that integrate visual and nonvisual sources of information about direction. In turn, gradual development of cortical circuitry permits functional body-centered representations to emerge between 3 and 7 months of age.

This association between spatial representations used in simple eye movement planning and other forms of spatial processing is buttressed by a recent investigation of saccade patterns in children with Williams Syndrome (WS). Adults with Williams Syndrome often have severely impaired abilities in spatial cognition but relatively spared abilities in language and face processing (e.g., Karmiloff-Smith, 1998). Indeed, Atkinson and colleagues have proposed that the visuospatial deficits found in WS may result from impairments in the dorsal cortical stream of visual processing (Atkinson, 2000). Brown and colleagues (Brown et al., in press) tested this hypothesis by examining patterns of saccades made by normal infants, infants with Down Syndrome (DS), and infants with WS on the double-step saccade task. WS infants displayed evidence of saccade planning deficits, and some made more eye-centered than body-centered saccade sequences. This is striking given that the WS children were 2 to 3 years old at the time of testing. These results provide partial support for the notion that body-centered saccade sequences depend to some degree on the extent to which dorsal stream visual processing circuits develop normally.

Summary

Under some circumstances, particularly when infants themselves are moved and when the visual cues in the environment are rich, environment-centered representations of direction can be used to guide the visual orienting behavior of infants 5 to 6 months of age. On the other hand, the results from the double-step saccade studies suggest that when objects in the environment move and the visual information is limited, the perception of spatial direction in young infants may be biased toward a simpler, eye-centered coordinate system. Indeed, Johnson and I have suggested that an eye-centered representation of visual direction is the most primitive possible form of spatial coding and is likely to be predominant in very young infants. Certainly, we do not yet know what factors give rise to the observed shift toward body-centered and environment-centered coding of direction, but a strong case can be made that cortical development, particularly in extrastriate areas in which visual and nonvisual information is systematically integrated, plays a central role. There is some evidence suggesting that dorsal stream circuits associated with motion processing mature somewhat earlier than ventral stream systems (Distler et al., 1996), but at present, little detailed information is available about the extent or timing of anatomical or physiological development in dorsal stream circuits in humans. So conclusive statements will have to await these vitally important data.

Perceiving Dynamic Direction

A second form of direction perception concerns the extraction of the trajectories of moving objects toward the observer or of the observer's direction of motion through the environment. Determining an observer's direction and speed of self-motion, or heading, is vital for a variety of species in controlling posture and locomotion and avoiding collisions. Perhaps the most important source of information about heading is the pattern of visual motion generated by an observer moving through a rigid environment called optic flow (Gibson, 1966, 1979). Extensive empirical investigations with human adults have shown that from optic flow patterns alone an observer can determine their heading and the direction, distance, and orientation of objects and surfaces in the environment (Warren, 1998). Under a variety of conditions, adult observers determine their direction of heading from optic flow to within 1° of visual angle (Royden, Crowell, & Banks, 1994; Warren, Morris, & Kalish, 1988), an accuracy that is more than sufficient for steering across a wide range of speeds (Cutting et al., 1992). Furthermore, recent neurophysiological studies have shown that optic flow selectively activates specific regions of the visual association cortex in non-human primates (Duffy & Wurtz, 1991) and homologous areas in human adults (de Jong et al., 1994). Consequently, studying how human infants perceive their direction of motion or heading from optic flow may help to answer more general questions about spatial perception and action planning early in life and what factors shape development in this domain.

Rudimentary sensitivity to some patterns of optic flow emerges early. For example, in the first weeks of life infants begin to respond with eye blinks and backward head movements to patterns of optic flow that specify an impending collision with an object approaching the face (Ball & Tronick, 1971; Yonas, Pettersen, & Lockman, 1979). However, the behavior develops rather slowly. Not until approximately 3 months of age do infants blink 60 to 75% of the time (Nañez, 1987; Yonas, Pettersen, & Lockman, 1979). Further, Nañez and Yonas (1994) observed that both 4- and 8-month-old infants showed greater blinking and backward head movements to optically expanding textures when the elements' motions were on a single depth plane rather than on multiple depth planes. Thus, in addition to discriminating information about an object's extent in depth, 4-month-olds appear also to discriminate information about the form of the approaching surface (Nañez & Yonas, 1994). Early reports (Ball & Tronick, 1971) suggested that infants discriminated whether objects were approaching the face on a collision course or would pass by, but in fact, little is known about the precision of young infants' sensitivity to small changes in the direction or trajectory of moving objects or, as we will see shortly, of their own movements through space.

A second domain in which sensitivity to visual motion and optic flow has been examined focuses on movements of the head, hips, and torso that are associated with the stabilization and control of posture. Lee and Aronson (1974) demonstrated that oscillating patterns of optic flow presented in a moving room apparatus could induce 13- to 16-month-old children to sway or even fall down. Subsequent research has focused on even younger infants who are not yet able to walk or who are just beginning to do so. There are reports that newborn infants make directionally appropriate lateral head movements in response to moving stripe patterns (Jouen & Lepecq, 1989) and that infants within the first 1 to 2 months of age respond to oscillating patterns of visual motion (Pope, 1984). Bertenthal and colleagues have carried out the most extensive studies of young infants' postural responses in relation to visual motion. These studies have indicated that visual motion produced by a moving room can induce directionally appropriate compensatory shifts of the body's center of pressure in 5-month-olds (Bertenthal & Bai, 1989; Bertenthal, Rose, & Bai, 1997). The magnitude and consistency of response are considerably lower than that observed in older, 7-, 9-, and 11-month-old infants. However, in the second half of the first year of life, the regularity and strength with which oscillating optic flow patterns evoke compensatory postural responses at the oscillating frequency increase (Ashmead & McCarty, 1991; Bertenthal & Bai, 1989; Bertenthal, Rose, & Bai, 1997) and become functionally specific to the direction of imposed visual motion (Ashmead & McCarty, 1991).

The evidence that young infants, who are generally unable to sit well without support, respond to the direction of visual movement in the moving room has suggested that the development of sensitivity to optic flow may not be the rate-limiting factor in the visual control of posture (Bertenthal, Rose, & Bai, 1997). Unfortunately, this claim cannot be evaluated for several reasons. The fact that very young infants can respond to forward or backward patterns of visual motion with forward and backward movement of the head and body tells us that young children are *sensitive* to some aspects of the direction of visual motion, that this sensitivity can influence movement in different action systems, and that there are developmental changes that occur in the coupling between perceptual information and motor responses. But these data by themselves do not allow us to quantify infants' abilities or answer specific questions about what actually is developing. For example, there is at present no evidence about how accurately infants can perceive their direction of self-motion from visual information. We do not yet know at what age infants' accuracy is sufficient for balance control or locomotion, nor do we know how that accuracy changes over time. These are questions that the moving room studies provoke but do not answer. Moreover, because the perception of one's direction of self-motion presumably involves the systematic integration of visual, vestibular, and other proprioceptive sources of information, carefully studying the pattern, time course, and neural substrates of its development may be related to other dimensions of spatial perception.

If development in the discrimination of heading is analogous to the detection of impending collisions or to the perception of object form, heading perception might be relatively accurate early in life and undergo relatively minimal change in subsequent months. On the other hand, if the discrimination of heading information depends on the development of spatial processing mechanisms in the cerebral cortex and on an infant's capacity to actively generate optic flow patterns through locomotion, accuracy may be rather poor in young prelocomotor infants and develop only gradually. My students and I sought to examine this question in a series of studies I will now describe. Preliminary reports of some of these findings have appeared elsewhere (Gilmore, 2001; Rettke, Gilmore, & Pupik, 2000).

Testing Discrimination of Self-Motion Information Using Habituation

The first series of experiments examined whether 4-month-old infants would discriminate optic flow patterns that simulated different directions of self-motion. An infant-controlled habituation procedure was used in which infants viewed an optic flow display until their looking times reached a habituation criterion. Discrimination was tested based on the extent to which infants' looking time changed following the presentation of familiar or novel directions of motion.

The first experiment we conducted tested the discrimination of optic flow patterns depicting 180° changes in direction (forward versus backward). In all of the studies, the display consisted of a series of computer-generated movies that simulated linear translation across a ground plane at a speed of 30 meters per second. Each movie consisted of 50 individual frames presented at 30 frames per second that looped continuously until the experimenter ended the trial with a computer key press. Each frame of the display consisted of white dots (72 candles per square meter) presented on a black background (0.1 candles per square meter) at a density of 0.11 dots per degree squared. At the specified viewing distance, each dot was 0.4° square, and the viewing region was 40° (horizontal) by 30° (vertical). The locations of the dots were chosen at random for each trial, subject to the constraint that dot positions were uniformly distributed along the region of the simulated ground plane that was visible at the start of a trial. Dots remained the same size throughout the animation sequence, thereby eliminating any cue associated with the optic expansion of individual elements. A simulated eye height of 90 centimeters and a horizon truncated at 5,000 centimeters were used to compute dot positions. Dots that disappeared from view during a frame reappeared on the next frame at the simulated horizon in order to create the illusion of continuous motion in depth. Figure 5.1 shows a schematic of the display.

During the habituation phase, all participants viewed repeated presentations of a display that simulated translational motion in a single direction. The habituation threshold was computed following the procedure outlined by Ashmead and Davis (1996). Specifically, following the fifth habituation trial, the computer fitted a second-order polynomial to the look time data. When the fitted look time following a given trial dropped below 50% of the value of the fitted look time for the first habituation trial, the computer determined that the habituation criterion had been reached. Afterward, the computer presented the first of four test trials, which depicted either fa-

Habituation

Test

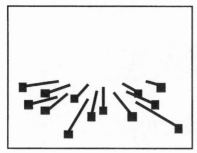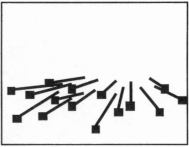

Figure 5.1. Schematic of optical flow display used in the heading discrimination studies using habituation. The dots are depicted in black, and the paths of the dots are indicated in order to improve the readability of the figure. In the actual display, the dots were white presented against a black background.

miliar or novel directions of motion. Thirty-one 4-month-old (107–129 days; 16 female) healthy, full-term infants participated.

Figure 5.2A summarizes the results. Four-month-old infants recovered looking time to the novel display when the change in direction was 180°. The mean look time to the test displays depicting a familiar direction of motion (M = 8.0 seconds, SD = 8.4) was smaller than looking time to the novel test displays (M = 13.3 seconds, SD = 11.9).

These data suggest that 4-month-old infants could discriminate optic flow displays depicting large changes in the direction of heading, at least under these circumstances. The result is consistent with other research in which infants at this age have been shown to discriminate objects moving forward from those moving backward (Schmuckler & Li, 1998; Yonas, Pettersen, & Lockman, 1979) by making different patterns of head movements and eye blinks. The results are also consistent with data showing that 5-month-olds make small but measurable changes in posture in response to forward-backward motion in a moving room (Bertenthal, Rose, & Bai, 1997). However, these data are the first to demonstrate that 4-month-old infants can discriminate displays depicting different directions of self-motion from motion cues alone—when the optic expansion of individual elements or parts is eliminated. Moreover, these results build upon previous findings by demonstrating that 4-month-olds are sensitive to direction of motion information contained in displays depicting only a ground surface. In particular, these results demonstrate that 4-month-olds' abilities to discriminate displays depicting different directions of motion are not confined to circumstances in which the visual information specifies a potential impending collision with the face.

Having demonstrated that infants discriminate between displays depict-

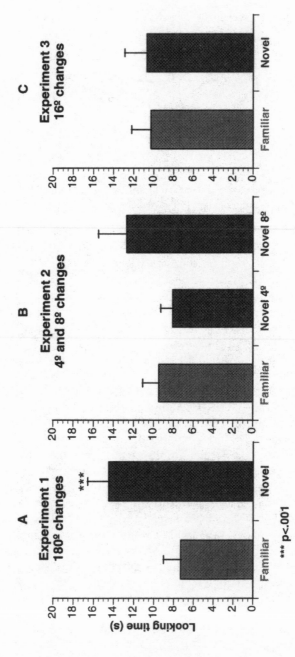

Figure 5.2. Summary of data from three habituation experiments. (A) Mean (+SE) look times to the familiar display (0° or 180°) and the novel (180° change) display. (B) Mean (+SE) look times to the familiar display (0°) and the novel (4° and 8° change) display. (C) Mean (+SE) look times to the familiar (0° or 16°) and the novel (16° change) display.

ing large differences in direction of motion, the next question was whether young infants could discriminate smaller changes in direction. Adults tested under similar stimulus conditions can detect changes in heading of less than 1° (Crowell & Banks, 1993; Warren, Morris, & Kalish, 1988). However, 4-month-olds should be less sensitive than adults to displays depicting changes in direction of heading information. Since there were no existing data upon which to base a specific prediction, infants' sensitivity to discriminate 4° and 8° changes of direction were tested. Discriminations of this magnitude are within adults' abilities to discriminate even under extremely limited conditions, such as when the number of moving elements is severely reduced (Warren, Morris, & Kalish, 1988). Furthermore, Banton and colleagues (Banton, Bertenthal, & Dobkins, 2001) have recently estimated that 18-week-old infants are sensitive to roughly 17° changes in the direction of a uniformly moving pattern of elements. Due to the distortion induced by the projection of points on the ground plane onto the projection surface, it turns out that the mean direction of moving elements in our displays is 0° (downward) in the forward motion condition, as one might expect, but 18° and 32° when the direction of heading is 4° and 8°, respectively. Consequently, if the discrimination of these optic flow displays is based on differences in the mean direction or orientation of moving elements, then heading changes of 4° and 8° should be discriminable by 4-month-old infants.

In our second experiment, 4-month-olds' abilities to discriminate 4° and 8° changes in heading were assessed by habituating infants to a display in which the simulated direction of motion was forward or at a heading of 0°. Infants were then tested with two novel directions of motion (4° and 8°) rather than one in order to acquire information about infants' abilities to discriminate two different magnitudes of headings. The logic of this design was that infants who could discriminate 4° changes should show look time recovery, relative to the last habituation trial, to both the 4° and 8° displays, while infants who could discriminate only the larger difference should show recovery only to the 8° change.

Twenty-four 4-month-old (115–139 days; 11 female) infants, recruited as described previously, participated. The results are described in Figure 5.2B. As the figure indicates, mean look times to the last habituation test display (M = 9.5 seconds, SD = 7.6) were not significantly lower than mean look times to either the 4° (M = 8.1 seconds, SD = 5.8) or 8° heading changes. In an attempt to gain more information about changes in heading direction that infants could discriminate, the design of Experiment 2 did not include a posthabituation repetition of the habituation pattern. As a result, the spontaneous recovery of look times could explain any apparent preferences for one of the novel directions. The apparent, but not statistically significant, increase in mean looking times to the 8° change in heading illustrates this difficulty. In order to rectify this issue and examine whether

4-month-old infants discriminate larger changes in direction, a third experiment was conducted with only a single magnitude of heading change (16°).

Twenty 4-month-old (121–135 days; 11 female) infants recruited as described previously participated. Infants were familiarized with a display depicting motion along 0° or 16° headings and were tested with displays depicting both the familiar and novel direction of heading. The results are plotted in Figure 5.2C. The mean looking time to the familiar direction (M = 10.3 seconds, SD = 8.5) did not differ from the mean looking time to the novel direction (M = 10.7 seconds, SD = 9.9).

Taken together, these data suggest that 4-month-olds' discriminate displays depicting 180° changes in heading direction under some circumstances but do not discriminate 4°, 8°, or 16° changes. In contrast, under similar display conditions, adults make similar discriminations easily (Crowell & Banks, 1993; Warren, Morris, & Kalish, 1988). Of course, these studies do not by themselves indicate whether infants actually perceived the patterns of optic flow as indicating different directions of self-motion. Nevertheless, the findings suggest that adultlike abilities to *discriminate* optic flow patterns simulating different directions of self-motion may not emerge early in life but instead undergo considerable postnatal development.

There are a number of reasons why discrimination performance might have been poor that merit discussion. One concerns the patterns of accretion and deletion of texture. It is possible that infants discriminated the forward from backward displays based on the different patterns of accretion and deletion of texture at the display boundaries. Indeed, this possibility reminds us that it is impossible from these experiments alone to determine exactly what feature or set of features infants were sensitive to in these displays. Still, the 4°, 8°, and 16° displays also differed from one another and the 0° display in terms of the pattern of accretion and deletion of texture. The fact that 4-month-olds did not discriminate the small heading displays suggests, at a minimum, that differential accretion or deletion of texture does not account for infants' performance in these studies.

Another factor specific to the habituation paradigm is memory demand. The habituation paradigm places demands on infants' memory since it is presumed to tap into stored representations about the familiar pattern. It is possible that these memory demands made it less likely that infants would discriminate displays depicting small changes in heading when the displays were separated in time by several seconds. The habituation data argue against this notion since there was no statistically significant effect of testing the novel pattern before the familiar pattern. Nevertheless, the memory demands of the habituation paradigm might have led to lower estimates of infants' sensitivity than would be possible using another technique. I will describe a method that overcomes this limitation in a subsequent section.

It is possible that the rapid speed of simulated self-motion (30 meters per second) underestimated infants' actual abilities by depicting moving elements whose speeds were outside of infants' abilities to detect accurately. Sensitivity to the speed and direction of visual motion is known to be quite poor in young infants relative to adults. The minimum (about 5° per second) and maximum (about 12° per second) speeds detectable by 8- to 10-week-olds in random dot patterns are an order of magnitude worse than adults (Wattam-Bell, 1996). By 15 to 20 weeks, infants detect motion up to 30° per second, but sensitivity remains substantially below adult levels. Unfortunately, there is minimal evidence about the development of velocity sensitivity in infants older than 15 to 20 weeks. Nevertheless, average dot speed in the habituation experiments was 20° per second, which is within the range of published speed sensitivities for infants of this age (Wattam-Bell, 1996). Moreover, infants discriminated the displays in the first experiment that depicted the same speed of motion in both conditions, so it seems unlikely that limitations on the ability to detect rapidly moving elements lead to the observed pattern of results. Adults' heading detection thresholds actually drop as the simulated speed of self-motion increases, reaching about 0.1° at the 30 meters per second (Crowell & Banks, 1993) simulated in our studies. So, at the very least, the current data imply that young infants have substantially poorer sensitivity to optic flow patterns than do adults.

Distinguishing the overall direction of a pattern of moving elements may be even more important for detecting changes in heading (Banton & Bertenthal, 1995, 1997), but surprisingly little is known about direction discrimination early in life. As mentioned previously, a more recent study (Banton, Bertenthal, & Dobkins, 2001) showed large improvements in the ability to discriminate uniform directions of motion between 6 and 18 weeks of age. Direction thresholds could not be obtained at 6 weeks but reached 17° by 18 weeks, roughly the age of the 4-month-olds we tested. Adults detect direction differences of less than 1° (de Bruyn & Orban, 1988), so direction discrimination undergoes considerable postnatal development. Nevertheless, the discrimination of direction changes in uniform motion patterns does not appear to account for the current optic flow results. Changes in the mean direction of the moving elements were 18°, 32°, and 64° for the 4°, 8°, and 16° heading conditions, respectively. The optic flow patterns were certainly not uniform in direction, but even if they were, on the basis of the previous uniform motion results, one would predict that 4-month-olds should discriminate displays showing smaller heading angles than 180°. In addition, the distribution of directions becomes increasingly uniform as the heading angle increases. Nevertheless, this additional potential cue did not facilitate the discrimination of displays depicting up to 16°

changes in heading. In sum, it seems unlikely that infants were unable to discriminate between these displays due wholly to some primary limitation on their ability to perceive the speed or direction of moving dots in the display.

The restriction of optic flow information to ground plane covering only the lower part of visual field might have diminished infants' performance. But this differential sensitivity is not shown in adults, who show comparable heading detection thresholds whether viewing simulated translation along a ground plane, through a cloud of dots, or relative to a frontoparallel plane (reviewed in Warren, 1998). It is also possible that by presenting infants with optic flow patterns in the central part of the visual field this paradigm underestimated their abilities. For example, there is some evidence that infants in a moving room situation respond most strongly to lateral movement of the side walls (Bertenthal & Bai, 1989), and several investigators have suggested that peripheral visual information dominates postural compensation mechanisms (e.g., Held, Dichgans, & Bauer, 1975). More recent research with adults suggests not only that optic flow presented in the center of the visual field induces greater postural sway (Stoffregen, 1985) but that judgments of heading are more accurate with radial flow fields presented in the center of the visual field, such as the kind presented in the infant studies, than lamellar flow fields presented in the periphery, such as those generated in the moving room (Crowell & Banks, 1993). Accordingly, it is unlikely that presenting optic flow patterns in the periphery would have improved infants' performance on this task, where discriminating changes in the direction of simulated heading is involved.

In a similar vein, the displays in the current series of studies simulated different directions of self-motion using only the movement of randomly positioned dots that remained a constant size. That is, the rich visual textures and shadows and interposition that are characteristic of locomotion through natural viewing environments were eliminated, and other cues, such as motion parallax, were reduced. It is possible that infants discriminate direction of motion information in a more robust fashion in natural, or at least richer, visual environments. Of course, patterns of optic flow are not the only cues to perceiving heading that have been proposed (e.g., Cutting et al., 1992) and tested in adults. But there is a large body of evidence that optic flow alone is sufficient for discrimination of direction of heading in adults and, in some cases, for steering (e.g., Warren, 1998). Further, we are not able, as of yet, to describe how multiple sources of spatial information might be integrated in adults, so how and when this process occurs in infancy remains an important unanswered question.

Estimating Discrimination Thresholds Using FPL

Despite the provocative findings from the habituation studies, they leave a number of unanswered questions. Most important is the smallest angle of heading change that young infants can detect. The habituation data suggest that this heading is somewhere between 16° and 180° at 30 meters per second of translational speed, but it is possible that memory demands or other factors led us to underestimate infants' abilities. In order to rectify some of the weaknesses with the habituation paradigm and provide a more efficient way of answering what angles infants could discriminate, we developed a forced-choice preferential looking (FPL) technique. FPL is a standard technique in infant visual psychophysics (Teller, 1979).

We measured whether infants would direct their gaze to one of two optic flow displays when the angle of motion depicted in one of the displays changed in a regular and repeating way. Both displays depicted forward and backward motion along a ground plane in an alternating fashion. Our habituation data had indicated that by 4 months infants could discriminate optic flow patterns specifying forward motion from those specifying backward motion. In order to isolate sensitivity to 180° changes in motion from the smaller angular changes, on every other forward/backward cycle, the angle of change depicted in one of the displays varied to some nonzero value. On the assumption that infants will tend to look first or more frequently at the side of the display that contains the more complex pattern of motion, the role of the observer is to try to determine which side depicts the changing direction of motion.

The display consisted of pairs of computer-generated movies depicting linear translational motion along a ground plane. The translational speed was 3.8 meters per second, a speed that approximated a fast running pace and, unlike the 30 meters per second speed used previously, is one that might actually have been experienced by some of our participants. The density of dots was 0.17 dots per degree squared, approximately 1.5 times that used in the habituation studies. Each optic flow movie consisted of alternating episodes of forward and backward motion in which the direction of motion changed at a temporal frequency of 0.6 hertz. Each movie depicted motion at a different angular heading with respect to the anterior-posterior axis. Each infant was shown a set of three nonzero angular magnitudes chosen from the set previously described. Each movie was displayed in a rectangular region 15° wide by 15° high separated by a central blank area 5° in width. Figure 5.3 shows a schematic of the display. Infants viewed a total of 36 trials in a single testing session. Adults viewed 48 trials showing changes in angle of 1.5°, 3°, 6°, and 12° and with the variations in side, direction, and number of replications as described for infants. For both groups, the order of presentation of the angles was random within each block of trials.

Participants were fourteen 3-month-old infants (82–107 days; mean 98 days; 9 female), nineteen 5-month-old infants (149–172 days; mean 159 days; 11 female), and two female adults with normal or corrected-to-normal visual acuity. Two adults with normal or corrected-to-normal visual

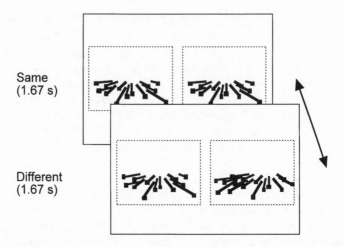

Same
(1.67 s)

Different
(1.67 s)

Figure 5.3. Schematic of display used in FPL studies of optic flow discrimination. Two optic flow patterns appeared simultaneously in two windows on the screen. The patterns simulated forward and backward motion along a ground plane. The patterns were identical on every other forward/backward cycle. The direction of motion simulated in one of the patterns varied on the alternate cycles. The magnitude of the direction difference varied from trial to trial. See text for additional detail.

acuity and who were generally aware of the hypotheses of the study also participated. A trained observer, who did not know which side contained the changed direction, made a forced choice decision as to whether the side of the changing motion was on the left or right. The observer was given an unlimited viewing duration and, following a key press to indicate the decision, feedback from the computer about whether a correct decision had been made.

All infants completed at least two blocks (24 trials), and the majority completed more than 30 trials. Both adult participants completed 48 trials. Judgments were typically made within 5 seconds of the display onset. Figure 5.4 shows the mean (+1SEM) proportion of correct judgments made by the observer as a function of the magnitude of direction simulated in the changing display. Data for the adult and 5-month-old groups indicate that the proportion of correct judgments made by the observer increased as the magnitude of simulated direction increased. Adults and 5-month-olds clearly differed. Note that at the 12° heading condition where adult performance was at ceiling, 5-month-olds were at chance. In contrast, the results for the 3-month-olds did not indicate that sensitivity increased with changes in the heading angle.

The advantage of the FPL method is that it allows specific threshold values to be estimated. We computed both group and individual thresholds.

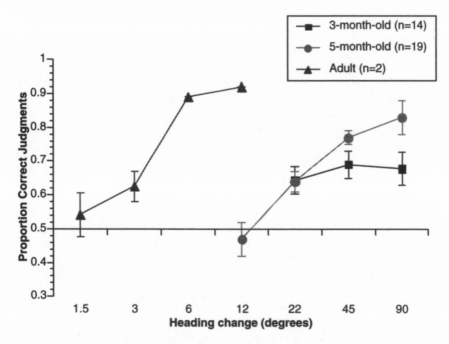

Figure 5.4. Data from FPL studies of optic flow discrimination. Average proportion correct judgments (+1 SEM) are depicted for three age groups, adults, 5-month-olds, and 3-month-olds. Each group viewed different but overlapping sets of displays varying only in the direction of simulated motion.

The group 75% correct discrimination threshold was computed by linear interpolation of the log proportion correct values that spanned 75%. This procedure indicated that the group threshold for the adults was 4.4°, and for the 5-month-olds it was 40.4°. Thresholds for the 3-month-old group could not be estimated. We also computed individual 75% thresholds for 5-month-old group by using linear regression through the three data points for each infant. These estimates ranged from 12° to 71.5°, with a mean of 41.7° and a median of 45.1°. Individual thresholds for the 3-month-old group could not be estimated.

These data suggest that even when the dot density is increased and the translational speed approximates a running pace, the heading discrimination threshold for 5-month-old infants is an order of magnitude greater than adults tested under similar conditions. These data suggest that the 4° and 8° changes depicted in the first pilot study were, in fact, beyond the ability of most infants to detect. Further, the fact that infants' thresholds for identical displays are considerably higher than adults' tested under the same display conditions indicates that considerable development must occur in the ability to discriminate optic flow patterns of this type. Adults' thresholds were somewhat larger than those estimated using other procedures, but some variability is expected, given differences in display size and the use of the forced choice looking procedure with judgments made in a relatively short period of time (less than 5 seconds). Indeed, in other work in my laboratory, we have shown that adults' discrimination thresholds approach 1° when the decision time is made longer.

Clearly, 3-month-old infants did not show systematic evidence of discriminating between these displays even at relatively large heading angles. This is likely to be due to the slower speed of moving elements in these displays, relative to those shown in the habituation studies. At a translational speed of 3.8 meters per second along a ground plane, the mean speed of moving elements was less than 5° per second, or below the published speed sensitivity for infants at this age (Wattam-Bell, 1996). The distribution of speeds is positively skewed for heading directions less than 90°, so *some* of the moving elements were probably above threshold for *some* of the infants, *some* of the time. But, overall, the slower mean speed of the moving elements probably accounts for the failure of the 3-month-old group to show systematic discrimination of these displays. The distribution of element speeds is highly dependent on the geometry of the visual environment. However, if sensitivity to the mean speed of motion in optic flow is an important factor in perceptual processing, it suggests that there are natural speeds of movement through certain types of visual environments that result in visual motion outside the range of detection of many young infants. The practical consequence of this may be that even if young infants could crawl or walk, those slow speeds of movement would not generate optic flow that is fast enough for them to detect.

Of course, we still do not know whether the visual discrimination of optic flow patterns is related to the use of optic flow to guide locomotion or maintain balance. Furthermore, even though the results of the habituation and FPL paradigms are broadly compatible, it is possible that the static viewing situation underestimated infants' true abilities. Actual self-movement is accompanied by vestibular and other proprioceptive information about the direction of speed of motion. It is possible, therefore, that infants failed to discriminate these displays because they were inconsistent with their own, correct, perceptions of the absence of self-motion. However, in laboratory settings, the addition of vestibular or proprioceptive information adds very little to the accuracy of adults' self-motion perception beyond that afforded by visual information alone (Telford, Howard, & Ohmi, 1995). Moreover, for this argument to hold, one would have to assume that infants perceived these optic flow patterns as specifying some possible pattern of self-motion, and without data from other measures, such as changes in body position. This conclusion is premature. There was no body movement in the first habituation study showing forward and backward movement, but infants discriminated those displays when the angle of heading change was large. So it is unlikely that the discrepancies between visual and proprioceptive information diminished infants' sensitivity to changes in heading direction. It would be instructive, however, to examine whether infants show increased sensitivity to changes in heading under conditions where they are actually moving through space. This question should be explored in future research.

In sum, the results of four different experiments using two different experimental paradigms converge on the same basic conclusion: Young infants do not accurately discriminate optic flow patterns that simulate relatively large changes in the direction of self-motion. The next section describes some data that may explain one reason why this might be so and how the discrimination of heading direction might be related to the integration of visual and nonvisual information involved in body-centered representations of space.

GENERAL DISCUSSION

Taken together, these data suggest that like sensitivity to visual information specifying distance, sensitivity to information about visual direction undergoes considerable development in the first 6 months of postnatal life. Evidence from a simple eye movement planning paradigm suggests that the earliest and most primitive form of processing about the static direction is derived from the 2D projection of visual information onto the retina. In contrast, coding static direction in head-, body-, or environment-centered coordinates requires the integration of this eye-centered information with additional information about the position and movements of the eyes, head, and body. Perhaps reflecting the requirement that these sources of information must be calibrated in order for precise representations of spatial direction in higher-order spatial coordinates to emerge, there is scant evidence that infants younger than 5 to 6 months of age invoke more complex representations of direction in planning actions. Similarly, despite previous evidence for rudimentary sensitivity to the direction of motion of moving objects toward or away from the face, or of surfaces toward or away from the viewer, the results from four separate studies suggest that 3- to 5-month-old infants do not accurately discriminate optic flow patterns that specify moderately small changes in the direction of self-motion. If the integration of visual and nonvisual sources of direction information is in a state of rapid change during the first several months of life, the consequence may be eye-centered saccade sequences in situations of reduced visual information, body-centered orienting errors in situations where objects or the observer is displaced, and limited capacities to discriminate direction of motion from optic flow.

Of course, these results leave a number of questions unanswered. One of the most intriguing is how direction perception changes after 6 to 7 months. The Gilmore and Johnson (1997a, 1997b) data suggest that eye-centered information continues to influence a large number of eye movement sequences even among 7-month-olds, but with the exception of the study on Williams and Down Syndrome children (Brown et al., in press), we know nothing about the developmental progression of this facet of direction perception. Similarly, we now have evidence that the discrimination of direction information is poor in 5-month-olds, but we do not have any data that describe how it changes over the next several months. The second year of life is likely to be a crucial time period for development in this domain because of the onset of most major locomotor milestones. My students and I are pursuing a number of techniques to address the development of heading direction sensitivity in older infants including measuring changes in body position in response to collisions with simulated contours, detecting changes in the direction of simulated motion, and estimating discrimination thresholds using operant techniques to maintain infants' interest and motivation.

Once we have established the normative time course of development in direction perception, we can then turn attention to the question of why direction perception changes in this way. In the discussion thus far, I have emphasized how biological factors, specifically the development of specific processing systems in the extrastriate areas of the cerebral cortex, might play a central role. It bears repeating that there is limited anatomical or physiological data about the development of neural systems involved in complex spatial processing. Nevertheless, the existing evidence suggests that increases in metabolic levels (Chugani & Phelps, 1986; Chugani, Müller, & Chugani, 1996) are somewhat delayed in these areas relative to those in primary visual cortex and that the most rapid period of synaptogenesis in primary visual cortex (Huttenlocher, 1990) corresponds to the same time frame in which we observe changes in infants' direction perception. Accordingly, it is likely that the functional immaturity in cortical circuits that specialize in complex spatial processing provides biological constraints on young infants' abilities to perceive certain aspects of visual direction. This statement is based on the assumption that there are specific neural substrates in which the integration of visual and nonvisual information occurs, that these substrates undergo considerable postnatal development, and that changes in the functional characteristics of these systems are reflected in infants' behavior. We have begun to identify some of these substrates in adult animals. They include regions of the parietal and frontal cortex and subcortical structures such as the superior colliculus. But the study of multisensory integration in the mature animal has only begun and therefore provides only a limited scaffold for developmental theories at present. Just as biological evidence has begun to influence theories in adult perceptual and cognitive psychology, this sort of evidence is likely to have a similar impact on our understanding of developmental processes in the years ahead.

At the same time, a complete account of the development of direction perception, or any other behavioral capacity, cannot rest solely on neurobiology but requires the systematic examination of changes in behavior within specific domains. For example, there are multiple interacting perceptual and cognitive factors that contribute to developmental changes in direction perception. Two examples are the extensive changes in visual acuity and the size of the effective visual field (Sireteanu, 1996) that occur postnatally. Both are likely to contribute to the spatial resolution and range of static direction perception. Similarly, changes in the extent to which infants can detect and process motion patterns that vary in speed, direction, and distribution are likely to be crucial for the capacity to distinguish moving objects from the motion of an observer and to determine precisely one's direction and speed of self-movement (Banton & Bertenthal, 1995, 1997; Banton, Bertenthal, & Dobkins, 2001). Indeed, the existing evidence suggests that the development of sensitivity to uniform patterns of motion, such as those generated by self-motion, differs from the emergence of sensitivity to relative patterns of motion, such as those generated by a stationary observer viewing a moving object (Banton & Bertenthal, 1997). How changes in low-level motion sensitivity in infants relates to higher-level discrimination of direction of self-motion is not yet known. The requirement that direction perception involves the integration of multiple sources of spatial information suggests that the processes of sensory integration and differentiation in early development also merit careful exploration.

Finally, and perhaps most important, it is crucial to consider what role visual experience might play in the development of spatial perception. In the first year of life, visual experience can take two distinct forms: active or passive. A large body of research has indicated that active visual experience associated with locomotor activity may play an important role in shaping young animals' abilities to perceive and act upon some forms of visual information about spatial relations, including some aspects of optic flow (Adolph, 1997, 2000; Bertenthal & Bai, 1989; Bertenthal, Campos, & Kermoian, 1994; Bertenthal, Rose, & Bai, 1997; Held & Hein, 1963). In contrast, locomotor experience may not influence the emergence of sensitivity to other spatial variables such as linear perspective or texture gradients (Arterberry, Yonas, & Bensen, 1989). Even prelocomotor infants produce visual experience tied to self-produced eye, head, and trunk movements. The role of these movements in normal development remains poorly understood.

Nevertheless, the possible role of passive visual experience has been of relatively little interest, in all likelihood due to the now-legendary demonstration that self-produced motion was superior to its passively experienced equivalent (Held & Hein, 1963) in shaping normal perceptual and motor development of kittens. The lack of interest in passive visual experience seems surprising given that human infants accrue a substantial amount of such experience in the first several months of life and that this time period coincides with rapid increases in functional brain activity and in visual capacities. Moreover, passive experience is deemed vital in the domain of speech perception and language development (Kuhl, 1994), but we do not actually know to what extent passive visual experience contributes to the normal emergence of visual function in humans. Of course, some might argue that infants actively explore the visual environment from birth using whatever movements are within their control, so no experience is truly or exclusively passive.

While this claim is correct in general, the fact remains that certain classes of visual patterns are associated with rather specific types of self-movements. For example, forward translational movement of the head results in radially expanding patterns of optic flow. It is clear that 3- to 5-month-old infants do not generate significant amounts of this sort of optic flow by means of their own self-movement. Consequently, it is possible, perhaps even likely, that sensitivity to some aspects of dynamic direction information may be relatively poor until infants begin to sit erect or crawl, thereby creating regular opportunities to perceive behaviorally relevant patterns of optic flow and tune perception and action accordingly. On the other hand, the data presented in this chapter suggest that some development in dynamic direction perception occurs between 3 and 5 months, a time period in which passive experience of some visual patterns dominates. It may be more productive, therefore, to think of passive visual experience as being associated with relatively slow rates of development and active experience with more rapid change. Alternatively, development associated with passive experience may allow the infant to develop the minimum degree of perceptual sensitivity that is necessary for the onset of a locomotor milestone such as independent sitting or crawling. Subsequent, more rapid development is then largely driven by active visual experience. Clearly, more focused examination of what forms of visual experience are generated by self versus others' movements early in life and additional research on the question of what roles passive and active experience jointly play in shaping the perception of information about direction, in particular, and spatial perception in general, are warranted.

CONCLUSION

The emergence of adultlike abilities to discriminate direction information about static visual targets and about an observer's heading from optic flow may have a prolonged developmental time course. This is probably due to the joint influence of perceptual, experiential, and neurological factors. Our results point toward a view in which a number of primitive, relatively inflexible but functionally effective perception-action systems control behavior early in life. These systems gradually give way to more mature, flexible, precise, and carefully calibrated systems for mediating perception and action that emerge sometime later. In the domain of discriminating heading direction, this implies that the visual discrimination of different directions of self-motion from optic flow is necessary, but not sufficient, for the use of that information to guide behavior. Indeed, it is possible, perhaps likely, that infants' abilities to discriminate some aspects of visual information relevant for locomotion precede their abilities to use that information to guide action. We note that this view is broadly consistent with recent data on the specificity of perception-action learning in locomotion to the particular body posture in which a mapping was acquired (Adolph, 1997; Adolph & Eppler, 1998).

Do very young infants accurately perceive the direction of visual targets or discriminate optic flow patterns specifying different directions of heading? Our results suggest that they do not do so especially well. When adult-like perception of direction information emerges and what factors influence its emergence remain challenges for future research.

NOTE

This chapter was prepared with financial assistance from the Pennsylvania State University and the National Science Foundation (BCS-0092452).

REFERENCES

Acredolo, L.P. (1979). Laboratory versus home: The effect of environment on the 9-month-old infant's choice of spatial reference system. *Developmental Psychology, 15,* 666–667.

Acredolo, L.P. (1990). Behavioral approaches to spatial orientation in infancy. *Annals of the New York Academy of Sciences, 608,* 596–612.

Adolph, K.E. (1997). Learning in the development of infant locomotion. *Monographs of the Society for Research in Child Development, 62* (3, Serial No. 251).

Adolph, K.E. (2000). Specificity of learning: Why infants fall over a veritable cliff. *Psychological Science, 11,* 94–299.

Adolph, K.E., & Eppler, M.A. (1998). Development of visually guided locomotion. *Ecological Psychology, 10,* 303–321.

Andersen, R.A. (1997). Multimodal integration for the representation of space in the posterior parietal cortex. *Philosophical Transactions of the Royal Society of London, 352,* 1441–1428.

Andersen, R.A., Snyder, L.H., Li, C.S., & Stricanne, B. (1993). Coordinate transformations in the representation of spatial information. *Current Opinion in Neurobiology, 3,* 171–176.

Arterberry, M., Yonas, A., & Bensen, A.S. (1989). Self-produced locomotion and the development of responsiveness to linear perspective and texture gradients. *Developmental Psychology, 25,* 976–982.

Ashmead, D.H., & Davis, D.L. (1996). Measuring habituation in infants: An approach using regression analysis. *Child Development, 67,* 2677–2690.

Ashmead, D.H., & McCarty, M.E. (1991). Postural sway of human infants while standing in light and dark. *Child Development, 62,* 1276–1287.

Aslin, R.N., & Shea, S.L. (1987). The amplitude and angle of saccades to double-step target displacements. *Vision Research, 27,* 1925–1942.

Atkinson, J. (1984). Human visual development over the first six months of life: A review and a hypothesis. *Human Neurobiology, 3,* 61–74.

Atkinson, J. (2000). *The developing visual brain.* Oxford: Oxford University Press.

Ball, W.A., & Tronick, E. (1971). Infant responses to impending collision: Optical and real. *Science, 171,* 818–820.

Banton, T., & Bertenthal, B.I. (1995). Infants' sensitivity to uniform motion. *Vision Research, 36,* 1633–1640.

Banton, T., & Bertenthal, B.I. (1997). Multiple developmental pathways for motion processing. *Optometry and Vision Science, 74,* 751–760.

Banton, T., Bertenthal, B.I., & Dobkins, K. (2001). Infant direction discrimination thresholds. *Vision Research, 41,* 1049–1056.

Becker, W., & Jürgens, R. (1979). An analysis of the saccadic system by means of double step stimuli. *Vision Research, 19,* 967–983.

Bertenthal, B.I., & Bai, D.L. (1989). Infants' sensitivity to optical flow for controlling posture. *Developmental Psychology, 25,* 936–945.

Bertenthal, B.I., Campos, J.J., & Kermoian, R. (1994). An epigenetic perspective on the development of self-produced locomotion and its consequences. *Current Directions in Psychological Science, 3,* 140–145.

Bertenthal, B.I., Rose, J.L., & Bai, D.L. (1997). Perception-action coupling in the development of visual control of posture. *Journal of Experimental Psychology: Human Perception and Performance, 23,* 1631–1643.

Bhatt, R.S., & Waters, S.E. (1998). Perception of three-dimensional cues in early infancy. *Journal of Experimental Child Psychology, 70,* 207–224.

Birch, E.E., Gwiazda, J., & Held, R. (1982). Stereoacuity development for crossed and uncrossed disparities in human infants. *Vision Research, 22,* 507–513.

Bremner, J.G. (1978). Egocentric versus allocentric spatial coding in nine-month-old infants: Factors influencing the choice of code. *Developmental Psychology, 14,* 346–355.

Bronson, G.W. (1982). Structure, status and characteristics of the nervous system at birth. In P. Stratton (Ed.), *Psychobiology of the human newborn* (pp. 99–118). Chichester: Wiley & Sons.

Brown, J., Johnson, M.H., Paterson, S., Gilmore, R.O., Gsödl, M., Longhi, E., & Karmiloff-Smith, A. (In press). Spatial representation and attention in toddlers with Williams Syndrome and Down Syndrome. *Neuropsychologia.*

Chugani, H.J., & Phelps, M.E. (1986). Maturational changes in cerebral function in infants determined by [18] FDG positron emission tomography. *Science, 231,* 840–843.

Chugani, H.T., Müller, R.A., & Chugani, D.C. (1996). Functional brain reorganization in children. *Brain Development, 18,* 347–356.

Conel, J.L. (1939–1967). *The postnatal development of the human cerebral cortex* (Vols. 1–8). Cambridge, MA: Harvard University Press.

Craton, L.G., & Yonas, A. (1990). The role of motion in infants' perception of occlusion. In T.E. James (Ed.), *Advances in psychology: 69. The development of attention: Research and theory* (pp. 21–46). Amsterdam, The Netherlands: North-Holland.

Crowell, J.A., & Banks, M.S. (1993). Perceiving heading with different retinal regions and types of optic flow. *Perception & Psychophysics, 53*, 325–337.

Crowell, J.A., & Banks, M.S. (1996). Ideal observer for heading judgments. *Vision Research, 36*, 471–490.

Cutting, J.E., Springer, K., Braren, P.A., & Johnson, S.H. (1992). Wayfinding on foot from information in retinal, not optical, flow. *Journal of Experimental Psychology: General, 121*, 41–72.

de Bruyn, B., & Orban, G.A. (1988). Human velocity and direction discrimination measured with random dot patterns. *Vision Research, 28*, 1323–1335.

de Jong, B.M., Shipp, S., Skidmore, B., Frackowiak, R.S.J., & Zeki, S. (1994). The cerebral activity related to the visual perception of forward motion in depth. *Brain, 117*, 1039–1054.

Distler, C., Bachevalier, J., Kennedy, C., Mishkin, M., & Ungerleider, L.G. (1996). Functional development of the corticocortical pathway for motion analysis in the macaque monky: A 14C-2-deoxyglucose study. *Cerebral Cortex, 6*, 164–195.

Duffy, C.J., & Wurtz, R.H. (1991). The sensitivity of MST neurons to optic flow stimuli. I. A continuum of response selectivity to large field stimuli. *Journal of Neurophysiology, 65*, 1329–1345.

Duhamel, J.R., Colby, C.L., & Goldberg, M.E. (1993). The updating of the representation of visual space in parietal cortex by intended eye movements. *Science, 255*, 90–92.

Duhamel, J.R., Goldberg, M.E., Fitzgibbon, E.J., Sirigu, A., & Grafman, J. (1992). Saccadic dysmetria in a patient with a right frontoparietal lesion: The importance of corollary discharge for accurate spatial behaviour. *Brain, 115*, 1387–1402.

Gibson, J.J. (1966). *The senses considered as perceptual systems.* Boston: Houghton Mifflin.

Gibson, J.J. (1979). *The ecological approach to visual perception.* Boston: Houghton Mifflin.

Gilmore, R.O. (2001). *Infants' discrimination of optic flow patterns specifying different directions of observer motion.* Poster presented at the Vision Sciences Society Conference, Sarasota, FL, May.

Gilmore, R.O., & Johnson, M.H. (1997a). Body-centered representations for visually-guided action emerge during early infancy. *Cognition, 65*, B1–B9.

Gilmore, R.O., & Johnson, M.H. (1997b). Egocentric action in early infancy: Spatial frames of reference for saccades. *Psychological Science, 8*, 224–230.

Groll, S.L., & Ross, L.E. (1982). Saccadic eye movements of children and adults to double-step stimuli. *Developmental Psychology, 18*, 108–123.

Hallett, P.E., & Lightstone, A.D. (1976a). Saccadic eye movements to flashed targets. *Vision Research, 114*, 107–114.

Hallett, P.E., & Lightstone, A.D. (1976b). Saccadic eye movements towards stimuli triggered by prior saccades. *Vision Research, 16*, 99–106.

Held, R. (1985). Binocular vision: Behavioral and neuronal development. In J. Mehler & R. Fox (Eds.), *Neonate cognition: Beyond the blooming, buzzing confusion* (pp. 37–44). Hillsdale, NJ: Lawrence Erlbaum.

Held, R., Birch, E., & Gwiazda, J. (1980). Stereoacuity in human infants. *Proceedings of the National Academy of Sciences (USA), 77*, 5572–5574.

Held, R., Dichgans, J., & Bauer, J. (1975). Characteristics of moving visual scenes influencing spatial orientation. *Vision Research, 15*, 357–365.

Held, R., & Hein, A. (1963). Movement produced stimulation in the development of visually guided behavior. *Journal of Comparative Physiological Psychology, 56*, 872–876.

Huttenlocher, P.R. (1990). Morphometric study of human cerebral cortex development. *Neuropsychologia, 28*, 517–527.

Huttenlocher, P.R., & Dabholkar, A.S. (1997). Regional differences in synaptogenesis in human cerebral cortex. *Journal of Comparative Neurology, 387*, 167–178.

Johnson, M.H. (1990). Cortical maturation and the development of visual attention in early infancy. *Journal of Cognitive Neuroscience, 2*, 81–95.

Jouen, F., & Lepecq, J.C. (1989). Sensitivity to optical flow among neonates. *Psychologie Francaise, 34*, 13–18.

Karmiloff-Smith, A. (1998). Is atypical development necessarily a window on the normal mind/brain? The case of Williams Syndrome. *Developmental Science, 1*, 273–277.

Kaufman, J., & Needham, A. (1999). Objective spatial coding by 6.5-month-old infants in a visual dishabituation task. *Developmental Science, 2*, 432–441.

Kellman, P.J., & Banks, M.S. (1998). Infant visual perception. In D. Kuhn & R.S. Siegler (Eds.), *Handbook of child psychology: Cognition, perception, and language* (Vol. 2, 5th ed., pp. 103–146). New York: John Wiley & Sons.

Kuhl, P.K. (1994). Learning and representation in speech and language. *Current Opinion in Neurobiology, 4*, 812–822.

Land, M.F., & Lee, D.N. (1994). Where we look when we steer. *Nature, 369*, 742–744.

Lee, D.N., & Aronson, E. (1974). Visual proprioceptive control of standing in human infants. *Perception and Psychophysics, 15*, 529–532.

LeVay, S., Wiesel, T.N., & Hubel, D.H. (1980). The development of ocular dominance columns in normal and deprived monkeys. *Journal of Comparative Neurology, 191*, 1–51.

Manny, R.E., & Fern, K.D. (1990). Motion coherence in infants. *Vision Research, 30*, 1319–1329.

Mays, R., & Sparks, D. (1980). Saccades are spatially, not retinocentrically coded. *Science, 208*, 1163–1165.

Milner, A.D., & Goodale, M.A. (1995). *The visual brain in action*. Oxford: Oxford University Press.

Nañez, J. (1987). Perception of impending collision in 3- to 6-week-old infants. *Infant Behavior and Development, 11*, 447–463.

Nañez, J.E., & Yonas, A. (1994). Effects of luminance and texture motion on infant defensive reactions to optical collision. *Infant Behavior & Development, 17,* 165–174.

Newcombe, N.S., & Huttenlocher, J. (2000). *Making space: The development of spatial representation and reasoning.* Cambridge, MA: MIT Press.

O'Dell, C.D., Quick, M.W., & Boothe, R.G. (1991). The development of stereoacuity in infant Rhesus monkeys. *Investigative Opthalmology and Visual Science* (Suppl.), *32,* 1044.

Pettigrew, J.D. (1974). The effect of visual experience on the development of visual specificity by kitten cortical neurons. *Journal of Physiology, 237,* 49.

Piaget, J., & Inhelder, B. (1948). *The child's conception of space* (F.J. Langdon & J.L. Lunzer, Trans.). London: Routledge & Kegan Paul.

Pope, M.J. (1984). *Visual proprioception in infant postural development.* Unpublished doctoral dissertation, University of Southampton, UK.

Rettke, H.R., Gilmore, R.O., & Pupik, C. (2000). *Infants' discrimination of heading from optic flow.* Poster presented at the XIIth International Conference on Infant Studies, Brighton, UK, July.

Rieser, J.J. (1979). Spatial orientation in six-month-old infants. *Child Development, 50,* 1078–1087.

Royden, C.S., Crowell, J.A., & Banks, M.S. (1994). Estimating heading during eye movements. *Vision Research, 34,* 3197–3214.

Schmuckler, M.A., & Li, N.S. (1998). Looming responses to obstacles and apertures: The role of accretion and deletion of background texture. *Psychological Science, 9,* 49–52.

Shinar, D., McDowell, E.D., & Rockwell, T.H. (1977). Eye movements in curve negotiation. *Human Factors, 19,* 63–71.

Sireteanu, R. (1996). Development of the visual field: Results from human and animal studies. In F. Vital-Durand, J. Atkinson, & O.J. Braddick (Eds.), *Infant vision* (pp. 17–31). Oxford: Oxford University Press.

Stein, J.F. (1992). The representation of egocentric space in the posterior parietal cortex. *Behavioral and Brain Sciences, 15,* 691–700.

Stoffregen, T.A. (1985). Flow structure versus retinal location in the optical control of stance. *Journal of Experimental Psychology: Human Perception & Performance, 11,* 554–565.

Telford, L., Howard, I.P., & Ohmi, M. (1995). Heading judgments during active and passive motion. *Experimental Brain Research, 104,* 502–510.

Teller, D.Y. (1979). The forced preferential looking procedure: A psychophysical technique for use with human infants. *Infant Behavior and Development, 2,* 77–86.

Timney, B. (1981). Development of binocular depth perception in kittens. *Investigative Ophthalmology and Visual Science, 21,* 493–496.

Ungerleider, L.G., & Mishkin, M. (1982). Two cortical visual systems: Separation of appearance and location of objects. In D.L. Ingle, M.A. Goodale, & R.J.W. Mansfield (Eds.), *Analysis of visual behavior* (pp. 549–586). Cambridge, MA: MIT Press.

von Hofsten, C., Kellman, P., & Putaansuu, J. (1992). Young infants' sensitivity to motion parallax. *Infant Behavior & Development, 15,* 245–264.

Warren, W.H. (1998). The state of flow. In T. Watanabe (Ed.), *High-level motion processing* (pp. 315–358). Cambridge, MA: MIT Press.

Warren, W.H., Morris, M.W., & Kalish, M. (1988). Perception of translational heading from optic flow. *Journal of Experimental Psychology: Human Perception and Performance, 14,* 646–660.

Wattam-Bell, J.R.B. (1996). Development of visual motion processing. In F. Vital-Durand, J. Atkinson, & O.J. Braddick (Eds.), *Infant vision* (pp. 79–94). Oxford: Oxford University Press.

Yonas, A., Arterberry, M.E., & Granrud, C.E. (1987). Space perception in infancy. In R. Vasta (Ed.), *Annals of child development* (Vol. 4, pp. 1–34). London: JAI.

Yonas, A., & Granrud, C.E. (1985). Development of visual space perception in young infants. In J. Mehler & R. Fox (Eds.), *Neonate cognition: Beyond the blooming buzzing confusion* (pp. 45–67). Hillsdale, NJ: Lawrence Erlbaum.

Yonas, A., Pettersen, L., & Lockman, J. (1979). Young infants' sensitivity to optical information for collision. *Canadian Journal of Psychology, 33,* 268–276.

Chapter 6

Linking Visual Cortical Development to Visual Perception

Stephen Grossberg

ABSTRACT

This chapter analyzes how the visual cortex autonomously develops, stabilizes its own development, and then gives rise to visual perception in the adult. Much evidence suggests that the visual cortex generates representations of perceptual boundaries and surfaces. The present chapter focuses on how the visual cortex develops the circuitry that generates perceptual boundaries. Boundary formation is also known as perceptual grouping, or the binding problem. Developing cortical circuits may be refined by visual experience. The model clarifies how developing circuits protect themselves against being catastrophically eroded by fluctuations in visual inputs. Remarkably, the processes that stabilize development in the infant lead to properties in the adult of perceptual grouping, attention, and learning. Thus, the laws of adult perception seem to be strongly constrained by stability constraints on infant development. This modeling perspective opens a path toward unifying three fields: infant cortical development, adult cortical neurophysiology and anatomy, and adult visual psychophysics. The model further clarifies why visual cortex, indeed all neocortex, is organized into layered circuits. It hereby contributes to an understanding of how the laminar organization of neocortex supports biological intelligence.

INTRODUCTION

A central question in cognitive science and neuroscience concerns how the visual cortex autonomously develops, stabilizes its own development, and then gives rise to visual perception in the adult. What is the link between processes of development in the infant and processes of perception and learning in the adult? What are the functional units that determine perception in the adult, and how do developmental processes give rise to these units?

During the past 20 years, a large body of experimental and theoretical evidence has lent accumulating support to the idea that the visual cortex devotes substantial processing resources to generating three-dimensional representations of perceptual boundaries and surfaces, notably representations that can separate figures from their backgrounds and complete the representations of partially occluded objects. It has been proposed that these boundary and surface representations are formed in the interblob and blob streams, respectively, that project between cortical areas V1 to V4 (see Grossberg [1994] for a review). These representations, in turn, then project to higher levels of the brain, notably inferotemporal cortex, where they are categorized, or unitized, into object representations. All of these cortical areas and their representations are, moreover, linked with each other through feedback pathways.

Perhaps the earliest modeling studies to propose that and how boundaries and surfaces are computed in these cortical streams were provided by the author and his colleagues (e.g., Cohen & Grossberg, 1984; Grossberg, 1984, 1987a, 1987b; Grossberg & Mingolla, 1985a, 1985b; Grossberg & Todorovic, 1988). Since that time, many experiments have lent support to this hypothesis (see Grossberg [1994, 1997] for reviews). A great deal of theoretical progress has also been made toward further characterizing these boundary and surface processes (e.g., Douglas et al., 1995; Finkel & Edelman, 1989; Grossberg, 1994, 1997; Grossberg & Kelly, 1999; Grossberg, Hwang, & Mingolla, 2001; Grossberg & McLoughlin, 1997; Grossberg & Pessoa, 1998; Heitger et al., 1998; Kelly & Grossberg, 2000; Li, 1998; McLoughlin & Grossberg, 1998; Mumford, 1992; Pessoa, Mingolla, & Neumann, 1995; Somers, Nelson, & Sur, 1995; Stemmler, Usher, & Niebur, 1995; Ullman, 1995). Another parallel processing stream, through cortical area MT, helps to compute object motion and cues useful for visual navigation. Motion processing will not be further discussed in this chapter. Relevant theoretical progress toward theoretically characterizing object motion and navigational processes can be found in Grossberg, Mingolla, and Viswanathan (2001) and Grossberg, Mingolla, and Pack (1999).

The present chapter will focus on aspects of how the visual cortex generates perceptual boundaries. This process is also known as *perceptual grouping*, or the *binding problem*. The present summary will not discuss three-dimensional boundary formation or the figure-ground problem. It will, instead, focus on some of the fundamental perceptual grouping mechanisms on which these three-dimensional processes are based. These perceptual grouping processes are known to play an important role in how infants perceive the world. For example, neonates appear to perceive a partly occluded object as disjoint parts. The ability to process these fragments as coherent objects via perceptual grouping develops rapidly within the first 2 to 4 months of life (Johnson, 2001; Johnson & Aslin, 1996; Kellman & Spelke, 1983).

A neural model is here reviewed of how such perceptual grouping circuits develop in the visual cortex. Many experiments over the past 30 years have illustrated how properties of cortical circuits may be influenced by visual experience. Whenever developing circuits may be "taught" by environmental inputs, a key concern is how these circuits protect themselves against being washed away by fluctuations in these inputs. The same problem arises during adult learning. This is often called the problem of "catastrophic forgetting." Catastrophic forgetting does not refer to the desirable refinement and adjustment of circuits in response to environmental fluctuations. Rather, it acknowledges that such fluctuations can cause an undesirable collapse in useful circuit properties in incompletely realized neural models. Most neural models, such as the popular back propagation model (see Grossberg [1988] for a review), do experience catastrophic forgetting because their mechanisms include biologically unrealistic elements.

The present model proposes neural mechanisms that enable developing cortical circuits to stabilize themselves using properties of their self-organized circuit interactions. Remarkably, the same processes that help to stabilize development in the infant lead to properties in the adult of perceptual grouping, attention, and learning. Many useful implications follow from this observation. One is that the laws of adult perception are strongly constrained by stability constraints on infant development. Because of this link between infant development and adult perception, the chapter discusses adult perceptual properties in some detail, since these are the targets to which infant development is aimed. Another implication of the model is that the visual cortex is not merely a bottom-up filtering device, as was suggested in the classical Nobel Prize–winning work of Hubel and Weisel (1977). Rather, even early stages of visual cortical processing actively carry out perceptual grouping, attentional selection, and adaptive reorganization of circuitry in response to changing environmental conditions.

The model further clarifies why visual cortex, indeed all neocortex, is organized into layered circuits. It hereby contributes to an understanding of how the laminar organization of neocortex supports biological intelligence. This laminar organization is shown to realize at least three interacting processes: (1) the developmental and learning processes whereby the cortex shapes its circuits to match environmental constraints in a *stable* way through time; (2) the binding process whereby cortex groups distributed data into coherent object representations that remain sensitive to analog properties of the environment; (3) the attentional process whereby cortex selectively processes important events. As noted above, the model proposes that the mechanisms that achieve property (1) imply properties of (2) and (3). The model also opens a path toward understanding how variations and specializations of these processes operate in other types of neocortex. This modeling perspective opens a path toward unifying three fields: infant cortical development, adult cortical neurophysiology and anatomy, and adult visual psychophysics.

The model is called a LAMINART model because it clarifies how mechanisms of adaptive resonance theory, or ART, can be realized within identified laminar cortical circuits. Earlier ART models were devoted to understanding how bottom-up and top-down cortical interactions work together for the control of cortical development, learning, perception, and cognition. Although these studies successfully explained and predicted a variety of behavioral and brain data, they did not show how these processes are realized within laminar cortical circuits. Grossberg (1999b) reviews some of these ART concepts and some of the data that they explain. The LAMINART model extends these results by proposing how bottom-up, top-down, and *horizontal* cortical circuits work together in *laminar* circuits and how they realize processes of development, learning, grouping, and attention. LAMINART hereby unifies concepts about ART learning and attention with concepts about perceptual grouping. This innovation was introduced in Grossberg, Mingolla, and Ross (1997) and by Grossberg (1999a).

Subsequent work on the LAMINART model has clarified how excitatory and inhibitory connections in the cortex can develop stably by maintaining a balance between excitation and inhibition in multiple cortical circuits (Grossberg & Williamson, 2001). It is known, for example (see below for references), that long-range excitatory horizontal connections between pyramidal cells in layer 2/3 of visual cortical areas play an important role in perceptual grouping. The model proposes how development enables the strength of these long-range excitatory horizontal connections to be (approximately) balanced against the strength of short-range disynaptic inhibitory interneurons that input to the same target pyramidal cells. These balanced connections are proposed to realize properties of perceptual grouping in the adult. Figure 6.1 summarizes how these balanced connections enable perceptual groupings to form between pairs, or greater numbers, of inducers in an image (the case of a Kanizsa square is here illustrated) but not outwardly from a single inducer, which would fill the percept with spurious boundaries.

The model also proposes that development enables the strength of excitatory connections from layer 6-to-4 is to be balanced against those of inhibitory interneuronal connections to the same layer 4 cells; see Figure 6.2. Due to this balance, the net excitatory effect of layer 6 on layer 4 is proposed to be modulatory. These (approximately) balanced excitatory and inhibitory connections exist within the on-center of an on-center off-surround network from layer 6-to-4. The off-surround cells can strongly inhibit their target cells, even though the on-center cells can only provide excitatory modulation to their target cells.

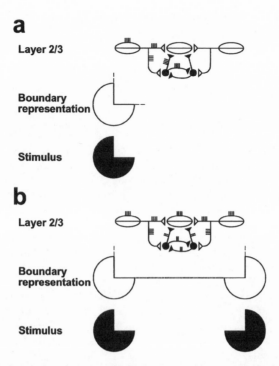

Figure 6.1. Schematic of the boundary grouping circuit in layer 2/3. Pyramidal cells with collinear, coaxial receptive fields (shown as ovals) excite each other via long-range horizontal axons (Bosking et al., 1997; Schmidt et al., 1997a), which also give rise to short-range, disynaptic inhibition via pools of interneurons, shown as filled-in black (McGuire et al., 1991). This balance of excitation and inhibition helps to implement what we call the *bipole property*. (a) Illustration of how horizontal input coming in from just one side is insufficient to cause above-threshold excitation in a pyramidal cell (henceforth referred to as the target) whose receptive field does not itself receive any bottom-up input. The inducing stimulus (e.g., a Kanizsa "pacman," shown here) excites the oriented receptive fields of layer 2/3 cells, which send out long-range horizontal excitation onto the target pyramidal. However, this excitation brings with it a commensurate amount of disynaptic inhibition. This creates a case of "one against one," and the target pyramidal is not excited above threshold. The boundary representation of the solitary pacman inducer produces only weak, subthreshold collinear extensions (thin dashed lines). (b) When two collinearly aligned induced stimuli are present, one on each side of the target pyramidal's receptive field, a boundary grouping can form. Long-range excitatory inputs fall onto the cell from both sides and summate. However, these inputs fall onto a shared pool of inhibitory interneurons, which, as well as inhibiting the target pyramidal, also inhibit each other (Tamas, Somogyi, & Buhl, 1998), thus normalizing the total amount of inhibition emanating from the interneuron pool, without any individual interneuron saturating. This summating excitation and normalizing inhibition together create a case of "two against one," and the target pyramidal is excited above threshold. This process occurs along the whole boundary grouping, which thereby becomes represented by a line of suprathreshold layer 2/3 cells (thick dotted line). Boundary strength scales in a graded analog manner with the strength of the inducing signals. Reprinted with kind permission from Grossberg, S., & Raizada, R.D.S. (2000). Contrast-sensitive perceptual grouping and object-based attention in the laminar circuits of primary visual cortex. *Vision Research, 40,* 1413–1432. Copyright 2000, Elsevier Science, Ltd., The Boulevard, Langford Lane, Kidlington OX5 1GB, UK.

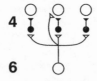

Figure 6.2. Schematic of the modulatory layer 6-to-layer 4 on-center off-surround path. Pyramidal cells in layer 6 give on-center excitation to layer 4 spiny stellates in the column above them but also make medium-range connections onto layer 4 inhibitory interneurons, shown as filled-in black (Ahmed et al., 1997; McGuire et al., 1984). These interneurons synapse onto the spiny stellates, creating a 6-to-4 off-surround, and also onto each other (connection not illustrated), thereby helping to normalize the total amount of inhibition (Ahmed et al., 1997). Note that the 6-to-4 off-surround inhibition spatially overlaps with the excitatory on-center, with the consequence that the 6-to-4 excitation is inhibited down into being modulatory, that is, priming or subthreshold (Callaway, 1998b; Stratford et al., 1996). Reprinted with kind permission from Grossberg, S., & Raizada, R.D.S. (2000). Contrast-sensitive perceptual grouping and object-based attention in the laminar circuits of primary visual cortex. *Vision Research, 40*, 1413–1432. Copyright 2000, Elsevier Science, Ltd., The Boulevard, Langford Lane, Kidlington OX5 1GB, UK.

The model proposes how this layer 6-to-4 circuit functions as a "selection circuit" because it can help to select the groupings that enter conscious attention. Grouping cells in layer 2/3 can activate the layer 6-to-4 selection circuit via excitatory connections from layer 2/3 to layer 6; see Figure 6.3a. When ambiguous and complex scenes are being processed, many possible groupings can start to form using the horizontal connections within layer 2/3. The selection circuit enables the strongest groupings to inhibit weaker groupings via the 6-to-4 off-surrounds of the strongest groupings.

The model clarifies how top-down attention can bias this selection process and thereby influence which groupings will enter conscious perception. In particular, it is proposed that top-down attentional signals from higher cortical areas, such as area V2, can also activate the layer 6-to-4 on-center off-surround network; see Figure 6.3b. Because both grouping and attention share the same selection circuit, this anatomical arrangement enables attention to influence which groupings are perceived. Attention hereby can modulate, or sensitize, cells in the attentional on-center, without fully activating them, because the excitatory and inhibitory signals in the on-center are balanced. Attention can also inhibit cells in the off-surround. In this way, attention can shift the excitatory/inhibitory balance that determines which groupings will enter consciousness. A dramatic example of this influence occurs when attention that is caste on one part of an object can flow selectively along the perceptual groupings that define the entire object. Roelfsema, Lamme, and Spekreijse (1998) have discovered such a flow of attention along a perceptual grouping during their neurophysiological recordings in macaque area V1. Because of this property, both infants and

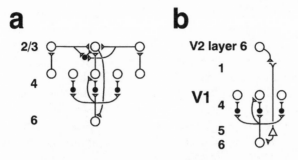

Figure 6.3. (a) Connecting the 6-to-4 on-center off-surround to the layer 2/3 grouping circuit: like-oriented layer 4 simple cells with opposite contrast polarities compete (not shown) before generating half-wave rectified outputs that converge onto layer 2/3 complex cells in the column above them. Like attentional signals from higher cortex, groupings that form within layer 2/3 also send activation into the *folded feedback* path to enhance their own positions in layer 4 beneath them via the 6-to-4 on-center and to suppress input to other groupings via the 6-to-4 off-surround. There exist direct layer 2/3-to-6 connections in macaque V1, as well as indirect routes via layer 5. (b) *Folded feedback* carries attentional signal from higher cortex into layer 4 of V1, via the modulatory 6-to-4 path. Corticocortical feedback axons tend preferentially to originate in layer 6 of the higher area and to terminate in the lower cortex's layer 1 (Salin & Bullier, 1995, p. 110), where they can excite the apical dendrites of layer 5 pyramidal cells whose axons send collaterals into layer 6. Several other routes through which feedback can pass into V1 layer exist. Having arrived in layer 6, the feedback is then "folded" back up into the feedforward stream by passing through the 6-to-4 on-center off-surround path (Bullier et al., 1996). Reprinted with kind permission from Grossberg, S., & Raizada, R.D.S. (2000). Contrast-sensitive perceptual grouping and object-based attention in the laminar circuits of primary visual cortex. *Vision Research, 40,* 1413–1432. Copyright 2000, Elsevier Science, Ltd., The Boulevard, Langford Lane, Kidlington OX5 1GB, UK.

adults can focus their attention selectively upon whole objects, rather than just random subsets of visual features.

The feedback circuits that govern the grouping and attentional selection processes are predicted to play a key role in helping to stabilize both development and adult learning within multiple cortical areas, including cortical areas V1 and V2. During development, the selection circuit (which itself is developing) helps to prevent the wrong combinations of cells from being coactivated and thus from being associated, or wired, together.

Balanced excitatory and inhibitory connections have other effects as well on cortical processing. Balanced connections help to explain the observed variability in the number and temporal distribution of spikes emitted by cortical neurons. Modeling studies have shown how balanced excitation and inhibition can produce the highly variable interspike intervals that are found in cortical data (Shadlen & Newsome, 1998; van Vreeswijk & Sompolinsky, 1998). The present model suggests that such variability may reflect mechanisms that are needed to ensure stable development and learning by cortical circuits. Given that "stability implies variability," the cortex is faced with the difficult problem that variable spikes are quite inefficient in driving responses from cortical neurons. On the other hand, when one analyzes how these balanced excitatory and inhibitory connections actually work to generate perceptual groupings, it becomes clear that the grouping circuits automatically have the property of preferentially responding to synchronized inputs. Figure 6.1 illustrates why synchronously activated cells will have a difficult time generating a perceptual grouping, whereas synchronously activated cells will not. According to Figure 6.1a, an asynchronous volley of horizontal signals from a single population of layer 2/3 cells will kill itself off due to balanced excitation and inhibition. According to Figure 6.1b, a synchronous volley from pairs of appropriately positioned cells will initiate grouping. Earlier studies have also shown how both perceptual grouping and attentional circuits can, in fact, actively resynchronize signals that have become partially desynchronized (Grossberg & Grunewald, 1997; Grossberg & Somers, 1991). The model hereby discloses a previously unsuspected link between properties of stable development, adult learning, grouping, attention, and synchronous cortical processing.

This contribution will focus primarily on how the types of horizontal connections and interlaminar connections develop within cortical layers 2/3, 4, and 6 that are mentioned above, primarily in cortical area V1, but by extension to V2 and higher cortical regions. These interactions are often cited as the basis of "nonclassical" receptive fields that are sensitive to the context in which individual features are found (Born & Tootell, 1991; Knierim & van Essen, 1992; Peterhans & von der Heydt, 1989; Sillito et al., 1995; von der Heydt, Peterhans, & Baumgartner, 1984). In this first modeling study, it is assumed that receptive fields of individual simple and complex cells in layers 4 and 2/3, respectively, have already substantially developed. Neurophysiologists classify simple and complex cells using a number of cell response properties. One of the most basic properties is that simple cells tend to respond to an oriented set of image features (oriented edge, shading, or texture gradient) with a prescribed contrast polarity (either dark-to-light or light-to-dark but not both). Simple cells are the first stage of processing for bottom-up inputs to the cortex from the lateral geniculate nucleus (LGN; see Figures 6.3a and 6.4a). Complex cells tend to respond to an oriented set of image features that may have either contrast polarity (either dark-to-light or light-to-dark). In the classical Hubel and Wiesel (1977) model of cortical organization, these properties were assumed to arise due to converging inputs from two or more simple cells that respond to either contrast polarity onto a shared population of complex cells. This processing step occurs between layer 4 and 2/3 in the model (Figures 6.3a and 6.4a). The Hubel and Wiesel picture cannot, however, be fully supported because there are known feedback interactions that link

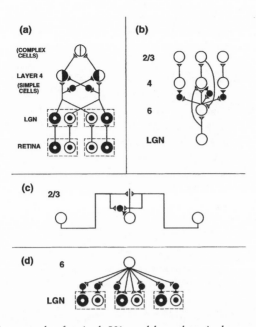

Figure 6.4. The adult network of retinal, V1, and lateral geniculate nucleus (LGN) neurons to which the developmental model converges. (a) Feedforward circuit from retina to LGN to cortical layer 4. *Retina*: Retinal ON cells have on-center off-surround organization (white disk surrounded by black annulus). Retinal OFF cells have an off-center on-surround organization (black disk surrounded by white annulus). *LGN*: The LGN ON and OFF cells receive feedforward ON and OFF cell inputs from the retina. *Layer 4*: LGN ON and OFF cell excitatory inputs to layer 4 establish oriented simple cell receptive fields. Like-oriented layer 4 simple cells with opposite contrast polarities compete before generating half-wave rectified outputs. Pooled simple cell outputs enable complex cells to respond to both polarities. They hereby full-wave rectify the image. See text for details. (b) Cortical feedback loop between layers 4, 2/3, and 6: LGN activates layer 6 as well as layer 4. Layer 6 cells excite layer 4 cells with a narrow on-center and inhibit them using layer 4 inhibitory interneurons that span a broader off-surround. Layer 4 cells excite layer 2/3 cells, which send excitatory feedback signals back to layer 6 cells via layer 5 (not shown). Layer 2/3 can hereby activate the feedforward layer 6-to-4 on-center off-surround network. (c) The horizontal interactions in layer 2/3 that initiate perceptual grouping: Layer 2/3 complex pyramidal cells monosynaptically excite one another via horizontal connections, primarily on their apical dendrites. They also inhibit one another via disynaptic inhibition that is mediated by model smooth stellate cells. Together these interactions can realize the "bipole property" that enables groupings to form inwardly across the space between two or more inducers, but not awardly from a single inducer. (d) Top-down corticogeniculate feedback from layer 6: LGN ON and OFF cells receive topographic excitatory feedback from layer 6 and more broadly distributed inhibitory feedback via LGN inhibitory interneurons that are excited by layer 6 signals. The feedback signals pool outputs over all cortical orientations and are delivered equally to ON and OFF cells. See the text for further details. Reprinted with kind permission from Grossberg, S., & Williamson, J. (2001). A neural model of how horizontal and interlaminar connections of visual cortex develop into adult circuits that carry out perceptual grouping and learning. *Cerebral Cortex, 11*, 37–58. Copyright 2001, Elsevier Science, Ltd., The Boulevard, Langford Lane, Kidlington OX5 1GB, UK.

cells in layers 2/3, 4, and 6 together, as illustrated in Figure 6.3a. These feedback signals cause the involved cells to share some of their response properties.

Two other models will be briefly reviewed in order to clarify how the simple and complex cell receptive fields themselves develop. Taken together, these three modeling studies provide a foundation for ongoing modeling work that is attempting to show how all the cortical layers develop (e.g., Seitz & Grossberg, 2001). The second model considers the basic question of how cortical area V1 manages to pack in all the simple cells that respond to different eyes or different orientations at different positions on the retina. Cells in cortical area V1 are arranged into columns that run vertically through the cortical layers. Local circuits link together cells within a column in the different cortical layers, as illustrated in Figures 6.3a and 6.4b. Cells in each column have similar orientational tuning and sensitivity to eye of origin, or ocular dominance. The cortex packs these columns together in an efficient way by using a two-dimensional *map* of orientation and ocular dominance (Hubel & Wiesel, 1962, 1963, 1968). This organization is called a map because cell tuning to orientation and ocular dominance varies in a systematic way as the cortex is traversed in a horizontal direction. Such maps exhibit properties that are called singularities, fractures, and linear zones (Blasdel, 1992a, 1992b; Obeymeyer & Blasdel, 1993). The model shows how these features of cortical maps develop (see Figure 6.14).

Because of the critical importance of simple cells and of cortical maps in understanding cortical function, a number of models have studied how simple cells develop their orientationally tuned receptive fields within maps of orientation and ocular dominance (e.g., Durbin & Mitchison, 1990; Grossberg, 1976a; Grossberg & Olson, 1994; Linsker, 1986a, 1986b; Miller, 1992, 1994; Obermayer, Blasdel, & Schulten, 1992; Obermayer, Ritter, & Schulten, 1990; Olson & Grossberg, 1998; Rojer & Schwartz, 1989, 1990; Sirosh & Miikkulainen, 1994; Swindale, 1980, 1982, 1992; von der Malsburg, 1973; Willshaw & von der Malsburg, 1976). The model described herein will show, in addition, how nearby pairs of simple cells develop that are sensitive to the same orientation but opposite contrast polarities (Liu et al., 1992). Such a model is called a Triple-O model because it shows how Orientation, Ocular dominance, and Opposite contrast polarities all develop together (Olson & Grossberg, 1998). Earlier models were either Single-O or Double-O models, and many did not represent the dynamics of the cells whose connections were undergoing development. The Triple-O model clarifies how nearby simple cells that are sensitive to opposite contrast polarities could, in principle, cooperate to activate a shared complex cell.

The third model suggests how nearby pairs of simple cells that are sensitive to opposite contrast polarities actually develop connections to shared complex cells (Grunewald & Grossberg, 1998). In addition to being tuned to position, size, orientation, and pooled contrast polarities, the complex cells in the model, and in vivo, are also tuned to binocular disparity, which is a well-known cue to object depth (Julesz, 1971). These complex cell properties help to explain how depth-sensitive perceptual groupings can form over objects that are seen in front of textured backgrounds and also how figure-ground properties emerge; see Grossberg (1994) for further discussion of how this happens. A key question for present purposes concerns how oppositely polarized simple cells, whose activations are *anticorrelated* in time (if a contrast at a given position is dark-to-light, it cannot also be light-to-dark, and conversely), can nonetheless develop connections to a shared complex cell and thereby become *correlated*.

Several mechanisms are proposed that work together to achieve this end. One mechanism causes *antagonist rebounds* to occur between simple cells that are sensitive to opposite contrast polarities but the same positions and orientations. For example, when a simple cell that has been on for awhile in response to a dark-to-light contrast shuts off, an opponent simple cell, which is sensitive to a light-to-dark contrast, briefly turns on. Such rebounds are proposed to be due to the chemical transmitters that carry signals between model cells. Certain of these transmitters are proposed to habituate, or inactivate, when they are released by signals in their pathways, or axons. These habituative transmitters also play a role in controlling how cortical maps of simple cells develop. It is also suggested how learned feedback from cortical area V1 to the LGN may carry out a matching process that helps to stabilize the development of disparity tuning in cortical complex cells and, by extension, the cortical map itself (see Figure 6.4d). This V1-to-LGN feedback is homologous to the attentional feedback that is proposed to occur from cortical area V2 to V1 (Figure 6.3b) and by extension other cortical areas as well. These various interactions clarify how complex cells can binocularly match left and right eye image features with the same contrast polarity, yet can also pool signals with opposite contrast polarities, consistent with psychophysical and neurobiological data about adult 3D vision (see Grossberg and McLoughlin, 1997 and McLoughlin and Grossberg, 1998 for an explanation of such data using these mechanisms). With this extended introduction in hand, the relevant modeling concepts will now be described in greater detail.

LINKING CORTICAL DEVELOPMENT TO ADULT PERCEPTION

Perceptual grouping is the process whereby the brain organizes image contrasts into emergent boundary structures that segregate objects and their backgrounds in response to texture, shading, and depth cues in scenes and images (Beck, Prazdny, & Rosenfeld, 1983; Julesz, 1971; Polat & Sagi,

1994; Ramachandran & Nelson, 1976). Perceptual grouping is a basic step in solving the "binding problem," whereby spatially distributed features are bound into representations of objects and events in the world. Illusory contours are a particularly vivid form of perceptual grouping since they illustrate how perceptual groupings can be completed over image locations that contain no contrastive scenic elements. Illusory contours are thus a popular and useful probe of how perceptual grouping occurs. Illusory contours are not just perceptual curiosities, however, since they also help to complete boundary representations over the retinal blind spot and veins, over missing pixels in textured images, and the like.

The first model to be reviewed (Grossberg & Williamson, 2001) suggests that many aspects of cortical design have evolved to carry out perceptual grouping. In particular, the model proposes how the laminar circuits of visual cortex enable it to develop connections capable of actively selecting and completing the perceptual grouping that best represents a visual scene and suppressing the weaker groupings that represent the scene less well. The winning grouping has the property of *coherence* in the sense that its constituent features are actively bound together, indeed even synchronized, by feedback interactions. The winning grouping that is chosen in this way can also represent *analog* properties of the world, such as the relative contrasts and spatial positions of objects in the scene. I have called this combination of properties *analog coherence*. Analog coherence is not an easy combination of properties to achieve computationally in a robust way, since an active selection process that leads to coherent binding can all too easily sharpen feature values so much that their analog properties are lost. The LAMINART model shows how the laminar circuits of neocortex can robustly achieve analog coherence and thereby solve the binding problem.

Models such as LAMINART that link brain to behavior need to show how interactions among many model cells give rise to emergent properties that match behavioral data. Several types of emergent properties are simulated by the model. As noted above, the model assumes that the classical receptive fields of simple and complex cells have already developed. This hypothesis is consistent with data showing that the oriented pattern of LGN-to-V1 connections develops prior to eye opening and structured visual input (e.g., Antonini & Stryker, 1993a; Chapman & Stryker, 1993; Chapman, Zahs, & Stryker, 1991; Stryker & Harris, 1986). The model focuses upon how the longer-range nonclassical connections between cortical columns develop both prior to eye opening and after structured visual inputs occur. It proposes rules whereby such cortical development is controlled. Several such rules work together to control stable growth of model connections by ensuring that balanced excitatory and inhibitory connections develop. The emergent properties of this developmental process are the adult anatomical and neurophysiological circuits into which the model develops. After model development stabilizes, visual inputs activate cells within the developed anatomy, thereby leading to a second type of emergent properties, namely, the cell activity patterns that match data about adult visual perception. These two types of emergent properties show how a single model can explain data about cortical development, anatomy, neurophysiology, and perception.

Classical Receptive Fields

The model assumes that three types of circuits with (primarily) classical receptive field properties develop, at least in part, before the circuits that subserve nonclassical receptive fields. We call the circuits that have already developed "predeveloped" circuits. The circuits that develop through model dynamics are called "selforganized" circuits. The model analyzes one important combination of intracortical and intercortical pathways. It does not attempt to model all cortical connections or the variations that exist across species. It also models the predeveloped circuits in the simplest possible way, since they are not the focus of this study (but see below for models of how the predeveloped circuits themselves develop), and the computational demands of the simulations are great even with these simplifications. Preliminary studies indicate, however, that the computational principles modeled herein can be elaborated and adapted to handle these variations.

Model analyses will be restricted to cortical area V1 and more particularly to the interblobs within V1 that are suggested to carry out early stages of perceptual grouping. Converging evidence suggests that area V2 replicates the structure of area V1, but at a larger spatial scale, notably with longer horizontal connections to carry out grouping (Felleman & van Essen, 1991; Grosof, Shapley, & Hawken, 1993; Kisvarday et al., 1995; van Essen & Maunsell, 1983; von der Heydt, Peterhans, & Baumgartner, 1984). These anatomical similarities make it plausible to assume that similar developmental processes may be operative in both V1 and V2. Due to the larger extent of horizontal connections in area V2, V2, rather than V1, may be carrying out the longer-range perceptual groupings that cross the blind spot, make illusory contours, and group discrete texture elements. In addition, V2 seems to be specialized for some of the processes that initiate depthful separation of figures from their backgrounds (see Grossberg [1994, 1997] for further analyses of figure-ground separation). The model's predeveloped and self-organized properties are intuitively described below. For a mathematical description, see Grossberg and Williamson (2001). Figure 6.4 schematizes the model's connections.

Direct LGN Inputs to Layer 4

In both the brain and the model, the retina activates the lateral geniculate nucleus, which, in turn, inputs to cortical area V1. LGN inputs directly excite layer 4 (Chapman, Zahs, & Stryker, 1991; Hubel & Wiesel, 1962; Reid & Alonso, 1995), as in Figures 6.4a and 6.4b. In modeling these data, a single, generic layer 4 is used for simplicity; see the pathways with open triangles in Figure 6.4a. These inputs play a key role in establishing the orientational tuning of V1 simple cells.

Model simple cells have predeveloped connections that respond to a given orientation and contrast polarity; that is, they respond best to visual inputs that have a prescribed orientation and whose luminance preference, across this oriented axis, goes either from dark-to-light or from light-to-dark but not both. Simple cells are represented by circular symbols with half-white and half-black hemidisks in Figure 6.4a. These properties arise as follows from model LGN inputs and intracortical interactions: LGN ON cells (cells that are turned on by input onset; see symbols with white disks and black annuli in Figure 6.4a) and LGN OFF cells (cells that are turned off by input onset; see symbols with black disks and white annuli in Figure 6.4a) both input to layer 4. They are organized into spatially offset arrays, with the ON cell inputs spatially displaced with respect to the OFF cell inputs, as in Figure 6.4a. Due to this input array, layer 4 simple cells can respond to an oriented input whose luminant area excites the ON cells and whose dark area excites the OFF cells.

Selectivity of simple cell responses to oriented contrasts is improved by mutually inhibitory interactions between cells that are sensitive to the same orientation but opposite contrast polarities (Ferster, 1988; Gove, Grossberg, & Mingolla, 1995; Liu et al., 1992; Palmer & Davis, 1981; Pollen & Ronner, 1981); see the pathways with black triangles in Figure 6.4a. Then when cells that code opposite contrast polarities are equally activated by a uniform input, they shut each other off by mutual inhibition. On the other hand, when an oriented input is presented, the simple cells that best match its position, orientation, and contrast polarity will be most activated. I review below how mutually inhibitory simple cells may develop that are sensitive to the same orientation and opposite contrast polarities, at the same time that a cortical map develops whose orientation and ocular dominance columns exhibit the fractures, singularities, and linear zones reported by Blasdel (1992a, 1992b) and Obermayer and Blasdel (1993).

Balanced LGN Inputs to Layer 4 via Layer 6

In both brain and model, LGN inputs also directly excite layer 6 (Ferster & Lindström, 1985), which then indirectly influences layer 4 via an oncenter off-surround network of cells (Ahmed et al., 1994, 1997; Grieve & Sillito, 1991a, 1991b, 1995). Cells in the on-center receive excitatory inputs from layer 6, whereas those in the spatially broader off-surround (that includes on-center cells) receive inhibitory inputs from layer 6 via inhibitory interneurons in layer 4. In Figure 6.4b, open triangles designate excitatory connections, and black triangles designate inhibitory connections.

The model explains why layer 4 receives both direct LGN inputs and indirect inputs via layer 6. The indirect inputs to layer 4 from layer 6 cannot activate layer 4 cells. Because of the (approximate) balance between excitation and inhibition in the on-center, layer 6 can at best weakly activate, or modulate, cells in layer 4. This modulatory property helps to ensure stable cortical development and adult learning within the model. Such a dual input to layer 4 is found in many neocortical areas (Felleman & van Essen, 1991; van Essen & Maunsell, 1983). The model suggests that the combination of direct and indirect inputs to layer 4 from LGN helps to preserve stable development and learning in all these areas, while also allowing them to be activated by bottom-up inputs. In particular, the model predicts that the balance between the on-center and the off-surround inputs from layer 6 to 4 has the consequence that direct activation of layer 6 can modulate, prime, or subliminally activate cells in layer 4 but cannot fire them vigorously. Although this prediction has not been directly tested, compatible data have been reported by Callaway (1998a), Hupé et al. (1997), and Wittmer, Dalva, and Katz (1997). The need to maintain this balance also predicts why direct inputs to layer 4 are needed, in addition to the indirect on-center inputs via layer 6, in many cortical areas. Since the indirect LGN-to-6-to-4 inputs cannot activate layer 4 cells without destabilizing cortical development and learning, the direct LGN-to-4 inputs are needed to initiate cortical firing. Model simulations support the prediction that if the excitatory on-center inputs from layer 6 get too strong relative to the off-surround inputs from layer 6 to 4, then development does not self-stabilize. Instead, the nonclassical receptive fields of the model proliferate uncontrollably. On the other hand, if the inhibition gets too strong, then it can inhibit the inputs arriving at layer 4 too much, thereby preventing the model cortex from becoming activated at all. Of course, one might argue that the direct LGN to layer 4 connections develop earlier in any case, but this explanation does not explain why this connection did not also develop the on-center off-surround network as a single input pathway.

Given that strong direct inputs from LGN to layer 4 do exist, the combined effect of both the direct and indirect pathways from LGN to layer 4 is to form an on-center off-surround network. When cells in such a network obey the membrane equations of neurophysiology, then they can maintain their sensitivity to input intensities that may vary over a large dynamic range (Douglas et al., 1995; Grossberg, 1973, 1980b; Heeger, 1993). This means that the *relative* input sizes can be detected by the target cells in layer 4, without saturation, over a wide dynamical range. This is because the membrane equations of neurophysiology that govern cell activation contain "shunting," or automatic gain control, terms that respond to properly balanced on-center and off-surround inputs by normalizing the activities of target cells without destroying their sensitivity to the relative sizes of the inputs; see Grossberg (1988) for a review of this property. In the present instance, such a network maintains the sensitivity of cells in layer 4 to inputs from the prior processing level, whether it be cells in V1 responding to LGN inputs, cells in V2 responding to inputs from V1, or any other combination of inputs.

In summary, the LAMINART model predicts that the mechanism whereby the balance between excitation and inhibition is maintained in the layer 6-to-4 circuit is of great importance for achieving stable cortical development and later visual perception. This issue has been hardly explored experimentally. This prediction implies that a key cortical design problem is the following: As more and more cells in the off-surround become activated by increasingly dense patterns of inputs, what prevents the total inhibition that is converging on a layer 4 cell from growing linearly? If there was just enough inhibition to balance the excitation when just a few inputs were active, then why would not the inhibition become much too strong when many inputs were active, thereby shutting down the network? On the other hand, if the inhibition is well balanced when many inputs are active, then why does not runaway excitation occur when just a few inputs are active?

Development of Self-Normalizing Inhibitory Interneurons in Layer 4

The model solves these problems by assuming that the inhibitory interneurons in layer 4 inhibit one another, as well as target cells in layer 4 (see Ahmed et al. [1994, 1997] for consistent data). In particular, the model suggests how layer 4 inhibitory interneurons learn connections to layer 4 spiny stellate excitatory cells as well as to other nearby layer 4 inhibitory interneurons. These connections start out with synaptic weights of zero magnitude, which are updated to learn the activity patterns of their target cells. The recurrent inhibition that develops between the inhibitory interneurons converts the network of inhibitory interneurons into a recurrent feedback network. Because the cells of this network obey membrane equations, this network of recurrent inhibitory interneurons tends to normalize the total activity across the interneuron population (Grossberg, 1973, 1980b). The total inhibition that converges on a layer 4 simple cell thus tends to be conserved as the total number of inputs varies, thereby maintaining the balance between excitation and inhibition and avoiding the problems stated above.

If this self-normalization property within the inhibitory interneuronal population is experimentally confirmed, then it will be an interesting example of how less order on one level of biological organization generates more order on a higher level. In particular, the crucial self-normalization property can be achieved simply by allowing the inhibitory interneurons to randomly develop to inhibit all cells within their range, rather than restricting the developing inhibitory pathways to reach only excitatory target cells. As a result of this less-ordered growth of inhibitory connections, the stability of the total network is facilitated.

Maintaining the balance between excitation and inhibition within the layer 6-to-4 on center does not imply that inhibition is weak. In fact, layer 4 cells that receive only off-surround inputs can be strongly inhibited. The model suggests how the on-center off-surround network from layer 6-to-4 can act as a *selection network* that selectively amplifies the strongest perceptual groupings in layer 2/3 via a 2/3-to-6-to-4 feedback loop, while actively suppressing LGN inputs to layer 4 that correspond to weaker groupings via the 6-to-4 off-surround; see Figure 6.1a. The inputs that have been supporting the weaker groupings are hereby inhibited and thus the groupings themselves. This is proposed to happen as follows.

Columnar Organization via Folded Feedback

Active model layer 4 cells are assumed to generate inputs to pyramidal cells in layer 2/3 via predeveloped pathways. These layer 2/3 cells initiate the formation of perceptual groupings via horizontal connections that self-organize during model development; see Figures 6.1a and 6.4. How these horizontal connections develop is described below. Before describing this, we first note what happens when layer 2/3 cells are activated. Throughout the developmental process, all cells that are activated in layer 2/3, whether by bottom-up or horizontal inputs, send excitatory feedback signals to layer 6 via layer 5 (Ferster & Lindström, 1985; Gilbert & Wiesel, 1979), as in Figure 6.1b. Layer 6, in turn, once again activates the on-center off-surround network from layer 6 to 4. This process is called *folded feedback* (Grossberg, 1999a), because feedback signals from layer 2/3 get transmitted in a feedforward fashion back to layer 4. The feedback is hereby "folded" back into the feedforward flow of bottom-up information within the laminar cortical circuits.

Folded feedback is predicted to be a mechanism that binds the cells throughout layers 2/3, 4, 5, and 6 into functional columns (Hubel & Wiesel, 1962, 1977; Mountcastle, 1957). The on-center off-surround network from layer 6 to 4 responds to its layer 2/3 inputs by helping to control which combinations of cells remain simultaneously active during development and thus which cells will wire together, because "cells that fire together wire together."

In particular, early during the development of model horizontal connections in layer 2/3, these connections are relatively unselective for colinear position and orientation, as in the data of Galuske and Singer (1996) and

Ruthazer and Stryker (1996). Without further selection among the possible connection patterns, cortical interactions could remain both spatially and orientationally dispersed. This is corrected in the model via the intracortical folded feedback loop. In particular, suppose that a combination of bottom-up inputs and horizontal connections activates one subset of layer 2/3 cells a little more than a nearby subset of cells. Then, other things being equal, the favored layer 2/3 cells more vigorously activate their layer 2/3-to-5-to-6 pathway and then their on-center off-surround layer 6-to-4 circuit. As a result, the cells whose activities form the strongest layer 2/3 grouping will suppress the activities of other cells via the layer 6-to-4 off-surround. The winning cells then get connected together via development, leading to a progressive increase in the projection range and orientation selectivity of these cells; see the simulations below. Such an increase in the projection range and orientation selectivity may explain why neonates appear to perceive a partly occluded object as disjoint parts but can process these fragments as coherent objects within the first 2 to 4 months of life (Johnson, 2001; Johnson & Aslin, 1996; Kellman & Spelke, 1983).

This refinement process exploits the fact that orientationally tuned simple cells can bias development to favor long-range horizontal connections that are colinear with the preferred orientations of spatially aligned simple cells (Fitzpatrick, 1996; Schmidt et al., 1997a). It is shown below how such oriented and colinear horizontal connections develop from an initial state in which no horizontal connections exist at all. It is also shown that, after development self-stabilizes, the same properties play a key role in generating perceptual groupings that exhibit properties of adult neurophysiological and psychophysical data. More recent modeling work simulates how the subplate can help to set up consistent initial orientational biases across layers even before layer 4 gets connected to layer 2/3 (Seitz & Grossberg, 2001).

Horizontal Connections and Perceptual Grouping

How these developing horizontal connections are prevented from generating runaway excitation and uncontrollable growth is one of the key properties of the model. A clue may be derived from properties of adult horizontal connections. In areas V1 and V2 of the adult, layer 2/3 pyramidal cells excite each other using monosynaptic long-range horizontal connections. They also inhibit each other using short-range disynaptic inhibitory connections that are activated by the excitatory horizontal connections (Hirsch & Gilbert, 1991; McGuire et al., 1991); see Figures 6.1a and 6.4c. The excitatory connections are hereby balanced by inhibitory connections. We show below how both types of connections can develop to generate perceptual groupings "inwardly" between two or more image contrasts that are aligned colinearly across space (Grosof, Shapley, & Hawken, 1993; Peterhans & von der Heydt, 1989; Redies, Crook, & Creutz-feldt, 1986; von der Heydt, Peterhans, & Baumgartner, 1984) but not "outwardly" from a single image contrast (Cannon & Fullenkamp, 1993; Hirsch & Gilbert, 1991; Knierim & van Essen, 1992; Somers, Nelson, & Sur, 1995; Stemmler, Usher, & Niebur, 1995). This is called the *bipole property* (Grossberg & Mingolla, 1985a, 1985b) and is illustrated in Figure 6.1. Illusory contours provide an excellent example of the bipole property: If a single image contrast could generate outward groupings, then our percepts would become crowded with webs of illusory contours spreading out from every feature in a scene. On the other hand, percepts of illusory contours between two or more colinear inducers are commonplace, as in the famous Kanizsa square (Kanizsa, 1979, 1985).

The model proposes how a balance between layer 2/3 excitation and inhibition develops that helps to stabilize cortical development and leads to the bipole property in the adult. For definiteness, call layer 2/3 pyramidal cells that receive bottom-up input from layer 4 "supported" cells, and those that do not, "unsupported" cells. In the model, if an unsupported cell receives a sufficient amount of horizontal excitation, then it will be driven above its firing threshold. The cell will then output horizontal excitation to itself as well as to other pyramidal cells. Turning off input support from layer 4 causes all layer 2/3 activities to decay to zero. Therefore, boundaries can group across a gap provided the gap is small enough and the grouping signals from the supported cells on each end of the gap are sufficiently strong to drive the unsupported cells that lie between them above threshold.

The horizontal excitation from a single supported cell cannot cause runaway excitation and outward grouping among unsupported cells because it activates balanced disynaptic inhibition from smooth stellate cells. In this situation, the disynaptic inhibition is proportional to the horizontal excitation because both pyramidal and smooth stellate cells receive the same horizontal input signal. The inhibition from smooth stellate cells to pyramidal cells can lag behind the direct excitation between pyramidal cells due to the time it takes the smooth stellate cells to integrate their inputs. Therefore, synchronized inputs to layer 2/3 facilitate grouping because they allow the horizontal signals to summate at the target pyramidal cells before inhibition from local smooth stellate cells takes effect. This property is consistent with the finding of Usher and Donnelly (1998) that visual groupings are facilitated when inducers are presented synchronously.

As in the case of the layer 4 off-surround, the model disynaptic inhibitory interneurons are predicted to inhibit each other as well as the pyramidal cells. This model hypothesis is consistent with anatomical data showing that inhibitory interneurons synapse on both pyramidal cells and other interneurons (Kisvarday, Beaulieu, & Eysel, 1993; McGuire et al., 1991). Hence, the total activation within such a population of inhibitory interneurons is predicted to be normalized. As a result, inhibition grows less quickly than summating activation of the pyramidal cells. The model hereby predicts that recurrent inhibition may be used to control the excitatory-inhibitory balance in both layer 2/3 and layer 4. Net activation of the target pyramidal cells is thus possible, and grouping can occur inwardly but not outwardly, thereby realizing the bipole property (Grossberg & Mingolla, 1985b), which has been used to explain and predict many perceptual grouping data (e.g., Born & Tootell, 1991; Dresp & Grossberg, 1997; Field, Hayes, & Hess, 1993; Gove, Grossberg, & Mingolla, 1995; Grossberg, 1994, 1997; Grossberg & Pessoa, 1998; Polat & Sagi, 1994; Shipley & Kellman, 1992; Watanabe & Cavanagh, 1992).

There is more neurophysiological evidence for the bipole property in cortical area V2 (e.g., von der Heydt & Peterhans, 1989; von der Heydt, Peterhans, & Baumgartner, 1984) than in V1. In V1, just a few unsupported cells have, to the present, been found that show full activation of unsupported cells by pairs of supporting cells. More V1 cells show a modulatory influence from neighboring pyramidal cells (e.g., Grosof, Shapley, & Hawken, 1993; Kapadia, et al., 1995; Redies, Crook, & Creutzfeldt, 1986; von der Heydt & Peterhans, 1989). These are challenging experiments to do in V1 because of the shorter horizontal connections there, and the existence of feedback from V2, which has longer horizontal connections. Unsupported V2 cells could be fully activated by stimuli that fall outside the V1 receptive fields and could modulate V1 cells by top-down feedback. For simplicity, the present model assumes that the bipole property holds in both V1 and V2.

Developmental Rules

These properties of adult grouping arise in the model by specializing two well-known developmental rules. The first rule is that axons are attracted to cell targets when the source and target cells are both active (Gundersen & Barrett, 1979, 1980; Letourneau, 1978; Lichtman & Purves, 1981; Purves & Lichtman, 1980). The second rule is that axons compete intracellularly for growth resources (Lichtman & Purves, 1981; Purves & Lichtman, 1980). In the present instance, the first rule enables horizontal connections to form if activations in a source pyramidal cell and a target pyramidal cell are sufficiently correlated—in particular, if the target cell satisfies the bipole property—and removed if they are not (Callaway & Katz, 1990, 1991; Dalva & Katz, 1994; Löwel & Singer, 1992). This rule is realized by an activity-dependent morphogenetic gradient whose strength decreases with distance from the target cell that emits it. The gradient influences horizontal growth only in active source cells. The developing cells sense the correlation between the chemicals that define the morphogenetic gradient and those that are activity dependent in the target cells. As contact between two cells is achieved, a synaptic learning law strengthens the synaptic contact by continuing to sense the correlation between presynaptic and postsynaptic activity.

The second rule prevents uncontrolled proliferation of horizontal connections by withdrawing connections from target cells that are receiving more poorly correlated signals than other target cells. The two rules work together to withdraw connections from cells that may be activated by weakly correlated image features or statistically insignificant noise.

Taken together, these model mechanisms for axonal growth and synaptic tuning dynamically stabilize cortical development as the developing cortical structure matches the statistics of its environmental inputs. If this match is disrupted later in life, then a new bout of development and/or learning can be triggered by the same mechanisms. Because of this property, the model can be used to clarify data about shared molecular substrates of neonatal development and adult learning (Bailey et al., 1992; Kandel & O'Dell, 1992; Mayford et al., 1992), plasticity of adult cortical representations after lesions (Chino et al., 1992; Darian-Smith & Gilbert, 1994; Das & Gilbert, 1995; Gilbert & Wiesel, 1992; Kapadia, Gilbert, & Westheimer, 1994; Merzenich et al., 1988; Schmidt et al., 1996), dynamical reorganization of long-range connections in the visual cortex (Gilbert & Wiesel, 1992; Zohary et al., 1994), and perceptual learning in the adult (Karni & Sagi, 1991; Poggio, Fahle, & Edelman, 1992). In fact, the model equations for activity-dependent controls of synaptic strength have already been used to explain properties of adult learning (e.g., Carpenter & Grossberg, 1991; Grossberg, 1980a).

Top-Down Feedback from V1 to LGN

Layer 6 of model area V1 sends top-down feedback to the LGN via an on-center off-surround network, as also occurs in vivo (Murphy & Sillito, 1987, 1996; Weber, Kalil, & Behan, 1989; see Figure 6.4d). The feedback on-center reinforces the activities of those LGN cells that have succeeded in activating V1 cells, notably V1 cells whose activations represent the strongest perceptual groupings. The feedback off-surround suppresses the activities of other LGN cells. As in the brain, this model feedback circuit increases the useful visual information that is transmitted from LGN to cortex by enhancing contextually significant differences between LGN responses (McClurkin, Optican, & Richmond, 1994), and also influences the length tuning of LGN cells (Murphy & Sillito, 1987). The LGN to V1 circuit is also known to be modulatory (Sillito et al., 1994).

Earlier modeling work predicted that this feedback pathway plays a role in stabilizing the development of bottom-up connections from LGN to V1, as well as the reciprocal top-down connections from V1 to LGN (Grossberg, 1976b, 1980a). Grunewald and Grossberg (1998) have modeled how the normal development of bottom-up disparity tuning can occur at V1 complex cells when such top-down feedback is operative and have shown how this development may break down when it is not. Further experimental study of this question is needed. For simplicity, in the model of how

UNSTRUCTURED VISION   STRUCTURED VISION

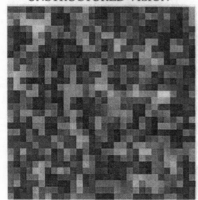 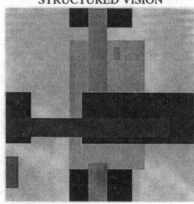

Figure 6.5. (*Left*) Example training image, consisting of Gaussian filtered random noise, used to model unstructured vision prior to eye opening. (*Right*) Example training image, consisting of seven randomly configured rectangles, with input values randomly distributed between 0 and 2, used to model structured vision after eye opening. Reprinted with kind permission from Grossberg, S., & Williamson, J. (2001). A neural model of how horizontal and interlaminar connections of visual cortex develop into adult circuits that carry out perceptual grouping and learning. *Cerebral Cortex, 11*, 37–58. Copyright 2001, Elsevier Science, Ltd., The Boulevard, Langford Lane, Kidlington OX5 1GB, UK.

horizontal and interlaminar cortical circuits develop, it was assumed that these top-down V1-to-LGN connections are predeveloped and are available to facilitate activation of the correct combinations of simple and complex cells.

DEVELOPMENTAL DATA AND SIMULATIONS

This section illustrates how the model of Grossberg and Williamson (2001) simulates data about the development of long-range horizontal connections in area V1. After development self-stabilizes, the resultant network can, without further change, simulate adult neurophysiological and psychophysical data about perceptual grouping. One such simulation will be shown below after developmental data are simulated.

As in the brain, the model undergoes two stages of development (Figure 6.5). One occurs prior to eye opening, when endogenous random geniculate and cortical activity determine the initial specificity of horizontal connections (Ruthazer & Stryker, 1996). The other occurs after eye opening, when patterned visual inputs can strengthen and refine these connections (Galuske & Singer, 1996).

Several anatomical studies have investigated how horizontal projections develop in the superficial layers of visual cortex into adult connections that connect columns of similar orientation preference (Callaway & Katz, 1990; Durack & Katz, 1996; Galuske & Singer, 1996). Callaway and Katz (1990) used neuronal tracing and intracellular staining to investigate the development of clustered horizontal connections in cat striate cortex, or area 17 (the analog of monkey area V1). They found an even, unclustered distribution up to 2 millimeters from the injection site during the first postnatal week, followed by an increase in the range and clustering of the projections in the second postnatal week, when the eyes are opened, and finally a long, slow refinement of projections due to the elimination of some connections until an adult level of clustering was reached in the sixth postnatal week.

Increase of Projection Range

The Galuske and Singer (1996) investigation of long-range projections in cat area 17 at different stages of postnatal development yielded a similar conclusion. Galuske and Singer (1996) also reported quantitative data about the projection range of pyramidal cells (Figure 6.6, *top*). Soon after eye opening, the projection range doubled over a period of 12 days (from P15 to P26). Presumably, the increase in projection range is due to the greater correlations in activity over large spatial distances that occurs in natural, structured images. Figure 6.6 (*bottom*) shows the simulated projection range in the model. Before eye opening, the short-range spatial correlations of the unstructured inputs are reflected in the relatively short-range extent of horizontal projections. Soon after eye opening, the long-range spatial correlations in the structured visual inputs cause the projection range to double, just as in the data of Galuske and Singer (1996). These results exploit the developmental rules described above by causing a larger projection range to grow when the statistics of visual imagery provided more long-range correlations. A similar effect in human infants, albeit delayed relative to the time scale of the cat, could explain how perceptual grouping takes hold between 2 and 4 months of age.

Increase of Orientation Selectivity

A similar pattern of exuberant growth followed by slow refinement of projections has also been found in the ferret. Because the ferret is born 3 weeks earlier in development than the cat, it has more stable orientation-selective cortical cell responses than the cat during the period in question (Durack & Katz, 1996; Ruthazer & Stryker, 1996). Ruthazer and Stryker (1996) reported quantitative data about the growing orientation selectivity of horizontal clustering over time, using a statistic called the Cluster Index (CI). The CI measures the log of the average nearest-neighbor distance between horizontal projections within a measurement window, di-

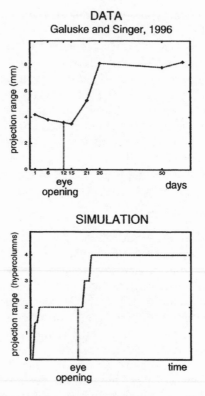

Figure 6.6. (*Top*) Projection range of pyramidal cells in cat visual cortex as a function of age. Projection range doubles after eye opening. Adapted from Galuske and Singer (1996). (*Bottom*) Projection range of model pyramidal cells during development. Model projection range also doubles after "eye opening." Reprinted with kind permission from Grossberg, S., & Williamson, J. (2001). A neural model of how horizontal and interlaminar connections of visual cortex develop into adult circuits that carry out perceptual grouping and learning. *Cerebral Cortex, 11*, 37–58. Copyright 2001, Elsevier Science, Ltd., The Boulevard, Langford Lane, Kidlington OX5 1GB, UK.

vided by the average distance between a randomly selected point in the window and the nearest horizontal projection. Therefore, a uniform distribution of horizontal projections would lead to a CI of log (1) = 0. As clustering becomes more refined, CI increases. Figure 6.7 (*top*) shows the CI obtained by Ruthazer and Stryker (1996) from 21 days postnatal up to adult age. Before eye opening, which is about 31 days postnatal, there is a positive CI, indicating a clustering bias, presumably favoring iso-orientation connections. After eye opening, the CI rapidly increases to reflect the strong, adult bias in favor of iso-orientation connections.

The model does not represent individual horizontal projections but rather the average strength of horizontal projections from an orientation column

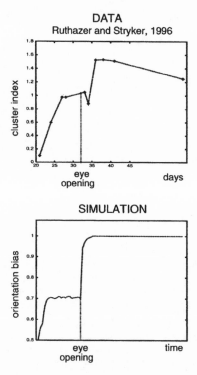

Figure 6.7. (*Top*) Mean Cluster Index (CI) in ferret area 17 as a function of age. From Ruthazer and Stryker (1996): "At P27 horizontal connections are significantly clustered, but single-unit recordings reveal poor orientation selectivity (25% of cells have orientation-selective responses), and optical imaging does not yet show an orientation map. Between P32 and P36, a secondary refinement of horizontal connections occurs along with the maturation of single-unit orientation selectivity and the emergence of the earliest optical orientation maps." Eye opening takes place at about P31. Adapted from Ruthazer and Stryker (1996). (*Bottom*) Clustering bias in model during development. The strength of horizontal connections to iso-orientation columns divided by the net strength of horizontal connections is plotted as a function of age. Like the data of Ruthazer and Stryker, the clustering bias increases after eye opening. Reprinted with kind permission from Grossberg, S., & Williamson, J. (2001). A neural model of how horizontal and interlaminar connections of visual cortex develop into adult circuits that carry out perceptual grouping and learning. *Cerebral Cortex, 11*, 37–58. Copyright 2001, Elsevier Science, Ltd., The Boulevard, Langford Lane, Kidlington OX5 1GB, UK.

to other orientation columns. Therefore, the model's format is unsuitable for computing a CI index. An analogous measurement of orientation preference was computed by dividing the strength of a column's horizontal connections to nearby columns with the same orientation preference by the strength of all the column's horizontal connections. This statistic is shown

DATA   SIMULATION

Fitzpatrick (1996)

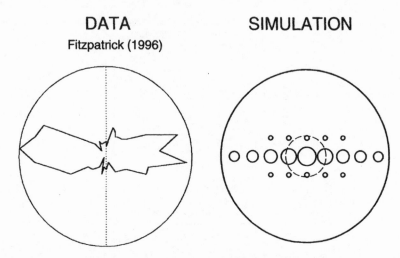

Figure 6.8 (*Left*) Polar plot of the projection field from a site in layer 2/3 of tree shrew striate cortex. The orientation of the projection field is in agreement with the orientation preference of its source neuron. Adapted from figure 11 of Fitzpatrick (1996). (*Right*) The projection field from a horizontally tuned column in layer 2/3 of the model after learning has equilibrated. The size of each circle represents the strength of the connection to each iso-orientation column. The dashed circle in the middle shows a layer 2/3 cell's classical receptive field, which is the spatial extent within which a point input causes the cell to "fire" (i.e., go above its output threshold). Reprinted with kind permission from Grossberg, S., & Williamson, J. (2001). A neural model of how horizontal and interlaminar connections of visual cortex develop into adult circuits that carry out perceptual grouping and learning. *Cerebral Cortex, 11*, 37–58. Copyright 2001, Elsevier Science, Ltd., The Boulevard, Langford Lane, Kidlington OX5 1GB, UK.

in Figure 6.7 (*bottom*). Like the CI index, it shows an initial moderate bias in favor of iso-orientation connections that dramatically increases after eye opening. In order to make the computer simulations tractable, the model presently represents only two orientations (vertical and horizontal), so Figure 6.7 shows the bias in favor of one orientation over the perpendicular orientation. If the model represented intermediate orientations as well, then the relative iso-orientation bias would be smaller because the presence of intermediate orientations would reduce the average orientation distance between iso- and non-iso-orientation columns.

After development, horizontal projections preferentially connect columns with similar orientation preferences that are aligned colinearly with their orientation preference (Fitzpatrick, 1996; Schmidt et al., 1997a). Figure 6.8 (*left*) shows a polar plot from Fitzpatrick (1996) of the projection field from a site in layer 2/3 of tree shrew striate cortex. The distance of each point from the center of the projection field represents the number of labeled terminals at that angle (in 10 degree increments). The orientation of the projection field is aligned with the orientation preference of its source neuron. Figure 6.8 (*right*) shows the analogous projection field from a horizontally tuned column in layer 2/3 of the model after development has equilibrated. The size of each circle represents the strength of the connection to each iso-orientation column. The anisotropy of the model's projection field is qualitatively consistent with Fitzpatrick's data. These results derive from the fact that visual cues are, with high probability, locally linear across space, so that the largest correlations would be generated by cells whose orientations match those of the input and are colinearly aligned across space. The developmental rules enable the network to sense these correlations and to selectively amplify the growth of those connections that best match them.

Projection Field versus Receptive Field

Neurophysiological recordings confirm that the anatomy that develops in the model has the cellular properties similar to those that have been recorded from adult animals. A remarkable property of this kind provides additional support for the bipole property. In particular, the extent of a cell's total anatomical projection field is much greater than that of its neurophysiologically recorded receptive field (Fitzpatrick, 1996). Fitzpatrick found that the projection fields in tree shrew extend for more than 2 millimeters from the injection site, a distance that corresponds to 15 degrees eccentricity, whereas the dimensions of neurophysiologically characterized receptive fields at that eccentricity are less than 5 degrees. A smaller classical receptive field than projection field was also shown by Das and Gilbert (1995), who compared cortical point spread (PS) distributions, measured with optical recording, which reflect both spiking and subthreshold activity, with spiking distributions measured with extracellular electrodes. A small oriented visual stimulus produced a PS distribution 20 times larger than the spiking distribution. Moreover, the close match of the PS distribution with columns whose orientation preference agrees with the orientation of the visual stimulus suggests that the distribution arises from iso-oriented long-range horizontal projections.

A similar property holds in the model after development equilibrates: Figure 6.8 (*right*) shows the size of a layer 2/3 cell classical receptive field (dashed-line circle) with respect to its projection field in the model. This discrepancy between projection field and receptive field can be traced to the model's bipole property: The classical receptive field reflects mainly bottom-up properties of the cortical network in the model, whereas the subthreshold activations reflect the fact that the bipole requirement for firing the cells via long-range horizontal connections was not satisfied. The developed model also exhibits the type of cortical point spread functions that have been found through optically recorded signals that are believed to arise from subthreshold dendritic activity in the superficial layers (Grinvald et al., 1994). See Grossberg and Williamson (2001) for further details.

PSYCHOPHYSICAL DATA AND SIMULATIONS

A crucial test of a model of visual cortical development concerns whether the developed model behaves perceptually like an adult cortex after development ends. This sort of test provides strong indirect evidence that the types of factors that influence how infants group image parts at different stages of development are actually being captured by the model. Without quantitative tests of such a linking hypothesis, it is difficult to feel any confidence in hypotheses about what brain mechanisms are responsible for observed changes in infant perception at different ages. In the present model, a key perceptual issue concerns whether the model can reproduce data about perceptual grouping. In particular, can the developed model generate illusory contours that are sensitive to changes in the strength and position of contour inducers in the same way that human observers are? This is a crucial test of perceptual grouping for at least two reasons: First, illusory contours require grouping to occur over positions that do not receive bottom-up inputs, so the model's *boundary completion* property is tested in this way. Second, analog changes in the emergent groupings as a function of input intensity and position—which I have called the property of *analog coherence*—is one of the key properties that laminar cortical circuitry has been predicted to generate. Two tests of these properties are summarized below.

Contour Sensitivity to Support Ratio

Figure 6.9 shows how the illusory contours formed by the model, either colinear to edges or perpendicular to line ends, vary in strength as the inducing features are parametrically varied. These simulations illustrate that the developed layer 2/3 connections do exhibit the property of analog coherence. Figure 6.9 (*top*) plots data of Shipley and Kellman (1992) that show the effect of increasing the length of the contour inducers while decreasing the gap between them, keeping the total length of inducers-plus-gap constant. Then, illusory contour clarity increases roughly linearly. In other words, "contour clarity increases with support ratio." Figure 6.9 (*top*) shows that the clarity of the model's illusory contours also increases linearly as the support ratio is increased. This result is due to the fact that as the gap between two inducers is made smaller, the grouping signal becomes stronger, due to the monotonically increasing magnitude of the layer 2/3 grouping kernel toward its center (see Figure 6.8).

The model matches the psychophysical data well, with the caveat that the model cannot form illusory contours when the support ratio falls below 0.5. This is due to simplifications in the model that were made for computational tractability. These simplifications limit the extent of the groupings it can make. In particular, model parameters were chosen so that its

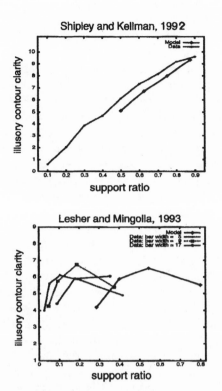

Figure 6.9. (*Top*) Shipley and Kellman (1992) obtained clarity ratings for illusory contours as a function of their support ratio. The stimulus was a 4-centimeter illusory Kanizsa square, induced by four pacman figures. As the support ratio increased (i.e., the size of the pacmen increases and the size of the gap decreases), the illusory contour clarity increased roughly linearly. Adapted from figure 5 of Shipley and Kellman (1992). The model results were obtained by measuring the strength of vertical grouping between two aligned rectangles (3 pixels wide). The length of the rectangles plus gap was 8 pixels. As the size of the gap was decreased from 4 pixels to 1 pixel by increasing the length of the rectangles, the average grouping strength in the gap increased. See text for a description of how the grouping strength was mapped into a metric of perceived illusory contour clarity. (*Bottom*) Lesher and Mingolla (1993) also obtained clarity ratings for illusory contours as a function of support ratio. However, they increased support ratio by increasing the number, and hence the density, of inducers in the following type of Kanizsa square display: The pacmen were built up from concentric rings of black contours whose number and density were increased across displays. As the number of inducing contours, and hence the support ratio, increases, the illusory contour clarity increases and then decreases. Adapted from figures 8a and 10c of Lesher and Mingolla (1993). The model's lusory contour strength was measured along a 4-pixel gap. Inducers were 2-pixel-wide bars, with the spacing between bars varied to yield 1, 2, 3, and 4 bars on each side of the gap, with interbar spacing of 3, 2, 1, and 0 pixels, respectively. Reprinted with kind permission from Grossberg, S., & Williamson, J. (2001). A neural model of how horizontal and interlaminar connections of visual cortex develop into adult circuits that carry out perceptual grouping and learning. *Cerebral Cortex, 11*, 37–58. Copyright 2001, Elsevier Science, Ltd., The Boulevard, Langford Lane, Kidlington OX5 1GB, UK.

developed horizontal projections extend only four hypercolumns away from the center. (A hypercolumn is a unit in the cortical map that contains the complete set of orientationally tuned and ocular dominance cells that represent a given position.) Another limitation is that the model only simulates grouping in V1 and does not take advantage of larger-scale processing in V2. Finally, the model does not include the retina-to-cortex cortical magnification factor (van Essen, Newsome, Maunsell, 1984), whereby scale expansion takes place as stimuli move into the periphery.

Figure 6.9 (*bottom*) summarizes psychophysical data obtained by Lesher and Mingolla (1993) showing that, if support ratio is increased in a different way, then an inverted U in illusory contour clarity strength is obtained. In this study, parallel bars with aligned ends were used to form four pacman figures with which to induce an illusory Kanizsa square percept. The square formed perpendicular to the bars through their aligned ends. Contour clarity of the illusory square was measured as the numbers of bars, and hence the support ratio, varied. The inducing pacmen had a circular radius of 128 pixels, and the gap between pacman pairs in which the Kanizsa square percept formed was 128 pixels. The support ratio was computed as the number of bar inducers (1, 2, 4, 8, 16 per pacman) times bar width, divided by the length of the side of the square (384 pixels). As the width of the bar inducers is increased, the number of possible inducers becomes limited, which is why there are only results for up to 16 inducers in the 9-pixel-width case and up to 8 inducers in the 17-pixel-width case.

Figure 6.9 (*bottom*) shows that the model simulates the inverted U in contour strength as a function of bar density. This inverted-U result is due to an interaction between the long-range excitatory horizontal connections in layer 2/3 and the medium-range inhibitory connections from layer 6-to-4. The Shipley and Kellman (1992) data, and our simulation thereof, show that decreasing the distance between inducers, up to a certain point, increases grouping strength as a result of layer 2/3 horizontal cooperation. As the inducers get even closer together, however, layer 6-to-4 inhibition increasingly inhibits the net excitation caused at layer 4 by each LGN input. Thus, although more inputs activate the cooperating layer 2/3 pyramidal cells, the net effect of each input on layer 2/3 gets smaller as the inducers get denser. This simulation shows that the self-organized connections preserve a good balance between layers 6, 4, and 2/3. As in the psychophysical data in Figure 6.9, the model's illusory contour strength is affected more strongly by variations in support ratio than in bar density.

Due to the implementational limitations of the model described above, the network simulated these data using bars that are relatively wide with respect to the length of the gap (2-pixel-wide bars, 4-pixel-long gap). Figure 6.9 (*bottom*) shows results obtained by the model with interbar gap size decreasing from 3 to 0, with the total length spanned by the inducers and gaps held roughly constant. The model's inverted-U curve is shifted to the right of the data curves, reflecting the fact that the model used inducers that were wider relative to the gap size. Note that, in the data as well, the curves shift to the right as the width of the inducers increases.

INTERACTIONS OF GROUPING, ATTENTION, AND RECOGNITION

Up to this point, the chapter has summarized a LAMINART model of how horizontal and interlaminar cortical connections in cortical areas V1 (and by extension, area V2) develop in a stable fashion. Stable development is controlled by the growth of balanced excitatory and inhibitory connections within layer 2/3 and between layers 6 and 4. The model grows connections that simulate key properties of developmental anatomical data and adult neurophysiological data about this process, and the developed network quantitatively simulates key data about adult perceptual grouping, notably data that depend upon nonclassical receptive field properties, thereby testing the linking hypothesis between brain mechanisms and perception. Many additional psychophysical data about both perceptual grouping and attentional modulation in the adult are simulated using the model in Grossberg and Raizada (2000) and Grossberg and Williamson (2001). With attentional connections also in place, the model may be summarized as in Figure 6.10.

As noted above, in both the brain and the model, layer 2/3 boundary signals feed back via connections to layer 6 via layer 5 (Ferster & Lindström 1985; Gilbert & Wiesel, 1979). Layer 6, in turn, activates the on-center off-surround network from layer 6-to-4 via folded feedback (Grossberg, 1999a). The feedback signals from layer 2/3 to layer 6 hereby get transmitted in a feedforward fashion back to layer 4 and thereupon to layer 2/3. Folded feedback links cells in layers 2/3, 6, 5, and 4 into functional columns (Hubel & Wiesel, 1962, 1977; Mountcastle, 1957). In so doing, it enables the strongest grouping signals in layer 2/3 to use the on-center off-surround network from layer 6-to-4 to reinforce the strongest groupings and to inhibit weaker groupings, during both early development and adult grouping and learning. As noted above, this feedback circuit helps to stabilize model development by shutting off cells that should not become connected for purposes of grouping. The full LAMINART model also has the following remarkable properties that illustrate how mechanisms that ensure stable cortical development also lead to useful properties of adult grouping, attention, and recognition.

Fast Feedforward Grouping and Recognition

Although the competitive selection circuit from layer 6-to-4 is needed to choose correct groupings in response to complex scenes with many almost

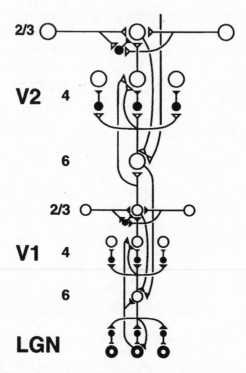

Figure 6.10. The LAMINART V1/V2 circuit. V2 repeats the laminar pattern of V1 circuitry, but at a larger spatial scale. In particular, the horizontal layer 2/3 connections have a longer range in V2, allowing above-threshold perceptual groupings between more widely spaced inducing stimuli to form (Amir, Harel, & Malach, 1993). V1 layer 2/3 projects up to V2 layers 6 and 4, just as LGN projects to layers 6 and 4 of V1. Higher cortical areas send feedback into V2, which ultimately reaches layer 6, just as V2 feedback acts on layer 6 of V1 (Sandell & Schiller, 1982). Feedback paths from higher cortical areas straight into V1 (not shown) can complement and enhance feedback from V2 into V1. Reprinted with kind permission from Grossberg, S., and Raizada, R.D.S. (2000). Contrast-sensitive perceptual grouping and object-based attention in the laminar circuits of primary visual cortex. *Vision Research, 40*, 1413–1432. Copyright 2000, Elsevier Science, Ltd., The Boulevard, Langford Lane, Kidlington OX5 1GB, UK.

equally strong groupings, the system can automatically generate a fast grouping of an unambiguous scene using a one-pass *feedforward* wave of activation through layers 4-to-2/3 in one area, then from layer 2/3 to layer 4 in the next area, and so on; see Figure 6.10. Such fast feedforward recognition has been experimentally shown to be possible in humans and monkeys (Thorpe, Fize, & Marlot, 1996). If the scene is complex and ambiguous, however, then inhibitory interactions between the competing groupings in the various layers (e.g., from layer 6-to-4 and within layer 2/3) attenuate the cortical output from layer 2/3 and thereby prevent strong outputs from being generated to higher cortical areas until a clear choice can be made. As weaker groupings are suppressed, the strongest groupings win the competition and become more active. The winning groupings can then more quickly reach their output threshold. This self-regulating design enables fast feedforward processing when the data are unambiguous, and a functionally determined delay for selecting a correct grouping via feedback when they are not. Thus, *after* the selection circuit enables orientationally selective receptive fields and horizontal connections to develop, it still plays an important role whenever ambiguity exists in the visual scene, since it then helps to choose the strongest groupings while also suppressing spurious correlations in cell activation that could otherwise degrade previously learned connections.

Selective Object Attention

As noted above, one of the key selection circuits that helps to choose perceptual groupings is realized by an on-center off-surround network from layer 6-to-4. This selection circuit is activated by *intra*cortical feedback from the horizontal groupings that start to form in layer 2/3 (Figure 6.4b). The same selection circuit is activated by top-down attention via *inter*cortical feedback from layer 6 of higher cortical areas (Figure 6.10). Because of this property, development and learning between different cortical regions can also be stabilized, as predicted by adaptive resonance theory (Grossberg, 1980b, 1999b). Simulations of the LAMINART model (Grossberg & Raizada, 2000) show how attention can selectively enhance an entire object while suppressing nearby distractors. This remarkable property was demonstrated in neurophysiological recordings in the awake monkey by Roelfsema, Lamme, and Spekreijse (1998). Object attention is achieved in the model through the sharing by both attention and grouping of the same selection circuit, whereby a correct grouping can be selected from among many possible groupings of a complex scene. Because attention and grouping both activate the same selection circuit, attention can propagate along an entire object's grouping after it reaches layer 2/3 via the 6-to-4-to-2/3 pathway.

Object Attention with Incomplete Boundaries

In humans, attention can selectively enhance an entire object when the object is defined by an image with lots of missing pixels, as can occur in high noise (Moore, Yantis, & Vaughan, 1998) or due to imperfections, such as a scotoma, in retinal processing. Model simulations have shown how grouping can preattentively complete the object boundary over the missing pixels via illusory contours; then attention can selectively enhance the completed object grouping.

Attentional Selection of Important Data

Using the top-down layer 6-to-6 attentional route, attention can leapfrog between multiple cortical areas. In this way, figure-ground and cognitive constraints from higher cortical areas can help to select groupings and to thereby search for desired objects in a scene. Attention can also tune the bottom-up adaptive filters in layer 4 of each area to be particularly sensitive to important information by using a layer 6-to-6-to-4 folded feedback pathway (Figure 6.10).

Why does not the top-down 6-to-6 route turn on the entire cortex like a bottom-up input would? If this happened, it would blur the distinction between intention and reality. Hallucinations would be commonplace. This does not happen because, as predicted by ART, the on-center in layer 6-to-4 has *balanced* excitation and inhibition. It can modulate, sensitize, or prime layer 4 to respond more vigorously to desired inputs, but it cannot, by itself, turn layer 4 on. This hypothesis is consistent with neurophysiological data of Hupé et al. (1997) who have shown that "feedback connections from area V2 modulate but do not create center-surround interactions in V1 neurons," and data from ferret visual cortex has shown that the layer 6-to-4 circuit is functionally weak (Wittmer, Dalva, & Katz, 1997). Such intercortical feedback connections from V2 to V1 can modulate the circuits of V1 with "higher-order" boundary completion and figure-ground perception properties of area V2 (Grossberg, 1994, 1997; Lamme, 1995; Zipser, Lamme, & Schiller, 1996) and/or other cortical areas (e.g., Hupé et al., 1998; Watanabe et al., 1998).

Why Two Bottom-Up Paths to Layer 4?

The predicted modulatory property of the layer 6-to-4 circuit helps to explain the otherwise mysterious existence of a direct input to layer 4 of V1 from the LGN (Figure 6.4b) and to layer 4 of V2 from layer 2/3 of V1 (Figure 6.10). Without the direct route to layer 4, cortex could never turn on at all, because the indirect 6-to-4 route, which can also be activated by bottom-up inputs, is merely modulatory. Why, in turn, is the indirect 6-to-4 route merely modulatory? Given that a similar arrangement seems to exist in *all* sensory and cognitive neocortex, why is this not a huge waste of wire? My proposed answer is: ART has proved mathematically that a modulatory feedback selection circuit is needed so that the cortex can stably develop its connections in the infant and can stably learn in the adult (Carpenter & Grossberg, 1991; Grossberg, 1976b, 1980b, 1999a, 1999b). The rules of stable development are thus predicted to define what we *mean* by adult attention, as well as adult grouping and learning.

DEVELOPMENT OF CORTICAL MAP

Triple-O Map Properties

Development of the primary visual cortex prior to visual experience produces orientationally tuned cortical neurons, classifiable according to the criteria of Hubel and Wiesel (1962) as either simple or complex. After several weeks of visual experience, these cortical cells evolve adult responsivity (DeAngelis, Ohzawa, & Freeman, 1993; Ghose, Freeman, & Ohzawa, 1994; Hubel & Wiesel, 1974). The prenatal segregation of geniculocortical afferents into ocular dominance columns also occurs independently of visual experience (Horton & Hocking, 1996). Monocular, but not binocular, deprivation during the first few weeks of visual experience can lead to drastic changes in the arrangement of ocular dominance patches (Hubel & Wiesel, 1977), but these changes may be blocked by the elimination of neural activity (Stryker & Harris, 1986), suggesting that an activity-dependent process is responsible for the development of ocular dominance.

Adult cortical cells are arranged into vertical columns with similar orientation tuning and ocular dominance, and these columns are arranged into smoothly changing two-dimensional maps of orientation and ocular dominance (Hubel & Wiesel, 1962, 1963, 1968). The properties of orientational tuning and of ocular dominance constitute two of the Os in the Triple-O map. The cortical map of orientation is arranged in swirling patterns around orientation centers in both cats (Bonhoeffer & Grinvald, 1991; Grinvald et al., 1994) and monkeys (Blasdel, 1992b; Blasdel & Salama, 1986), but the patchy pattern of ocular dominance in cats (Anderson, Olavarria, & Sluyters, 1988; LeVay, Stryker, & Shatz, 1978; Löwel & Singer, 1987; Löwel et al., 1988) differs somewhat from the stripelike pattern in monkeys (Blasdel, 1992a, 1992b; Hubel & Wiesel, 1977; Hubel, Wiesel, & Stryker, 1978; LeVay, Hubel, & Wiesel, 1975; LeVay et al., 1985; Obermayer & Blasdel, 1993). In both species, these patterns are evident at a spatial scale of about 1 millimeter.

The third O in the Triple-O concept concerns the existence of opponent simple cells at a much smaller spatial scale. That is, there exist nearby cortical simple cells that exhibit opposite spatial phase (Pollen & Ronner, 1981), and these cells may be connected by functionally inhibitory connections (DeAngelis, Ohzawa, & Freeman, 1991; Liu et al., 1992; Palmer & Davis, 1981). An arrangement of simple cells with complementary ON and OFF zones into mutually inhibitory pairs helps to explain the source of local intracortical inhibition, which provides functional antagonism between ON and OFF zones in simple cell receptive fields (Hubel & Wiesel, 1962). This complementary representation also helps to explain the robust expression of orientation tuning following blockade of ON retinal ganglion cells by the application of APB (Schiller, 1982). These facts are summarized well by models in which ON and OFF geniculate afferents synapse onto pairs of mutually inhibitory simple cells (e.g., Gove, Grossberg, & Mingolla, 1995; Shulz, Debanne, & Fregnac, 1993).

Complex cells also respond to oriented stimuli but do not have well-segregated ON and OFF receptive field subregions. Complex cells are found in almost every layer of V1 (Gilbert, 1977), which is consistent with the intracortical feedback loops that exist, say, between layers 4, 2/3, and 6. Several models of how individual complex cells achieve their orientation tuning without segregated ON and OFF regions have been described that pool simple cell responses with differing spatial phases at a single complex cell (Emerson, Korenberg, & Citron, 1992; Gove, Grossberg, & Mingolla, 1995; Grossberg & Mingolla, 1985a, 1985b; Jacobson et al., 1993 Spitzer & Hochstein, 1985).

Shared Properties of Cortical Map Development Models

A number of models have demonstrated how individual simple cell response characteristics and global maps can be simultaneously self-organized by local processes. One of the earliest models showed how a neural network with weights modified by an associative learning rule can produce orientation tuning when presented with oriented inputs (Grossberg, 1976b; von der Malsburg, 1973). Linsker (1986a, 1986b, 1986c) subsequently demonstrated self-organization of orientationally tuned cells without oriented inputs. Other modeling work has shown how ocular dominance maps can arise from uncorrelated inputs (Kohonen, 1982, 1989; Miller, Keller, & Stryker, 1989; Rojer & Schwartz, 1989, 1990; Swindale, 1980), how maps of orientation can form (Swindale, 1982), how maps of orientation and ocular dominance may develop simultaneously (Durbin & Mitchison, 1990; Obermayer, Blasel, Schulten, 1992; Obermayer, Ritter, & Schulten, 1990; Sirosh & Miikkulainen, 1994; Swindale, 1992), and how the development of orientationally tuned simple cells and their arrangement into cortical maps may progress synchronously (Miller, 1992, 1994). Each of these models computes its maps with somewhat different equations. Some models, for example, focus on the learning that alters neural connections without modeling the dynamics of the cells themselves (e.g., Miller, 1992, 1994). The fact that all of these models realize three computational principles (Grossberg & Olson, 1994)—a source of noise, a band pass filter, and normalization across all feature dimensions—clarifies what all these different models have in common from a computational viewpoint. Grossberg and Olson (1994) showed that these three factors are sufficient to generate cortical maps that exhibit the singularities, fractures, and linear zones that are found in vivo (Blasdel, 1992a, 1992b).

The neural model for cortical map development that is briefly reviewed here (Olson & Grossberg, 1998) builds upon these earlier developmental models. This model demonstrates the self-organization of cortical maps of ocular dominance and orientation, while simultaneously developing neighboring orientationally tuned simple cells that are sensitive to opposite contrast polarities and that exhibit either even-symmetric or odd-symmetric receptive fields. These paired simple cells provide a natural explanation for such facts as how subcortical application of APB influences cortical orientation tuning and how cortical complex cells come to pool signals from oppositely polarized simple cells within a developing cortical map.

Opponent Simple Cells and Habituative Rebounds

In order to achieve these results, the dynamics of both cortical cells and their intercellular interactions needed to be explicitly modeled. In particular, the model starts with arrays of spatially contiguous cortical cells that interact in pairs. (More loosely organized cell groupings would also work, but cell pairs are the simplest case.) These cells have no significant orientational preference before development occurs; they are activated by bottom-up inputs whose connection strengths are randomly chosen. The cell pairs do, however, have the property that offset of activity in one cell of a pair can lead to a transient antagonistic rebound of activity in the opponent cell of the pair. The cells in each pair are called ON cells and OFF cells because *offset* of an input to an ON cell can trigger transient activation in the corresponding OFF cell. This rebound is caused by an interaction of three factors: Some of the cells interact via opponent competition; the chemical transmitters in some of the network pathways habituate in an activity-dependent way; and some of the cells receive an internal source of tonic activation. When these three factors are properly arranged in circuits (e.g., Figure 6.11), then when an ON cell is activated by a bottom-up input, the transmitter that is released by the input activates the cell, but it also habituates, or depresses, in an activity-dependent way (Abbott et al., 1997; Grossberg, 1972, 1976b). When the input to the ON cell turns off, the transmitter habituation lasts for awhile afterward. The OFF cell transmitter is not habituated to the same extent because the OFF cell was not active during this time.

The bottom-up input is not the only input that can activate these transmitters. A tonically active input to both ON and OFF cell is also present and activates the ON and OFF cells equally; that is, it is a *nonspecific* input. When the input to the ON cell shuts off, the tonic input can activate the OFF cell more than the ON cell, because the ON cell transmitter is more habituated, or depressed. After opponent competition between the cells occurs, there is a net OFF activation, leading to an antagonistic rebound of activity. The rebound is transient—that is, lasts only for a short amount

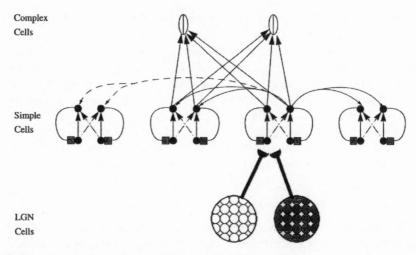

Figure 6.11. Pairs of unoriented cells (that will become simple cells) interact via opponent competition (dashed lines between simple cells) and habituative transmitters (square synapses). In addition, longer-range on-center recurrent excitation (horizontal solid lines between simple cells) and still longer-range off-surround recurrent inhibition (horizontal dashed lines between simple cells) exist. Inputs that are received from the lateral geniculate nucleus (LGN) ON cells (open circles) and OFF cells (gray disks). Adaptive weights under learning in the geniculocortical pathways (hemidisk synapses). Complex cells respond to a weighted sum of simple cell responses at the same cortical locations. All teractions are shown only with respect to one cell. Reprinted with kind permission from Olson, S.J., & Grossberg, S. (1998). A neural network model for the development of simple and complex cell receptive fields within cortical maps of orientation and ocular dominance. *Neural Networks, 11*, 189–208. Copyright 1998, Elsevier Science, Ltd., The Boulevard, Langford Lane, Kidlington OX5 1GB, UK.

of time—because the equal tonic inputs to both the ON and OFF cells gradually habituate the transmitters to both cells equally as well. Then the opponent competition between the cells shuts them both off.

Such antagonistic rebounds have elsewhere been used to explain psychophysical data about visual aftereffects (Francis & Grossberg, 1996; Grunewald & Lankheet, 1996), persistence (Francis, Grossberg, & Mingolla, 1994), and binocular rivalry (Grossberg, 1987b), among others. Ringach et al. (1996) have reported direct neurophysiological evidence for rebound phenomena using reverse correlation techniques to analyze orientational tuning in neurons of cortical area V1.

Recurrent On-Center Off-Surround Network Dynamics

When embedded in a model whose mechanisms realize the three computational properties listed above—namely, a source of noise, a band pass filter, and normalization across all feature dimensions—these opponent cells develop into simple cells with similar orientation tuning but sensitivity to opposite contrast polarities. These additional mechanisms include medium-range recurrent excitation and long-range recurrent inhibition that interact with the short-range opponent mechanism (Figure 6.11). These longer-range interactions tend to normalize the total activity across the simple cells. They also contrast-enhance the inputs that are received from the lateral geniculate nucleus ON cells (open circles) and OFF cells (black disks). When a random input first activates the LGN, it is filtered by the (then) random, and small, adaptive weights in the pathways between the LGN and the simple cells. The simple cells that receive the largest inputs win the contrast-enhancing competition that is realized by the recurrent on-center off-surround interaction. This interaction selects the winning cells and contrast-enhances their activity. Once the winning simple cells are selected, their activity helps to drive learning in the adaptive weights, or long-term memory traces, that exist within the synapses that abut them (see the hemidisks in Figure 6.11).

How do antagonist rebounds influence this learning process? When the input to a selected simple cell shuts off, an antagonistic rebound activates its corresponding OFF cell. At the same time, input offset also causes antagonistic rebounds of activity in the LGN. The adaptive weights in the pathways between the rebounded LGN cells and the rebounded simple cells learn the correlation between their activations. An antagonistic rebound in the LGN represents the same spatial pattern of activation as its ON response, but with an opposite contrast polarity. As a result, while the LGN-to-ON cell weights learn to code a prescribed orientation, the LGN-to-OFF cell weights learn to code the same orientation, but with an opposite contrast polarity. This property is schematized in Figure 6.12.

This opponent learning is more complicated than stated here, because OFF cell learning must also respond to direct LGN inputs to the OFF cells that are due to external inputs that have opposite contrast polarity from those that activate the ON cells. Computer simulations have demonstrated that the rebounded activity is sufficient to bias this learning to achieve the desired result; namely, the network can develop pairs of nearby simple cells that are sensitive to opposite contrast polarities but the same orientation (Figure 6.13). A second important result is that nonoverlapping, oriented ON and OFF subregions develop in the model geniculocortical cell weights. This property helps to explain how simple cells in primary visual cortex receive direct excitatory connections from distinct regions of the LGN (Liu et al., 1992; Reid & Alonso, 1995). These distinct ON and OFF subregions provide direct oriented input to cortical simple cells (Ferster, Chung, & Wheat, 1996; Hawken & Parker, 1984; Reid & Alonso, 1995; Schiller, 1982). The Triple-O model thus suggests how prenatal development leads to the segregation of initially intermingled ON and OFF inputs to cortical cells into oriented excitatory subregions.

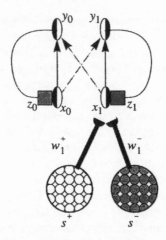

Figure 6.12. Local connectivity of opponent simple cells consists of a pair of input cells $x_i(j,k)$, feedback cells $y_i(j,k)$, and habituating transmitters $z_i(j,k)$ that make up two channels, corresponding to units with subscript 0 and to units with subscript 1, respectively. Each simple cell $x_i(j,k)$ receives LGN ON (+) and OFF (−) signals along weighted pathways. Vertical feedforward excitation (solid arrows) within and reciprocal feedforward inhibition (dashed arrows) between the channels produce an antagonistic relationship between simple cells. Positional indices (j,k) have been dropped. Reprinted with kind permission from Olson, S.J., & Grossberg, S. (1998). A neural network model for the development of simple and complex cell receptive fields within cortical maps of orientation and ocular dominance. *Neural Networks, 11*, 189–208. Copyright 1998, Elsevier Science, Ltd., The Boulevard, Langford Lane, Kidlington OX5 1GB, UK.

Instar Synaptic Learning Law

Model adaptive weights are modified according to an associative learning rule that is called the *instar* learning rule or *gated steepest descent* learning rule (Grossberg, 1976a, 1976b; see also Kohonen, 1989; Obermayer, Blasdel, & Schulten, 1992; Singer, 1983). According to this learning rule, changes in the weights are made only when the postsynaptic simple cell is active. Then the weights slowly change to track the input signals that they sense within their pathways. The instar learning rule normalizes the weights when activity in the presynaptic and postsynaptic neural fields is normalized by their on-center off-surround interactions. Normalization tends to render the sum of the weights that impinge on each cortical cell to be approximately constant.

Map Properties: Singularities, Linear Zones, and Fractures

When all the mechanisms in the model interact together, map properties emerge that are similar to those reported experimentally. In particular, the

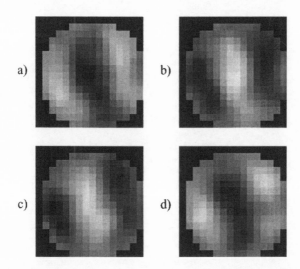

Figure 6.13. Opponency of learned adaptive weights. Model development leads to opposite polarity ON and OFF adaptive weights in opponent simple cells. (a) and (b) represent the ON and OFF weights corresponding to a given simple cell; (c) and (d) represent the ON and OFF weights corresponding to the opponent simple cell. Note that where ON cell weights are strong, OFF cell weights are weak, and conversely. Reprinted with kind permission from Olson, S.J., & Grossberg, S. (1998). A neural network model for the development of simple and complex cell receptive fields within cortical maps of orientation and ocular dominance. *Neural Networks, 11*, 189–208. Copyright 1998, Elsevier Science, Ltd., The Boulevard, Langford Lane, Kidlington OX5 1GB, UK.

developed map exhibits the swirling, gradually changing character of biological orientation maps as well as the key features of these maps: singularities (regions of low orientation selectivity around which all other orientations are grouped), linear zones (regions in which orientation changes relatively linearly with cortical distance), and fractures (regions in which orientation changes rapidly along one spatial direction and slowly or not at all in the orthogonal direction). Each of these key features is present in the simulated orientation map shown in Figure 6.14.

In addition, ocular dominance maps, which reflect eye preference of cortical cells, also develop. An index of ocular dominance was computed by subtracting the total weight contributed by the ipsilateral eye from the total weight contributed by the contralateral eye at each cortical position. Figure 6.15 shows the orientation map superimposed on the map of ocular dominance. Regions dominated by the contralateral eye are colored white, and regions dominated by the ipsilateral eye are colored gray. As with cortical maps, this model map of ocular dominance is made up of interlaced dark and light patches corresponding to regions dominated by each eye. Ocular dominance and orientation preference are related in much the same way as

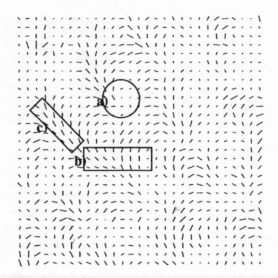

Figure 6.14. Orientation map. Subset of the simulated binocular orientation map. Key features of the biological orientation maps are present here: (a) singularities, (b) linear zones, and (c) fractures. Reprinted with kind permission from Olson, S.J., & Grossberg, S. (1998). A neural network model for the development of simple and complex cell receptive fields within cortical maps of orientation and ocular dominance. *Neural Networks, 11,* 189–208. Copyright 1998, Elsevier Science, Ltd., The Boulevard, Langford Lane, Kidlington OX5 1GB, UK.

they are in cortical maps: Regions dominated by one eye or the other tend to line up with regions of low orientation selectivity, and regions of high orientation selectivity tend to be aligned with the borders of the ocular dominance bands (Blasdel, 1992b). Earlier modeling work has shown that using a spatial anisotropic filter can produce striped ocular dominance maps that even more closely resemble the patterns observed experimentally in monkeys (Grossberg & Olson, 1994; Rojer & Schwartz, 1989, 1990; Swindale, 1980). This could be accomplished within the present modeling framework either through the use of an anisotropic pattern of lateral connections among simple cells or through an anisotropic pattern of geniculocortical connectivity. It remains to be seen if this enhancement naturally arises, for example, when the model in Figure 6.11 is embedded into the laminar model of Figure 6.4, including its anisotropic horizontal connections. Other properties of the Triple-O model include the development of both even-symmetric and odd-symmetric simple cells with well-segregated ON and OFF subregions. Because of the spatial arrangement of these simple cells, complex cells that are activated by a weighted average of simple cells across a small region do not have well-segregated ON and OFF subregions and also pool responses from simple cells that are sensitive to opposite contrast polarities.

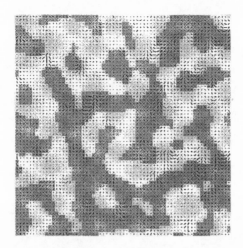

Figure 6.15. Orientation preference and ocular dominance maps. Orientation preference at each position is indicated by a line segment at the preferred orientation with length proportional to orientation selectivity. Regions dominated by the contralateral eye are colored white; regions dominated by the ipsilateral eye are gray. Reprinted with kind permission from Olson, S.J., & Grossberg, S. (1998). A neural network model for the development of simple and complex cell receptive fields within cortical maps of orientation and ocular dominance. *Neural Networks, 11*, 189–208. Copyright 1998, Elsevier Science, Ltd., The Boulevard, Langford Lane, Kidlington OX5 1GB, UK.

This pooling process plays an important role in cortical models of visual perception. Because complex cells pool half-wave rectified output signals from pairs of oppositely polarized but similarly oriented simple cells, they compute an oriented, full-wave rectification of the image. Such an operation has become standard in models that explain data about human texture segregation (Chubb & Sperling, 1989; Grossberg & Mingolla, 1985b; Grossberg & Pessoa, 1998; Sutter, Beck, & Graham, 1989). Because complex cells pool signals from opposite contrast polarities, they can generate object boundaries around objects lying in front of textured backgrounds. In particular, a gray object lying in front of a black-and-white textured background will generate gray-to-white (light-to-dark) and gray-to-black (dark-to-light) contrasts along its perimeter. Because complex cells can respond to both contrast polarities, they can help to generate a boundary that encloses the entire gray object (see Figure 6.4a).

RAPID DEVELOPMENT OF DISPARITY-SENSITIVE COMPLEX CELLS

The Triple-O model does not show how connections from simple cells to complex cells develop. Nor does it indicate how complex cells can rap-

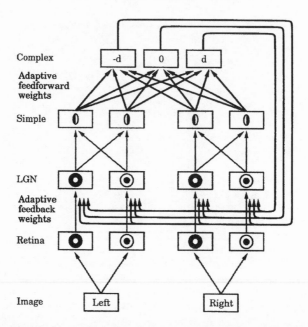

Figure 6.16. Model of how disparity-sensitive complex cells may develop. The dark lines indicate pathways that are adaptive and that contribute to this development. Symbols (-d, 0, d) stand for complex cells that will become sensitive to different disparities. Reprinted with kind permission from Grunewald, A., & Grossberg, S. (1998). Self-organization of binocular disparity tuning by reciprocal corticogeniculate interactions. *Journal of Cognitive Neuroscience, 10,* 199–215. Copyright 1998 by the Massachusetts Institute of Technology.

idly become sensitive to binocular disparity as a result of these connections. The study by Grunewald and Grossberg (1998) models how these events may occur. This model (Figure 6.16) suggests that both feedforward and feedback interactions among retinal, LGN, and cortical simple and complex cells contribute to the rapid development of highly tuned disparity-selective neural responses from the coarse level of stereopsis that is found in infants (Birch, Gwiazda, & Held, 1983; Blakemore, Hawken, & Mark, 1982; Blakemore & van Sluyters, 1974; Daw, 1994; Daw & Wyatt, 1976; Freeman & Ohzawa, 1992; Held, Birch, & Gwiazda, 1980; Leventhal & Hirsch, 1980; Movshon & Düsteler, 1977; Shimogo et al., 1986). Some of the key modeling mechanisms that help to explain this developmental process will now be reviewed. Of particular interest are the top-down corticogeniculate connections of the model, which help to assure that binocular disparity tuning can develop quickly without a loss of instability; that is, these top-down connections enable fast learning to occur without catastrophic forgetting and thereby illustrate how adaptive resonance theory principles can operate at even the earliest levels of visual processing (Grossberg, 1999b).

Competition and Habituative Rebound in Disparity Development

Monocularly activated simple cells from both eyes may initially activate a broad expanse of complex cells, as depicted in Figure 6.16. Contrast-enhancing competition across the complex cells determines a local winner, which tends to be the complex cell population that best matches the binocular disparity of the simple cells from both eyes that activate it. These winning complex cells can then learn, using instar learning, the pattern of activities that is active within the pathways from the active simple cells. As in the Triple-O model, the disparity-tuning model exploits dynamic rebounds between opponent ON and OFF simple cells that are due to imbalances in habituative transmitter gates. When these rebounds occur between oppositely polarized simple cells that are tuned to the same orientation, they help to explain how pairs of oppositely polarized simple cells, whose activity is *anti*correlated through time, can become associated during development with a shared complex cell. The main idea is that after a simple ON cell activates a particular complex cell, that complex cell's activity lingers for awhile after the simple cell shuts off. When the simple cell shuts off, an oppositely polarized simple cell is activated by an antagonistic rebound. This newly activated simple cell is then simultaneously active while the complex cell is still active. As a result, connections from this simple cell can be strengthened at the complex cell. This transient learning episode is enough to direct development of connections from both simple cells to the shared complex cell. In this way, complex cells develop that can pool opposite polarities of image contrast. At the same time, the simple-to-complex cell connections learn to binocularly fuse only stimuli for which both eyes process the same contrast polarity. Figure 6.17 illustrates a computer simulation of how disparity tuning evolves in time, including the fact that pairs of light-dark (LD) polarity and dark-light (DL) polarity simple cells develop the same disparity tuning.

Corticogeniculate Matching in Stabilizing Disparity Tuning

The development of complex cell receptive fields and their disparity tuning in the model is impaired in the absence of either antagonistic rebounds or corticogeniculate feedback. The rebound response ensures that opposite-polarity simple cells develop the correct connections to the same complex cell. Corticogeniculate feedback prevents the learning of multiple disparity peaks and shifts in these peaks through time.

How is learning stabilized by corticogeniculate feedback in response to

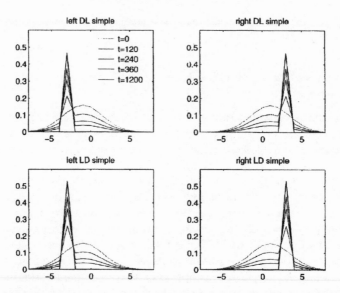

Figure 6.17. The development of individual bottom-up kernels to complex cells of far, or uncrossed, disparity preference. The *top* panels show the kernels between DL simple cells and the complex cell. On the *left* is shown the kernel between the left DL simple cells and the complex cell, and on the *right* between the right DL simple cells and the complex cell. The *bottom* panels show the kernels between LD simple cells and the same complex cell. Note that the DL and LD kernels are indistinguishable. Over time the kernels become narrower, and their preference shifts away from the central, zero-disparity location. Reprinted with kind permission from Grunewald, A., & Grossberg, S. (1998). Self-organization of binocular disparity tuning by reciprocal corticogeniculate interactions. *Journal of Cognitive Neuroscience, 10,* 199–215. Copyright 1998 by the Massachusetts Institute of Technology.

a changing visual environment? As in the LAMINART model, top-down ART matching properties seem to play an important role in this cortico-geniculate pathway. In particular, whenever a complex cell emerges as a winner, a top-down matching, or confirmation, signal is sent to the LGN (Sillito et al., 1994; Varela & Singer, 1987). When the confirmation signal matches the LGN activity pattern, then the matched LGN activities are amplified and synchronized. A mismatch between the confirmation signal pattern and the LGN input pattern leads to a reduction of LGN activity. This selective attenuation of mismatched LGN cells helps to stabilize the learning process and to trigger selection of a new complex cell winner if the match is bad enough. The data of Sillito et al. (1994) possess all of the predicted properties of the ART matching rule in this situation. In addition, Murphy, Duckett, and Sillito (1999) have shown that the connections in the corticogeniculate pathways share the orientation preference of the cortical cells that are involved.

When the ART model was introduced in Grossberg (1976b), it was predicted that corticogeniculate feedback carries out a matching process in order to stabilize the development of cortical binocular tuning during the visual cortical period and also that the top-down adaptive weights that control the matching process are also learned. The results from the Sillito lab are consistent with these predictions. It remains to be tested whether the bottom-up connections tend to get dynamically stabilized by the top-down corticogeniculate matching process. Gove, Grossberg, and Mingolla (1995) have predicted that elimination of the top-down matching process can cause the illusory brightness that is perceived in an Ehrenstein illusion to look dark, rather than bright. Grunewald and Grossberg (1998) have shown that the model can be used to explain psychophysical and neurobiological data concerning the dynamics of binocular disparity processing, including correct registration of disparity in response to dynamically changing stimuli, binocular summation of weak stimuli, and fusion of anticorrelated stimuli when they are delayed but not when they are simultaneous (Cogan, Lomakin, & Rossi, 1993; Julesz, 1960). Simultaneous anticorrelated stereograms cannot be fused because only like-contrasts fuse. Delayed anticorrelated stereograms can be fused because the antagonistic rebound reverses contrast polarity, so the delayed response can be fused with the later response. More generally, the model's binocular circuit forms part of a larger theory of binocular vision that has been used to explain many data concerning 3D vision and figure-ground separation (Grossberg, 1987b, 1994, 1997; Grossberg & Kelly, 1999; Grossberg & McLoughlin, 1997; Grossberg & Pessoa, 1998; Kelly & Grossberg, 2000; McLoughlin & Grossberg, 1998).

CONCLUDING REMARKS

The present chapter reviews how key anatomical data about visual cortical development can be explained by recent neural models. The model cortical networks that emerge from these developmental processes can also explain a wide range of data about visual neuroscience and perception, notably data about binocular vision, perceptual grouping, and attention. This linkage of developmental, anatomical, neurophysiological, and perceptual data shows that the developmental hypotheses of the model are sufficient to generate cortical structures that can achieve key perceptual competences. In particular, the model's ability to simulate data about adult perceptual grouping after development is complete lends support to the hypothesis that the development of horizontal connections in cortical areas like V1 and V2 may be responsible for the rapid change in a human infant's ability, between the second and fourth month of life, to group image fragments into more complete object representations (Johnson, 2001; Johnson & Aslin, 1996; Kellman & Spelke, 1983).

Three types of models were reviewed here: the development of the cortical map of simple cells, which are the first stage of cortical processing; the development of complex cells, which receive inputs from simple cells; and the development of horizontal connections between complex cells, as well as the development of interlaminar connections that process inputs on their way to simple cells. The simulations of perceptual grouping and attention that derived from the third model assumed that the simple cells and complex cells had themselves already developed. Taken together, the three models clarify how the simple and complex cell properties themselves developed that were used to explain perceptual grouping and attention data. More generally, these component models provide a good foundation for the next steps of modeling cortical development in which all of these processes will be unified into a single comprehensive developmental model. Steps toward such a synthesis, along with an analysis of how the cortical subplate helps to coordinate development across the cortical layers, have already begun (Seitz & Grossberg, 2001).

None of the present developmental studies have considered how three-dimensional boundary and surface representations develop (although the development of disparity-sensitive complex cells is a step in that direction); how properties of figure-ground separation or motion perception develop; how processes or form and motion interact together; how boundary and surface representations are used for learned visual object recognition; or how these processes are realized within laminar circuits of visual cortex. Neural models of all these processes have, however, been described that are just a step away from these goals and that utilize neural mechanisms similar to those described here (e.g., see Baloch & Grossberg, 1997; Bradski & Grossberg, 1995; Grossberg, 1994, 1997, 1999b; Grossberg & McLoughlin, 1997; Grossberg, Mingolla, & Viswanathan, 2001; Grossberg & Pessoa, 1998; Grossberg & Williamson, 1999; Kelly & Grossberg, 2000; McLoughlin & Grossberg, 1998). Thus, the outlines of a general theory of visual perception are already discernible, along with some of the developmental mechanisms that lead to adult perception and recognition as we know it.

NOTE

Supported in part by the Defense Advanced Research Projects Agency and the Office of Naval Research (ONR N00014-95-1-0409), the National Science Foundation (NSF IRI-97-20333), and the Office of Naval Research (ONR N00014-95-1-0657). The author thanks Diana Meyers and Robin Amos for their valuable assistance in the preparation of the manuscript and figures.

REFERENCES

Abbott, L.F., Varela, J.A., Sen, K., & Nelson, S.B. (1997). Synaptic depression and cortical gain control. *Science, 275*, 220–224.

Ahmed, R., Anderson, J.C., Douglas, R.J., Martin, K.A.C., & Nelson, J.C. (1994). Polyneuronal innervation of spiny stellate neurons in cat visual cortex. *Journal of Comparative Neurology, 341*, 39–49.

Ahmed, R., Anderson, J.C., Martin, K.A.C., & Nelson, J.C. (1997). Map of the synapses onto layer 4 basket cells of the primary visual cortex of the cat. *Journal of Comparative Neurology, 380*, 230–242.

Amir, Y., Harel, M., & Malach, R. (1993). Cortical hierarchy reflected in the organization of intrinsic connections in macaque monkey visual cortex. *Journal of Comparative Neurology, 334*, 19–46.

Anderson, P., Olavarria, J., & Sluyters, R. (1988). The overall pattern of ocular dominance bands in cat visual cortex. *Journal of Neuroscience, 8*, 2183–2200.

Antonini, A., & Stryker, M.P. (1993a). Functional mapping of horizontal connections in developing ferret visual cortex: Experiments and modeling. *Journal of Neuroscience, 14*, 7291–7305.

Antonini, A., & Stryker, M.P. (1993b). Rapid remodeling of axonal arbors in the visual cortex. *Science, 260*, 1819–1821.

Bailey, C.H., Chen, M., Keller, F., & Kandel, E.R. (1992). Serotonin-mediated endocytosis of a pCAM: An early step of learning-related synaptic growth in aplysia. *Science, 256*, 645–649.

Baloch, A., & Grossberg, S. (1997). A neural model of high-level motion processing: Line motion and formotion dynamics. *Vision Research, 37*, 3037–3059.

Beck, J., Prazdny, K., & Rosenfeld, A. (1983). A theory of textural segmentation. In J. Beck, B. Hope, & A. Rosenfeld (Eds.), *Human and machine vision* (pp. 1–38). New York: Academic Press.

Birch, E.E., Gwiazda, J., & Held, R. (1983). The development of vergence does not account for the onset of stereopsis. *Perception, 12*, 331–336.

Blakemore, C., Hawken, M.F., & Mark, R.F. (1982). Brief monocular deprivation leaves subthreshold synaptic input on neurons of the cat's visual cortex. *Journal of Physiology (London), 327*, 489–505.

Blakemore, C., & van Sluyters, R.C. (1974). Reversal of the physiological effects of monocular deprivation in kittens: Further evidence for a sensitive period. *Journal of Physiology (London), 265*, 195–216.

Blasdel, G.G. (1992a). Differential imaging of ocular dominance and orientation selectivity in monkey striate cortex. *Journal of Neuroscience, 12*, 3115–3138.

Blasdel, G.G. (1992b). Orientation selectivity, preference, and continuity in monkey striate cortex. *Journal of Neuroscience, 12*, 3139–3161.

Blasdel, G., & Salama, G. (1986). Voltage sensitive dyes reveal a modular organization in monkey striate cortex. *Nature, 321*, 579–585.

Bonhoeffer, T., & Grinvald, A. (1991). Iso-orientation domains in cat visual cortex are arranged in pinwheel-like patterns. *Nature, 353*, 429–431.

Born, R.T., & Tootell, R.B. (1991). Single-unit and 2-deoxyglucose studies of side inhibition in macaque striate cortex. *Proceedings of the National Academy of Sciences (USA), 88*, 7071–7075.

Bosking, W., Zhang, Y., Schofield, B., & Fitzpatrick, D. (1997). Orientation selectivity and the arrangement of horizontal connections in tree shrew striate cortex. *Journal of Neuroscience, 17*, 2112–2127.

Bradski, G., & Grossberg, S. (1995). Fast learning VIEWNET architectures for recognizing 3-D objects from multiple 2-D views. *Neural Networks, 8*, 1053–1080.

Bullier, J., Hupé, J.M., James, A., & Girard, P. (1996). Functional interactions between areas V1 and V2 in the monkey. *Journal of Physiology (Paris), 90*, 217–220.

Callaway, E.M. (1998a). Local circuits in primary visual cortex of the macaque monkey. *Annual Review of Neuroscience, 21*, 47–74.

Callaway, E.M. (1998b). Prenatal development of layer-specific local circuits in primary visual cortex of the macaque monkey. *Journal of Neuroscience, 18*, 1505–1527.

Callaway, E.M., & Katz, L.C. (1990). Emergence and refinement of clustered horizontal connections in cat striate cortex. *Journal of Neuroscience, 10*, 1134–1153.

Callaway, E.M., & Katz, L.C. (1991). Effects of binocular deprivation on the development of clustered horizontal connections in cat striate cortex. *Proceedings of the National Academy of Sciences (USA), 88*, 745–749.

Cannon, M.W., & Fullenkamp, S.C. (1993). Spatial interactions in apparent contrast: Individual differences in enhancement and suppression effects. *Vision Research, 33*, 1685–1695.

Carpenter, G., & Grossberg, S. (1991). *Pattern recognition by self-organizing neural networks*, Cambridge, MA: MIT Press.

Chapman, B., & Stryker, M.P. (1993). Development of orientation selectivity in ferret visual cortex and effects of deprivation. *Journal of Neuroscience, 13*, 5251–5262.

Chapman, B., Zahs, K.R., & Stryker, M.P. (1991). Relation of cortical cell orientation selectivity to alignment of receptive fields of the geniculocortical afferents that arborize within a single orientation column in ferret visual cortex. *Journal of Neuroscience, 11*, 1347–1358.

Chino, Y.M., Kaas, J.H., Smith, E.L., Langston, A.L., & Cheng, H. (1992). Rapid reorganization of cortical maps in adult cats following restricted deafferentation in retina. *Vision Research, 32*, 789–796.

Chubb, C., & Sperling, G. (1989). Two motion perception mechanisms revealed through distance-driven reversal of apparent motion. *Proceedings of the National Academy of Sciences (USA), 86*, 2985–2989.

Cogan, A.I., Lomakin, A.J., & Rossi, A.F. (1993). Depth in anticorrelated stereograms: Effects of spatial density and interocular delay. *Vision Research, 33*, 1959–1975.

Cohen, M.A., & Grossberg, S. (1984). Neural dynamics of brightness perception: Features, boundaries, diffusion, and resonance. *Perception and Psychophysics, 36*, 428–456.

Dalva, M.B., & Katz, L.C. (1994). Rearrangements of synaptic connections in visual cortex revealed by laser photostimulation. *Science, 265*, 255–258.

Darian-Smith, C., & Gilbert, C.D. (1994). Axonal sprouting accompanies functional reorganization in adult cat striate cortex. *Nature, 368*, 737–740.

Das, A., & Gilbert, C.D. (1995). Long-range horizontal connections and their role in cortical reorganization revealed by optical recording of cat primary visual cortex. *Nature, 375*, 780–784.

Daw, N.W. (1994). Mechanisms of plasticity in the visual cortex. *Investigative Ophthalmology and Visual Science, 35*, 4168–4179.

Daw, N.W., & Wyatt, H.J. (1976). Kittens reared in a unidirectional environment: Evidence for a critical period. *Journal of Physiology (London), 257*, 155–170.

DeAngelis, G.C., Ohzawa, I., & Freeman, R.D. (1991). Depth is encoded in the visual cortex by a specialized receptive field structure. *Nature, 352*, 156–159.

DeAngelis, G.C., Ohzawa, I., & Freeman, R.D. (1993). Spatiotemporal organization of simple-cell receptive fields in the cat's striate cortex. I. General characteristics and postnatal development. *Journal of Neurophysiology, 69*, 1091–1117.

Douglas, R.J., Koch, C., Mahowald, M., Martin, K.A.C., & Suarez, H.H. (1995). Recurrent excitation in neocortical circuits. *Science, 269*, 981–985.

Dresp, B., & Grossberg, S. (1997). Contour integration across polarities and spatial gaps: From local contrast filtering to global grouping. *Vision Research, 37*, 913–924.

Durack, J.C., & Katz, L.C. (1996). Development of horizontal projections in layer 2/3 of ferret visual cortex. *Cerebral Cortex, 6*, 178–183.

Durbin, R., & Mitchison, G. (1990). A dimension reduction framework for understanding cortical maps. *Nature, 343*, 644–647.

Emerson, R.C., Korenberg, M.J., & Citron, M.C. (1992). Identification of complex-cell intensive nonlinearities in a cascade model of cat visual cortex. *Biological Cybernetics, 66*, 291–300.

Felleman, D.J., & van Essen, D.C. (1991). Distributed hierarchical processing in the primate cerebral cortex. *Cerebral Cortex, 60*, 121–130.

Ferster, D. (1988). Spatially opponent excitation and inhibition in simple cells of the cat visual cortex. *Journal of Neuroscience, 8*, 1172–1180.

Ferster, D., Chung, S., & Wheat, H. (1996). Orientation selectivity of thalamic input to simple cells of cat visual cortex. *Nature, 380*, 249–252.

Ferster, D., & Lindström, S. (1985). Synaptic excitation of neurons in area 17 of the cat by intracortical axon collaterals of cortico-geniculate cells. *Journal of Physiology, 367*, 233–252.

Field, D.J., Hayes, A., & Hess, R.F. (1993). Contour integration by the human visual system: Evidence for a local "association field." *Vision Research, 33*, 173–193.

Finkel, L.H., & Edelman, G.M. (1989). Integration of distributed cortical systems by reentry: A computer simulation of interactive functionally segregated visual areas. *Journal of Neuroscience, 9*, 3188–3208.

Fitzpatrick, D. (1996). The functional organization of local circuits in visual cortex: Insights from the study of tree shrew striate cortex. *Cerebral Cortex, 6*, 329–341.

Francis, G., & Grossberg, S. (1996). Cortical dynamics of form and motion integration: Persistence, apparent motion and illusory contours. *Vision Research, 35,* 149–173.

Francis, G., Grossberg, S., & Mingolla, E. (1994). Cortical dynamics of feature binding and reset: Control of visual persistence. *Vision Research, 34,* 1089–1104.

Freeman, R.D., & Ohzawa, I. (1992). Development of binocular vision in the kitten's striate cortex. *Journal of Neuroscience, 12,* 4721–4736.

Galuske, R.A.W., & Singer, W. (1996). The origin and topography of long-range intrinsic projections in cat visual cortex: A developmental study. *Cerebral Cortex, 6,* 417–430.

Ghose, G.M., Freeman, R.D., & Ohzawa, I. (1994). Local intracortical connections in the cat's visual cortex: Postnatal development and plasticity. *Journal of Neurophysiology, 72,* 1290–1303.

Gilbert, C.D. (1977). Laminar differences in receptive field properties of cells in cat primary visual cortex. *Journal of Physiology, 268,* 391–421.

Gilbert, C.D., & Wiesel, T.N. (1979). Morphology and intracortical projections of functionally characterized neurons in the cat visual cortex. *Nature, 280,* 120–125.

Gilbert, C.D., & Wiesel, T.N. (1992). Receptive field dynamics in adult primary visual cortex. *Nature, 356,* 150–152.

Gove, A., Grossberg, S., & Mingolla, E. (1995). Brightness perception, illusory contours, and corticogeniculate feedback. *Visual Neuroscience, 12,* 1027–1052.

Grieve, K.L., & Sillito, A.M. (1991a). The length summation properties of layer VI cells in the visual cortex and hypercomplex cell end zone inhibition. *Experimental Brain Research, 84,* 319–325.

Grieve, K.L., & Sillito, A.M. (1991b). A re-appraisal of the role of layer VI of the visual cortex in the generation of cortical end inhibition. *Experimental Brain Research, 87,* 521–529.

Grieve, K.L., & Sillito, A.M. (1995). Non-length-tuned cells in layers II/III and IV of the visual cortex: The effect of blockade of layer VI on responses to stimuli of different lengths. *Experimental Brain Research, 104,* 12–20.

Grinvald, A., Lieke, E.E., Frostig, R.D., & Hildesheim, R. (1994). Cortical point-spread function and long-range lateral interactions revealed by real-time optical imaging of macaque monkey primary visual cortex. *Journal of Neuroscience, 14,* 2545–2568.

Grosof, D.H., Shapley, R.M., & Hawken, M.J. (1993). Macaque V1 neurons can signal "illusory" contours. *Nature, 365,* 550–552.

Grossberg, S. (1972). A neural theory of punishment and avoidance. II. Quantitative theory. *Mathematical Biosciences, 15,* 39–67.

Grossberg, S. (1973). Contour enhancement, short-term memory, and constancies in reverberating neural networks. *Studies in Applied Mathematics, 52,* 217–257. Reprinted in Grossberg, S. (1982). *Studies of mind and brain.* Dordrecht, The Netherlands: D. Reidel Publishing.

Grossberg, S. (1976a). Adaptive pattern classification and universal recoding. I: Parallel development and coding of neural feature detectors. *Biological Cybernetics, 23,* 121–134.

Grossberg, S. (1976b). Adaptive pattern classification and universal recoding. II:

Feedback, expectation, olfaction, and illusions. *Biological Cybernetics, 23,* 187–202.

Grossberg, S. (1980a). Biological competition: Decision rules, pattern formation, and oscillations. *Proceedings of the National Academy of Sciences (USA), 77,* 2338–2342.

Grossberg, S. (1980b). How does a brain build a cognitive code? *Psychological Review, 87,* 1–51.

Grossberg, S. (1984). Outline of a theory of brightness, color, and form perception. In E. Degreef & J. van Buggenhaut (Eds.), *Trends in mathematical psychology* (pp. 5559–5586). Amsterdam: Elsevier Science.

Grossberg, S. (1987a). Cortical dynamics of three-dimensional form, color and brightness perception. I: Monocular theory. *Perception and Psychophysics, 41,* 87–116.

Grossberg, S. (1987b). Cortical dynamics of three-dimensional form, color and brightness perception. II: Binocular theory. *Perception and Psychophysics, 41,* 117–158.

Grossberg, S. (1988). Nonlinear neural networks: Principles, mechanisms, and architectures. *Neural Networks, 1,* 17–61.

Grossberg, S. (1994). 3-D vision and figure-ground separation by visual cortex. *Perception and Psychophysics, 55,* 48–120.

Grossberg, S. (1997). Cortical dynamics of 3-D figure-ground perception of 2-D pictures. *Psychological Review, 104,* 618–658.

Grossberg, S. (1999a). How does the cerebral cortex work? Learning, attention, and grouping by the laminar circuits of visual cortex. *Spatial Vision, 12,* 163–186.

Grossberg, S. (1999b). The link between brain learning, attention, and consciousness. *Consciousness and Cognition, 8,* 1–44.

Grossberg, S., & Grunewald, A. (1997). Cortical synchronization and perceptual framing. *Journal of Cognitive Neuroscience, 9,* 117–132.

Grossberg, S., Hwang, S., & Mingolla, E. (2001). *Thalamocortical dynamics of the McCollough effect: Boundary-surface alignment through perceptual learning.* Technical Report TR-01-004, Boston University.

Grossberg, S., & Kelly, F. (1999). Neural dynamics of binocular brightness perception. *Vision Research, 39,* 3796–3816.

Grossberg, S. & McLoughlin, N. (1997). Cortical dynamics of three-dimensional surface perception: Binocular and half-occluded scenic images. *Neural Networks, 10,* 1583–1605.

Grossberg, S., & Mingolla, E. (1985a). Neural dynamics of form perception: Boundary completion, illusory figures, and neon color spreading. *Psychological Review, 92,* 173–211.

Grossberg, S., & Mingolla, E. (1985b). Neural dynamics of perceptual grouping: Textures, boundaries, and emergent segmentations. *Perception and Psychophysics, 38,* 141–171.

Grossberg, S., Mingolla, E., & Pack, C. (1999). A neural model of motion processing and visual navigation by cortical area MST. *Cerebral Cortex, 9,* 878–895.

Grossberg, S., Mingolla, E., & Ross, W.D. (1997). Visual brain and visual perception: How does the cortex do perceptual grouping? *Trends in Neurosciences, 20*, 106–111.

Grossberg, S., Mingolla, E., & Viswanathan, L. (2001). Neural dynamics of motion integration and segmentation within and across apertures. *Vision Research, 41*, 2521–2553.

Grossberg, S., & Olson, S. (1994). Rules for the cortical map of ocular dominance and orientation columns. *Neural Networks, 7*, 883–894.

Grossberg, S., & Pessoa, L. (1998). Texture segregation, surface representation, and figure-ground separation. *Vision Research, 38*, 137–161.

Grossberg, S., & Raizada, R.D.S. (2000). Contrast-sensitive perceptual grouping and object-based attention in the laminar circuits of primary visual cortex. *Vision Research, 40*, 1413–1432.

Grossberg, S., & Somers, D. (1991). Synchronized oscillations during cooperative feature linking in a cortical model of visual perception. *Neural Networks, 4*, 453–466.

Grossberg, S., & Todorovic, D. (1988). Neural dynamics of 1-D and 2-D brightness perception: A unified model of classical and recent phenomena. *Perception and Psychophysics, 43*, 241–277.

Grossberg, S., & Williamson, J. (1999). A self-organizing neural system for learning to recognize textured scenes. *Vision Research, 39*, 1385–1406.

Grossberg, S., & Williamson, J. (2001). A neural model of how horizontal and interlaminar connections of visual cortex develop into adult circuits that carry out perceptual grouping and learning. *Cerebral Cortex, 11*, 37–58.

Grunewald, A., & Grossberg, S. (1998). Self-organization of binocular disparity tuning by reciprocal corticogeniculate interactions. *Journal of Cognitive Neuroscience, 10*, 199–215.

Grunewald, A., & Lankheet, M.J.M. (1996). Orthogonal motion after-effect illusion predicted by a model of cortical motion processing. *Nature, 384*, 358–360.

Gundersen, R.W., & Barrett, J.N. (1979). Neuronal chemotaxis: Chick dorsal-root axons turn toward high concentrations of nerve growth factor. *Science, 206*, 1079–1080.

Gundersen, R.W., & Barrett, J.N. (1980). Characterization of the turning response of dorsal root neurites toward nerve growth factor. *Journal of Cell Biology, 87*, 546–554.

Hawken, M.J., & Parker, A.J. (1984). Contrast sensitivity and orientation selectivity in lamina IV of the striate cortex of old world monkeys. *Experimental Brain Research, 54*, 367–372.

Heeger, D.J. (1992). Normalization of cell responses in cat striate cortex. *Visual Neuroscience, 9*, 181–197.

Heeger, D.J. (1993). Modeling simple-cell direction selectivity with normalized, half-squared, linear operators. *Journal of Neurophysiology, 70*, 1885–1898.

Heitger, F., von der Heydt, R., Peterhans, E., Rosenthaler, L., & Kubler, O. (1998). Simulation of neural contour mechanisms: Representing anomalous contours. *Image and Visual Computation, 16*, 407–421.

Held, R., Birch, E.E., & Gwiazda, J. (1980). Stereoacuity of human infants. *Proceedings of the National Academy of Sciences (USA), 77*, 5572–5574.

Hirsch, J.A., & Gilbert, C.D. (1991). Synaptic physiology of horizontal connections in the cat's visual cortex. *Journal of Neuroscience, 11,* 1800–1809.

Horton, J.C., & Hocking, D.R. (1996). An adult-like pattern of ocular dominance columns in striate cortex of newborn monkeys prior to visual experience. *Journal of Neuroscience, 16,* 1791–1807.

Hubel, D.H., & Wiesel, T.N. (1962). Receptive fields, binocular interaction and functional architecture in the cat's visual cortex. *Journal of Physiology, 160,* 106–154.

Hubel, D.H., & Wiesel, T.N. (1963). Shape and arrangement of columns in cat's striate cortex. *Journal of Physiology, 195,* 215–243.

Hubel, D.H., & Wiesel, T.N. (1968). Receptive fields and functional architecture of monkey striate cortex. *Journal of Physiology (London), 195,* 215–243.

Hubel, D.H., & Wiesel, T.N. (1974). Sequence regularity and geometry of orientation columns in the monkey striate cortex. *Journal of Comparative Neurology, 158,* 267–293.

Hubel, D.H., & Wiesel, T.N. (1977). Functional architecture of macaque monkey visual cortex. *Philosophical Transactions of the Royal Society of London, Series B, 198,* 1–59.

Hubel, D.H., Wiesel, T.N., & Stryker, M. (1978). Anatomical demonstration of orientation columns in macaque monkey. *Journal of Comparative Neurology, 177,* 361–380.

Hupé, J.M., James, A.C., Girard, D.C., & Bullier, J. (1997). Feedback connections from V2 modulate intrinsic connectivity within V1. *Society for Neuroscience Abstracts, 406.15,* 1031.

Hupé, J.M., James, A.C., Payne, B.R., Lomber, S.G., & Bullier, J. (1998). Cortical feedback improves discrimination between figure and background by V1, V2 and V3 neurons. *Nature, 394,* 784–787.

Jacobson, L.D., Gaska, J.P., Chen, H., & Pollen, D.A. (1993). Structural testing of multi-input linear-nonlinear cascade models for cells in macaque striate cortex. *Vision Research, 33,* 609–626.

Johnson, S.P. (2001). Visual development in human infants: Binding features, surfaces, and objects. *Visual Cognition, 8,* 565–578.

Johnson, S.P., & Aslin, R.N. (1996). Perception of object unity in young infants: The roles of motion, depth, and orientation. *Cognitive Development, 11,* 161–180.

Julesz, B. (1960). Binocular depth perception of computer-generated patterns. *Bell System Technical Journal, 38,* 1001–1020.

Julesz, B. (1971). *Foundations of cyclopean perception.* Chicago: University of Chicago Press.

Kandel, E.R., & O'Dell, T.J. (1992). Are adult learning mechanisms also used for development? *Science, 258,* 243–246.

Kanizsa, G. (1979). *Organization in vision.* New York: Praeger.

Kanizsa, G. (1985). Seeing and thinking. *Revista di Psicologia, 49,* 7–30.

Kapadia, M.K., Gilbert, C.D., & Westheimer, G. (1994). A quantitative measure for short-term cortical plasticity in human vision. *Journal of Neuroscience, 14,* 451–457.

Kapadia, M.K., Ito, M., Gilbert, C.D., & Westheimer, G. (1995). Improvement in visual sensitivity by changes in local context: Parallel studies in human observers and in V1 of alert monkeys. *Neuron, 15*, 843–856.

Karni, A., & Sagi, D. (1991). Where practice makes perfect in textural discrimination: Evidence for primary visual cortex plasticity. *Proceedings of the National Academy of Sciences (USA), 88*, 4966–4970.

Kellman, P.J., & Spelke, E.S. (1983). Perception of partially occluded objects in infancy. *Cognitive Psychology, 15*, 483–524.

Kelly, F., & Grossberg, S. (2000). Neural dynamics of 3-D surface perception: Figure-ground separation and lightness perception. *Perception and Psychophysics, 62*, 1596–1618.

Kisvarday, Z.F., Beaulieu, C., & Eysel, U.T. (1993). Network of GABAergic large basket cells in cat visual cortex (area 18): Implication for lateral disinhibition. *Journal of Comparative Neurology, 327*, 398–415.

Kisvarday, Z.F., Toth, E., Rausch, M., & Eysel, U.T. (1995). Comparison of lateral excitatory and inhibitory connections in cortical orientation maps of the cat. *Society of Neuroscience Abstracts, 21*, pt. 2, 907.

Knierim, J.J., & van Essen, D.C. (1992). Neuronal responses to static texture patterns in area V1 of the alert macaque monkey. *Journal of Neurophysiology, 67*, 961–980.

Kohonen, T. (1982). Self-organized formation of topologically correct feature maps. *Biological Cybernetics, 43*, 59–69.

Kohonen, T. (1989). *Self-organization and associative memory* (3rd ed.). New York: Springer-Verlag.

Lamme, V.A.F. (1995). The neurophysiology of figure-ground segregation in primary visual cortex. *Journal of Neuroscience, 15*, 1605–1615.

Lesher, G.W., & Mingolla, E. (1993). The role of edges and line-ends in illusory contour formation. *Vision Research, 33*, 2253–2270.

Letourneau, P.C. (1978). Chemotactic response of nerve fiber elongation to nerve growth factor. *Developmental Biology, 66*, 183–196.

LeVay, S., Connolly, M., Houde, J., & Van Essen, D. (1985). The complete pattern of ocular dominance stripes in the striate cortex and visual field of the macaque monkey. *Journal of Neuroscience, 5*, 486–501.

LeVay, S., Hubel, D., & Wiesel, T. (1975). The pattern of ocular dominance columns in macaque visual cortex revealed by a reduced silver stain. *Journal of Comparative Neurology, 159*, 559–576.

LeVay, S., Stryker, M., & Shatz, C. (1978). Ocular dominance columns and their development in layer IV of the cat's visual cortex: A quantitative study. *Journal of Comparative Neurology, 179*, 223–244.

Leventhal, A.G., & Hirsch, H.V.B. (1980). Receptive field properties of different classes of neurons in visual cortex of normal and dark-reared cats. *Journal of Neurophysiology, 43*, 1111–1132.

Li, Z. (1998). A neural model of contour integration in the primary visual cortex. *Neural Computation, 10*, 903–940.

Lichtman, J.W., & Purves, D. (1981). Regulation of the number of axons that innervate target cells. In D.R. Garrod & J.D. Feldman (Eds.), *Development in the nervous system* (pp. 233–243). Cambridge: Cambridge University Press.

Linsker, R. (1986a). From basic network principles to neural architecture. Emergence of spatial-opponent cells. *Proceedings of the National Academy of Sciences (USA), 83,* 7508–7512.

Linsker, R. (1986b). From basic network principles to neural architecture. Emergence of orientation-selective cells. *Proceedings of the National Academy of Sciences (USA), 83,* 8390–8394.

Linsker, R. (1986c). From basic network principles to neural architecture: Emergence of orientation columns. *Proceedings of the National Academy of Sciences (USA), 83,* 8779–8783.

Liu, Z., Gaska, J.P., Jacobson, L.D., & Pollen, D.A. (1992). Interneuronal interaction between members of quadrature phase and anti-phase pairs in the cat's visual cortex. *Vision Research, 32,* 1193–1198.

Löwel, S., Bischof, H., Leutenecker, B., & Singer, W. (1988). Topographic relations between ocular dominance and orientation columns in the cat striate cortex. *Experimental Brain Research, 71,* 33–46.

Löwel, S., & Singer, W. (1987). The pattern of ocular dominance columns in flat mounts of the cat visual cortex. *Experimental Brain Research, 68,* 661–666.

Löwel, S., & Singer, W. (1992). Selection of intrinsic horizontal connections in the visual cortex by correlated neuronal activity. *Science, 255,* 209–212.

Mayford, M., Barzilai, A., Keller, F., Schacher, S., & Kandel, E.R. (1992). Modulation of an NCAM-related adhesion molecule with long-term synaptic plasticity in *Aplysia. Science, 256,* 638–644.

McClurkin, J.W., Optican, L.M., & Richmond, B.J. (1994). Cortical feedback increases visual information transmitted by monkey parvocellular lateral geniculate nucleus neurons. *Visual Neuroscience, 11,* 601–617.

McGuire, B.A., Gilbert, C.D., Rivlin, P.K., & Wiesel, T.N. (1991). Targets of horizontal connections in macaque primary visual cortex. *Journal of Comparative Neurology, 305,* 370–392.

McGuire, B.A., Hornung, J.P., Gilbert, C.D., & Wiesel, T.N. (1984). Patterns of synaptic input to layer 4 of cat striate cortex. *Journal of Neuroscience, 4,* 3021–3033.

McLoughlin, N., & Grossberg, S. (1998). Cortical computation of stereo disparity. *Vision Research, 38,* 91–99.

Merzenich, M.M., Recanzone, E.G., Jenkins, W.M., Allard, T.T., & Nudo, R.J. (1988). Cortical representational plasticity. In P. Rakic and W. Singer (Eds.), *Neurobiology of neocortex* (pp. 41–67). New York: Wiley.

Miller, K.D. (1992). Development of orientation columns via competition between on- and off-center inputs. *NeuroReport, 3,* 73–76.

Miller, K.D. (1994). A model for the development of simple cell receptive fields and the ordered arrangement of orientation columns through activity-dependent competition between ON- and OFF-center inputs. *Journal of Neuroscience, 14,* 409–441.

Miller, K.D., Keller, J.B., & Stryker, M.P. (1989). Ocular dominance column development: Analysis and simulation. *Science, 245,* 605–615.

Moore, C.M., Yantis, S., & Vaughan, B. (1998). Object-based visual selection: Evidence from perceptual completion. *Psychological Science, 9,* 104–110.

Mountcastle, V.B. (1957). Modality and topographic properties of single neurons of cats somatic sensory cortex. *Journal of Neurophysiology, 20,* 408–434.

Movshon, J.A., & Düsteler, M.R. (1977). Effects of brief periods of unilateral eye closure on the kitten's visual system. *Journal of Neurophysiology, 40,* 1255–1265.

Mumford, D. (1992). On the computational architecture of the neocortex. II. The role of cortico-cortical loops. *Biological Cybernetics, 66,* 241–251.

Murphy, P.C., Duckett, S.G., & Sillito, A.M. (1999). Feedback connections to the lateral geniculate nucleus and cortical response properties. *Science, 286,* 1552–1554.

Murphy, P.C., & Sillito, A.M. (1987). Corticofugal feedback influences the generation of length tuning in the visual pathway. *Nature, 329,* 727–729.

Murphy, P.C., & Sillito, A.M. (1996). Functional morphology of the feedback pathway from area 17 of the cat visual cortex to the lateral geniculate nucleus. *Journal of Neuroscience, 16,* 1180–1192.

Obermayer, K., & Blasdel, G.G. (1993). Geometry of orientation and ocular dominance columns in monkey striate cortex. *Journal of Neuroscience, 13,* 4114–4129.

Obermayer, K., Blasdel, G.G., & Schulten, K. (1992). Statistical-mechanical analysis of self-organization and pattern formation during the development of visual maps. *Physical Review A, 45,* 7568–7589.

Obermayer, K., Ritter, H., & Schulten, K. (1990). A principle for the formation of the spatial structure of retinotopic maps, orientation and ocular dominance columns. *Proceedings of the National Academy of Sciences (USA), 87,* 8345–8349.

Olson, S.J., & Grossberg, S. (1998). A neural network model for the development of simple and complex cell receptive fields within cortical maps of orientation and ocular dominance. *Neural Networks, 11,* 189–208.

Palmer, L.A., & Davis, T.L. (1981). Receptive field structure in cat striate cortex. *Journal of Neurophysiology, 46,* 260–276.

Pessoa, L., Mingolla, E., & Neumann, H. (1995). A contrast and luminance-driven multiscale network model of brightness perception. *Vision Research, 35,* 2201–2223.

Peterhans, E., & von der Heydt, R. (1989). Mechanisms of contour perception in monkey visual cortex. II. Contours bridging gaps. *Journal of Neuroscience, 9,* 1749–1763.

Poggio, T., Fahle, M., & Edelman, S. (1992). Fast perceptual learning in visual hyperacuity. *Science, 256,* 1018–1021.

Polat, U., & Sagi, D. (1994). The architecture of perceptual spatial interactions. *Vision Research, 34,* 73–78.

Pollen, D.A., & Ronner, S.F. (1981). Phase relationships between adjacent simple cells in the visual cortex. *Science, 212,* 1409–1411.

Purves, D., & Lichtman, J.W. (1980). Elimination of synapses in the developing nervous system. *Science, 210,* 153–157.

Ramachandran, V.S., & Nelson, J.I. (1976). Global grouping overrides point-to-point disparities. *Perception, 5,* 125–128.

Redies, C., Crook, J.M., & Creutzfeldt, O.D. (1986). Neural responses to borders with and without luminance gradients in cat visual cortex and dLGN. *Experimental Brain Research, 61,* 469–481.

Reid, R.C., & Alonso, J.-M. (1995). Specificity of monosynaptic connections from thalamus to visual cortex. *Nature, 378,* 281–284.

Ringach, D., Carandini, M., Sapiro, G., & Shapley, R. (1996). Cortical circuitry revealed by reverse correlation in the orientation domain. *Perception, 25* (Supp. 31).

Roelfsema, P.R., Lamme, V.A.F., & Spekreijse, H. (1998). Object-based attention in the primary visual cortex of the macaque monkey. *Nature, 395,* 376–381.

Rojer, A.S., & Schwartz, E.L. (1989). A parametric model of synthesis of cortical column patterns. *International Joint Conference on Neural Networks, 2,* 603.

Rojer, A.S., & Schwartz, E. (1990). Cat and monkey cortical columnar patterns modeled by band-pass-filtered 2D white noise. *Biological Cybernetics, 62,* 381–391.

Ruthazer, E.S., & Stryker, M.P. (1996). The role of activity in the development of long-range horizontal connections in area 17 of the ferret. *Journal of Neuroscience, 15,* 7253–7269.

Salin, P., & Bullier, J. (1995). Corticocortical connections in the visual system: Structure and function. *Physiological Reviews, 75,* 107–154.

Sandell, J.H., & Schiller, P.H. (1982). Effect of cooling area 18 on striate cortex cells in the squirrel monkey. *Journal of Neurophysiology, 48,* 38–48.

Schiller, P.H. (1982). Central connections on the retinal ON- and OFF-pathways. *Nature, 297,* 580–583.

Schiller, P. (1992). The on and off channels of the visual system. *Trends in Neuroscience, 15,* 86–92.

Schmidt, K.E., Goebel, R., Löwel, S., & Singer, W. (1997a). The perceptual grouping criterion of colinearity is reflected by anisotropies of connections in the primary visual cortex. *European Journal of Neuroscience, 9,* 1083–1089.

Schmidt, K.E., Schlote, W., Bratzke, H., Rauen, T., Singer, W., & Galuske, R.A.W. (1997b). Patterns of long range intrinsic connectivity in auditory and language areas of the human temporal cortex. *Society for Neuroscience Abstracts, 415.13,* 1058.

Schmidt, L.M., Rosa, M.G.P., Calford, M.B., & Ambler, J.S. (1996). Visuotopic reorganization in the primary visual cortex of adult cats following monocular and binocular retinal lesions. *Cerebral Cortex, 6,* 388–405.

Seitz, A., & Grossberg, S. (2001). Coordination of laminar development in V1 by the cortical subplate. *Society for Neuroscience Abstracts, 619.12.*

Shadlen, M.N., & Newsome, W.T. (1998). The variable discharge of cortical neurons: Implications for connectivity, computation, and information coding. *Journal of Neuroscience, 18,* 3870–3896.

Shimojo, S., Bauer, J., O'Connell, K.M., & Held, R. (1986). Prestereoptic binocular vision in infants. *Vision Research, 26,* 501–510.

Shipley, T.F., & Kellman, P.J. (1992). Strength of visual interpolation depends on the ratio of physically specified to total edge length. *Perception and Psychophysics, 52,* 97–106.

Shulz, D., Debanne, D., & Fregnac, Y. (1993). Cortical convergence of on- and off-pathways and functional adaptation of receptive field organization in cat area 17. *Progress in Brain Research, 95,* 191–205.

Sillito, A.M., Grieve, K.L., Jones, H.E., Cudeiro, J., & Davis, J. (1995). Visual cortical mechanisms detecting focal orientation discontinuities. *Nature, 378,* 492–496.

Sillito, A.M., Jones, H.E., Gerstein, G.L., & West, D.C. (1994). Feature-linked synchronization of thalamic relay cell firing induced by feedback from the visual cortex. *Nature, 369,* 479–482.

Singer, W. (1983). Neuronal activity as a shaping factor in the self-organization of neuron assemblies. In E. Basar, H. Flohr, H. Haken, & A.J. Mandell (Eds.), *Synergetics of the brain* (pp. 89–101). New York: Springer-Verlag.

Sirosh, J., & Miikkulainen, R. (1994). Cooperative self-organization of afferent and lateral connections in cortical maps. *Biological Cybernetics, 71,* 66–78.

Somers, D.C., Nelson, S.B., & Sur, M. (1995). An emergent model of orientation selectivity in cat visual cortical simple cells. *Journal of Neuroscience, 15,* 5448–5465.

Spitzer, H., & Hochstein, S. (1985). A complex-cell receptive-field model. *Journal of Neurophysiology, 53,* 1266–1286.

Stemmler, M., Usher, M., & Niebur, E. (1995). Lateral interactions in primary visual cortex: A model bridging physiology and psychophysics. *Science, 269,* 1877–1880.

Stratford, K.J., Tarczy-Hornoch, K., Martin, K.A.C., Bannister, N.J., & Jack, J.J.B. (1996). Excitatory synaptic inputs of spiny stellate cells in cat visual cortex. *Nature, 382,* 258–261.

Stryker, M.P., & Harris, W.A. (1986). Binocular impulse blockade prevents the formation of ocular dominance columns in cat visual cortex. *Journal of Neuroscience, 6,* 2117–2133.

Sutter, A., Beck, J., & Graham, N. (1989). Contrast and spatial variables in texture segregation: Testing a simple spatial-frequency channels model. *Perception and Psychophysics, 46,* 312–332.

Swindale, N. (1980). A model for the formation of ocular dominance column stripes. *Proceedings of the Royal Society of London, Series B, 208,* 243–264.

Swindale, N. (1982). A model for the formation of orientation columns. *Proceedings of the Royal Society of London, Series B, 215,* 211–230.

Swindale, N. (1992). A model for the coordinated development of columnar systems in primate striate cortex. *Biological Cybernetics, 66,* 217–230.

Tamas, G., Somogyi, P., & Buhl, E.H. (1998). Differentially interconnected networks of GABAergic interneurons in the visual cortex of the cat. *Journal of Neuroscience, 18,* 4255–4270.

Thorpe, S., Fize, D., & Marlot, C. (1996). Speed of processing in the human visual system. *Science, 381,* 520–522.

Ullman, S. (1995). Sequence seeking and counter streams: A computational model for bi-directional information flow in the visual cortex. *Cerebral Cortex, 5,* 1–11.

Usher, M., & Donnelly, N. (1998). Visual synchrony affects binding and segmentation in perception. *Nature, 394,* 179–182.

van Essen, D.C., & Maunsell, J.H.R. (1983). Hierarchical organization and functional streams in the visual cortex. *Trends in Neurosciences, 6,* 370–375.

van Essen, D.C., Newsome, W.T., & Maunsell, J.H.R. (1984). The visual representation in striate cortex of macaque monkey: Asymmetries, anisotropies and individual variability. *Vision Research, 24,* 429–448.

van Vreeswijk, C., & Sompolinsky, H. (1998). Chaotic balanced state in a model of cortical circuits. *Neural Computation, 10,* 1321–1371.

Varela, F.J., & Singer, W. (1987). Neuronal dynamics in the visual corticothalamic pathway revealed through binocular rivalry. *Experimental Brain Research, 66,* 10–20.

von der Heydt, R., & Peterhans, E. (1989). Mechanisms of contour perception in monkey visual cortex. I. Lines of pattern discontinuity. *Journal of Neuroscience, 9,* 1731–1748.

von der Heydt, R., Peterhans, E., & Baumgartner, G. (1984). Illusory contours and cortical neuron responses. *Science, 224,* 1260–1262.

von der Malsburg, C. (1973). Self-organization of orientation sensitive cells in the striate cortex. *Kybernetik, 14,* 85–100.

Watanabe, T., & Cavanagh, P. (1992). Depth capture and transparency of regions bounded by illusory and chromatic contours. *Vision Research, 32,* 527–532.

Watanabe, T., Sasaki, Y., Miyauchi, S., Putz, B., Fujimake, N., Nielsen, M., Takino, R., & Miyakawa, S. (1998). Attention-regulated activity in human primary visual cortex. *Journal of Neurophysiology, 79,* 2218–2221.

Weber, J., Kalil, R.E., & Behan, M. (1989). Synaptic connections between corticogeniculate axons and interneurons in the dorsal lateral geniculate nucleus of the cat. *Journal of Comparative Neurology, 289,* 156–164.

Willshaw, D., & von der Malsburg, C. (1976). How patterned neural connections can be set up by self-organization. *Proceedings of the Royal Society of London, Series B, 194,* 431–445.

Wittmer, L.L., Dalva, M.B., & Katz, L.C. (1997). Reciprocal interactions between layer 4 and layer 6 cells in ferret visual cortex. *Society for Neuroscience Abstracts, 651.5,* 1668.

Zipser, K., Lamme, V.A.F., & Schiller, P.H. (1996). Contextual modulation in primary visual cortex. *Journal of Neuroscience, 16,* 7376–7389.

Zohary, E., Cerebrini, S., Britten, K.H., & Newsome, W.T. (1994). Neuronal plasticity that underlies improvement in perceptual performance. *Science, 263,* 1289–1292.

Author Index

Subject Index

About the Contributors

BARBARA CLANCY is an Assistant Professor at the University of Central Arkansas, where she teaches neuroscience and studies neurons implicated in disorders associated with perinatal injury and dementias. She was a post-doctoral fellow at Cornell University, working with Barbara Finlay on the hypothesis that dissimilar areas of developing brains may follow common connectivity "rules." While there, she also worked with Barbara Finlay and Richard Darlington on evolutionary-based modeling, a statistical technique that allows research done in laboratory animals to be related to the study of the developing human brain. She obtained her Ph.D. under Larry Cauller at the University of Texas at Dallas and was also a postdoctoral fellow at the University of Alabama at Birmingham, where she worked with Michael J. Friedlander exploring the function of cells in the white matter of the cortex.

NIGEL W. DAW has been Professor of Visual Sciences and of Neurobiology at Yale University Medical School since 1992. Most of his career prior to that was spent at Washington University in St. Louis. He studies the neurophysiology of the visual system, with particular interests in the development of visual properties, the effects of visual deprivation, mechanisms of direction selectivity, and color vision and the role of synaptic transmitters and second messengers in these properties. He is the author of the text *Visual Development*. He was the recipient of the Friedenwald Award of the Association for Research in Vision and Ophthalmology for this work in 1994.

MICHELLE DE HAAN is a Lecturer in the Developmental Cognitive Neuroscience Unit at the Institute of Child Health, University College, London. She received her B.A. in psychology in 1991 from McMaster University, Canada, and her Ph.D. with a major in child psychology and minor in neuroscience in 1996 from the University of Minnesota. She then took a position as research scientist at the Medical Research Council Cognitive Development Unit, London, for two years, where she investigated the development and neural bases of face recognition during infancy using event-related potentials. Her current research focuses on development and neural bases of visual cognition and memory in typical and atypical populations.

BARBARA L. FINLAY received her Ph.D. in brain and cognitive science at the Massachusetts Institute of Technology in 1976. She has worked on many aspects of visual system development and function, emphasizing evolutionary issues. She is presently the W.R. Kenan Jr. Professor of Psychology at Cornell University and also holds an appointment in the Department of Neurobiology and Behavior.

RICK O. GILMORE is Assistant Professor of Psychology at Penn State University. He earned his B.A. in cognitive science from Brown University and Ph.D. in psychology from Carnegie Mellon University. His research focuses on the development of spatial perception, action planning, memory, and problem solving in early infancy.

STEPHEN GROSSBERG is Wang Professor of Cognitive and Neural Systems and Professor of Mathematics, Psychology, and Biomedical Engineering at Boston University. He is the founder and director of the Center for Adaptive Systems, founder and chairman of the Department of Cognitive and Neural Systems, founder and first president of the International Neural Network Society, and founder and coeditor in chief of the journal *Neural Networks*. Grossberg has also been an editor of many other journals. He was general chairman of the Institute of Electrical and Electronics Engineers (IEEE) First International Conference on Neural Networks. He received the 1991 IEEE Neural Network Pioneer Award, the 1992 International Neural Network Society (INNS) Leadership Award, and the 1992 Thinking Technology Award of the Boston Computer Society. He was elected a fellow of the American Psychological Association in 1994 and of the Society of Experimental Psychologists in 1996. He and his colleagues have pioneered and developed a number of the fundamental principles, mechanisms, and architectures that form the foundation for contemporary modeling of brain and behavior, particularly those that enable individuals to adapt successfully in real time to unexpected environmental changes. Grossberg received his graduate training at Stanford University and Rockefeller University and was a professor at the Massachusetts Institute of Technology before assuming his present position at Boston University.

BRIAN HOPKINS is a Professor in the Department of Psychology at Lancaster University, where he has been for the last six years. Prior to that he was Professor in the Faculty of Human Movement Sciences at the Vrije Universiteit Amsterdam. His research interests cover the pre- and postnatal development of movement and posture and within that context the development of laterality.

SCOTT P. JOHNSON is an Assistant Professor in the Department of Psychology at Cornell University, where he has been for the last four years. Prior to that he spent two years as an Assistant Professor at Texas A&M University and two years as a Lecturer in Psychology at Lancaster University. His research interests concern infant perceptual and cognitive development, with an emphasis on visual perception, object concepts, and early learning.

MARCY A. KINGSBURY received her B.A. in psychobiology from Hamilton College in 1993. She went directly on to graduate school in Barbara Finlay's laboratory in the Department of Psychology at Cornell University, where she studied how cerebral cortical connections develop in the absence of visual input. Upon receiving her Ph.D. in 2000, Kingsbury moved to San Diego, California, and began working as a postdoctoral fellow in Jerold Chun's laboratory in the Department of Pharmacology at the University of California, San Diego (UCSD). While at UCSD, she was awarded a position on the Neuroplasticity of Aging Training Grant to study the importance of lysophospholipid signaling in the development of the cerebral cortex. More recently, she has been studying how genetic instability in developing cerebral cortical neurons may contribute to neuronal diversity and/or disease.

HILLARY R. RODMAN is a member of the faculty of the Department of Psychology at Emory University as well as a member of the Division of Visual Science of the Yerkes Primate Center and the Undergraduate Program in Neuroscience and Behavioral Biology. She received an M.A. and Ph.D. in psychology and neuroscience from Princeton University and postdoctoral training in the Department of Neuroscience at the University of California, San Diego. Rodman's main interests include the development and plasticity of cerebral cortex and the neurobiology of individual and species differences in vision and cognition. One focus of Rodman's research had been the use of a rhesus monkey model of the human "blindsight" phenomenon to study the anatomical circuits responsible for the marked recovery or sparing of function seen after early cortical damage in humans and other primates. Another emphasis has been to understand the development of temporal lobe mechanisms of object recognition, concentrating on the ontogeny of corticocortical feedback circuits and neural signals related to social recognition in normal subjects. Finally, Rodman seeks to be an advocate for the application of comparative perspectives on brain organization for the purposes of better discovering brain-behavior relationships within and across species, subjects, and evolution.